T0329543

Interventional Stroke Therapy

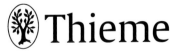

Interventional Stroke Therapy

Edited by

Olav Jansen, MD, PhD
Professor
Schleswig-Holstein University Hospital
Department of Neuroradiology
Kiel, Germany

Hartmut Brueckmann, MD, PhD
Professor
University of Munich–Grosshadern Medical Center
Department of Clinical Radiology
Division of Neuroradiology
Munich, Germany

Thieme
New York • Stuttgart

Library of Congress Cataloging-in-Publication Data
Interventionelle Therapie des Schlaganfalls. English.
  Interventional stroke therapy / edited by Olav Jansen, Hartmut Br?ckmann.
     p. ; cm.
  Includes bibliographical references and index.
  ISBN 978-3-13-169921-3
  I. Jansen, Olav. II. Br?ckmann, Hartmut. III. Title.
  [DNLM: 1. Stroke—therapy. WL 356]

  616.8'106--dc23
                                        2012042324

This book is an authorized translation of the first German edition published and copyrighted 2011 by Georg Thieme Verlag, Stuttgart, Germany. Title of the German edition: Interventionelle Therapie des Schlaganfalls

Translator: Terry C. Telger, Fort Worth, TX, USA

Important note: Medicine is an ever-changing science undergoing continual development. Research and clinical experience are continually expanding our knowledge, in particular our knowledge of proper treatment and drug therapy. Insofar as this book mentions any dosage or application, readers may rest assured that the authors, editors, and publishers have made every effort to ensure that such references are in accordance with **the state of knowledge at the time of production of the book.**

Nevertheless, this does not involve, imply, or express any guarantee or responsibility on the part of the publishers in respect to any dosage instructions and forms of applications stated in the book. **Every user is requested to examine carefully** the manufacturers' leaflets accompanying each drug and to check, if necessary in consultation with a physician or specialist, whether the dosage schedules mentioned therein or the contraindications stated by the manufacturers differ from the statements made in the present book. Such examination is particularly important with drugs that are either rarely used or have been newly released on the market. Every dosage schedule or every form of application used is entirely at the user's own risk and responsibility. The authors and publishers request every user to report to the publishers any discrepancies or inaccuracies noticed. If errors in this work are found after publication, errata will be posted at www.thieme.com on the product description page.

© 2013 Georg Thieme Verlag
Rüdigerstrasse 14, 70469 Stuttgart, Germany
http://www.thieme.de
Thieme Medical Publishers, Inc.,
333 Seventh Avenue,
New York, NY 10001, USA
http://www.thieme.com

Cover design: Thieme Publishing Group
Typesetting by Maryland Composition, USA
Printed in Italy by L.E.G.O., Vicenza

ISBN 978-3-13-169921-3
eISBN 978-3-13-169931-2

Preface

The first endovascular recanalization was performed 30 years ago by Hermann Zeumer. His technique for the local intra-arterial fibrinolysis of vertebrobasilar and middle cerebral artery occlusions was a major milestone in the development of interventional treatments for stroke.

Advances in both the diagnosis and treatment of stroke have followed in quick succession during the past three decades.

Initially, cranial CT could distinguish only between hemorrhage and ischemia and could supply information on the etiology of strokes. MRI, developed approximately 10 years after cranial CT, was initially important only for the evaluation of brainstem infarctions. But some 20 years ago MRI gained the ability to provide high-contrast diffusion-weighted images of a fresh cerebral infarction. The capabilities and individual components of "stroke MRI" significantly advanced our understanding of the pathophysiology of stroke and especially ischemic stroke. Today, the options of CT angiography and perfusion CT (*stroke CT*) have made computed tomography the first-line imaging study in stroke patients–especially for the relatively common ischemic strokes in the anterior circulation.

There has been equally rapid growth in the range of available interventional devices and techniques, fibrinolytic agents, platelet-aggregation inhibitors, and platelet-receptor inhibitors.

The wide range of techniques available for the diagnosis and interventional treatment of acute stroke prompted us to publish an "inventory" of these options in the form of a textbook. While we know that the techniques are still in flux, this is an opportune time to review current methods in detail, rate their efficacies, and make progress toward uniformity.

Fortunately, we had access to a strong "network" of neuroradiologists in which highly experienced colleagues were able to collaborate in the creation of this book.

The book is intended for all colleagues who seek concise, clinically relevant information in their day-to-day practice of diagnosing and treating stroke patients.

Kiel and Munich
Winter, 2013

Olav Jansen
Hartmut Brueckmann

Contributors

Editors

Olav Jansen, MD, PhD
Professor
Schleswig-Holstein University Hospital
Department of Neuroradiology
Kiel, Germany

Hartmut Brueckmann, MD, PhD
Professor
University of Munich-Grosshadern Medical Center
Department of Clinical Radiology
Division of Neuroradiology
Munich, Germany

Contributing Authors

Joachim Berkefeld, MD
Johann Wolfgang Goethe University Hospital
Department of Neuroradiology
Frankfurt am Main, Germany

Ansgar Berlis, MD
Augsburg Medical Center
Department of Diagnostic Radiology and Neuroradiology
Augsburg, Germany

Tibias Boeckh-Behrens, MD
Technical University of Munich
Rechts der Isar Hospital
Department of Radiology
Division of Neuroradiology
Munich, Germany

Arnd Doerfler
University of Erlangen Medical Center
Department of Neuroradiology
Erlangen, Germany

Bernd Eckert, MD
Asklepios Hospital Altona
Department of Neuroradiology
Hamburg, Germany

Gunther Fesl, MD
University of Munich-Grosshadern Medical Center
Department of Clinical Radiology
Division of Neuroradiology
Munich, Germany

Holger Goerike, MD
Conradia Imaging Center
Hamburg, Germany

Gerhard F. Hamann, MD
Dr. Horst Schmidt Hospital
Department of Neurology
Wiesbaden, Germany

Markus Holtmannspoetter, MD
Rigshospitalet Diagnostik
Department of Radiology
Copenhagen, Denmark

Joachem Klisch, MD
Helios Hospital Erfurt
Department of Diagnostic and Interventional Radiology
and Neuroradiology
Erfurt, Germany

Michael Knauth, MD
Göttingen University Hospital
Department of Neuroradiology
Göttingen, Germany

Andreas Kreusch
Göttingen University Hospital
Department of Neuroradiology
Göttingen, Germany

Wiebke Kurre, MD
Supervising Physician at Department of Diagnostic and
Interventional Radiology
Katharinenhospital
Stuttgart, Germany

Thomas Liebig, MD
Cologne University Hospital
Department of Diagnostic Radiology and Neuroradiology
Cologne, Germany

Jennifer Linn, MD
University of Munich-Grosshadern Medical Center
Department of Clinical Radiology
Division of Neuroradiology
Munich, Germany

Nina Lummel, MD
University of Munich-Grosshadern Medical Center
Department of Clinical Radiology
Division of Neuroradiology
Munich, Germany

Thomas E. Mayer, MD
Jena University Hospital
Center for Radiology
Division of Neuroradiology
Jena, Germany

Dominik Morhard, MD
Munich-Harlaching Municipal Hospital
Department of Diagnostic and Interventional Radiology,
Neuroradiology, and Nuclear Medicine
Munich, Germany

Christian Riedel, MD
Schleswig-Holstein University Hospital
Kiel Campus
Department of Neuroradiology
Kiel, Germany

Axel Rohr, MD
Schleswig-Holstein University Hospital
Kiel Campus
Department of Neuroradiology
Kiel, Germany

Gernot Schulte-Altedorneburg, MD
Munich-Harlaching Municipal Hospital
Department of Diagnostic and Interventional Radiology,
Neuroradiology, and Nuclear Medicine
Munich, Germany

Tobias Struffert, MD
University of Erlangen Medical Center
Department of Neuroradiology
Erlangen, Germany

Marc Tietke, MD, DDS.
Helios Hospital Schwerin
Department of Radiology and Neuroradiology
Schwerin, Germany

Abbreviations

A1	A1 segment of the anterior cerebral artery	FDA	Food and Drug Administration
ACA	Anterior cerebral artery	FLAIR	Fluid-attenuated inversion recovery
ACST	Asymptomatic Carotid Surgery Trial	FOV	Field of view
ACT	Activated clotting time	GESICA	Grupo de Estudio de la Sobrevida en la Insuficiencia Cardiac en Argentina
ADC	Apparent diffusion coefficient		
AICA	Anterior inferior cerebellar artery	h	Hour
AP	Anteroposterior	HMCAS	Hyperdense middle cerebral artery sign
APSAC	Anisoylated plasminogen-streptokinase activator complex	i.a.	Intra-arterial
		IAT	Intra-arterial thrombolysis
aPTT	Activated partial thromboplastin time	ICA	Internal carotid artery
ASK	Australian Streptokinase Study	ICSS	International Carotid Stenting Study
ASPECT	Alberta Stroke Program Early CT Score	ICU	Intensive care unit
atm	Atmospheres	INR	International normalized ratio
AV fistula	Arteriovenous fistula	IU	International units
BASICS	Basilar Artery International Cooperation Study	i.v.	Intravenous
		IVT	Intravenous thrombolysis
b.w.	Body weight	lys-plas	Human-derived Lys-plasminogen
CASES	Canadian Activase for Stroke Effectiveness Study	M1	M1 segment of the middle cerebral artery
		MAST-E	Multicenter Acute Stroke Trial–Europe Study Group 1996
CCA	Common carotid artery		
CE	Communauté Européenne (certification mark)	MAST-I	Multicenter Acute Stroke Trial–Italy 1995
		mbar	Millibars
CI	Confidence interval	MCA	Middle cerebral artery
CNS	Central nervous system	MIP	Maximum intensity projection
CREST	Carotid Revascularization Endarterectomy vs. Stenting Trial	MPR	Multiplanar reconstruction
		MPRAGE	Magnetization-prepared rapid acquisition gradient echo
CSF	Cerebrospinal fluid		
CT	Computed tomography	MRA	Magnetic resonance angiography
CTA	Computed tomographic angiography	MRI	Magnetic resonance imaging
CTP	CT perfusion imaging	mRS	Modified Rankin Scale, Modified Rankin Score
CVST	Cerebral venous and sinus thrombosis		
DAC	Distal access catheter	MT	Mechanical thrombectomy
DSA	Digital subtraction angiography	MTT	Mean transit time
DSC-PWI	Dynamic susceptibility-weighted perfusion MRI	NASCET	North American Symptomatic Carotid Endarterectomy Trial
DWI	Diffusion-weighted imaging	NIHSS	National Institutes of Health Stroke Scale
DW MRI	Diffusion-weighted magnetic resonance imaging	NINDS	National Institute of Neurological Disorders and Stroke
ECA	External carotid artery	NMDA	N-methyl-d-aspartate
ECASS	European Cooperative Acute Stroke Study	PA	Posteroanterior
ECG	Electrocardiography	PAI-1	Plasminogen activator inhibitor-1
ECASS	European Cooperative Acute Stroke Study	PCA	Posterior cerebral artery
ECST	European Carotid Surgery Trial	PI	Platelet inhibitor
EMEA	European Medicines Evaluation Agency	PICA	Posterior inferior cerebellar artery
EVA	Endarterectomy versus Angioplasty in Patients with Symptomatic Severe Carotid Stenosis	PSV	Peak systolic velocity
		PTA	Peripheral transluminal angioplasty
		PTT	Partial thromboplastin time
FII, FVII	Coagulation factor II, factor VII (etc.)	PWI	Perfusion-weighted imaging

RSAR	Removable stent-assistant revascularization	**TIA**	Transient ischemic attack
rtPA	Recombinant tissue plasminogen activator	**TOF MRA**	Time-of-flight magnetic resonance angiography
s	Seconds		
SITS-MOST	Safe Implementation of Thrombolysis in Stroke–Monitoring Study	**tPA**	Tissue-type plasminogen activator
		TTD	Time to drain
SK	Streptokinase	**TTP**	Time to peak
SWAN	Susceptibility-weighted angiography	**U**	Units
SWI	Susceptibility-weighted imaging	**UK**	Urokinase
SPACE	Stent-Protected Angioplasty versus Carotid Endarterectomy	**WASID**	Warfarin-Aspirin for Symptomatic Intracranial Disease

Contents

Contents

Neuroimaging of Stroke

1 Internal Carotid Artery Occlusion

O. Jansen

Introduction

Segmental Anatomy of the Internal Carotid Artery

The intradural portion of the internal carotid artery (ICA) is divided into four segments that are named and numbered as (from distal to proximal):
- *C1 segment:* the segment below the division of the carotid artery into the middle and anterior cerebral arteries (the "carotid T")
- *C2 segment:* the distal horizontal segment of the cavernous part of the ICA
- *C3 segment:* the vertical segment of the cavernous part
- *C4 segment:* the proximal horizontal segment of the cavernous part

The more proximal portions of the ICA are referred to in clinical parlance (from distal to proximal) as the petrous part; the subpetrous, cervical, or suprabulbar ICA; and finally the carotid bulb and origin of the ICA.

Definition of Carotid Artery Occlusion

> **Note**
>
> Every occlusion site correlates with an underlying cause that is typical for that location.

For example, occlusions of the ICA at its origin or at the carotid bulb are almost always caused by atherosclerotic stenosis. Most occlusions of the cervical ICA are caused by an acute carotid dissection, which always terminates at the entrance to the petrous part of the vessel. An acute occlusion of the petrous part is rare but may be caused by atherosclerosis at that level. The same applies to acute occlusions of the cavernous part (C2–C4), which are generally caused by the occlusion of a local, preexisting atherosclerotic stenosis.

On the other hand, acute occlusions of the C1 segment or the carotid T are almost always due to embolism from a cardiac source or, less commonly, a carotid source. The carotid T is the first site of relative narrowing in the carotid circulation where an embolus of substantial size may become lodged at the arterial junction, causing an acute vascular occlusion, and may subsequently grow due to proximal and/or distal thrombosis. As a result, these carotid T or C1 occlusions typically present with a large thrombus burden.

Traumatic or spontaneous intracranial carotid dissections are a very rare cause of acute carotid occlusions. Spontaneous intracranial carotid dissections, which are even rarer than traumatic dissections, may occur in patients with fibromuscular dysplasia or may be secondary to vasculitis.

Frequency of Carotid Artery Occlusions

Acute occlusions of the ICA, whether intra- or extracranial, have been recognized as the cause of ~5% of all strokes. Like acute basilar artery thrombosis, they are quite rare but may have severe manifestations due to the potential magnitude of the acute cerebral perfusion deficit, especially with a carotid-T occlusion, as well as the severity of acute neurologic deficits and the potential size of the resulting brain infarction.

In patients with a well-formed circle of Willis that would allow for the development of a collateral circulation, acute carotid occlusions proximal to the C1 segment may be asymptomatic or may produce fluctuating clinical symptoms. The latter presentation reflects a deficiency of collateral flow that is blood pressure–dependent and may lead to a hemodynamic infarction pattern.

Imaging Studies

Computed Tomography

As in all patients with acute stroke, noncontrast computed tomography (CT) is the initial imaging study of choice for patients with an acute carotid artery occlusion

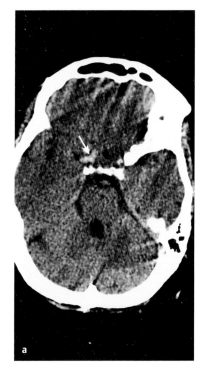 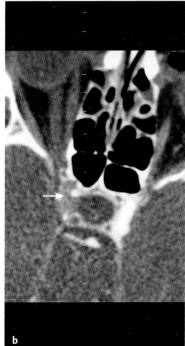 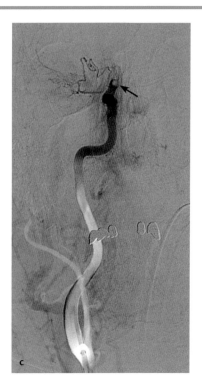

Fig. 1.1a–c Acute embolic occlusion of the carotid T.
a The hyperdense embolus is clearly visualized on cranial CT (*arrow*).
b CTA (source image) documents lack of opacification of the carotid siphon (*arrow*).

c DSA demonstrates the occlusion site in the C1 segment of the ICA and defines the proximal end of the thrombus (*arrow*).

(see Chapter 2). It can exclude hemorrhagic stroke and other causes of an acute neurologic deficit.

If the acute carotid occlusion is located proximal to the C1 segment, CT scans usually show no abnormalities other than possible early infarct signs (see Chapter 2 for more details). If collateral flow is deficient and clinical symptoms have been present for some time, CT images of these proximal carotid occlusions may demonstrate a chain of small infarctions in the terminal carotid branches above the level of the ventricles (cella media).

By contrast, the intravascular thrombi causing an acute occlusion of the carotid T and/or C1 segment almost always produce a hyperdense artery sign on noncontrast CT (see Chapter 2). This is particularly true when we note that the large thrombus burden of these occlusions allows for direct visualization of the thrombus even in relatively thick CT slices (**Fig. 1.1a**).

CT Angiography

CT angiography (CTA) is the CT technique of choice for the detection of carotid occlusion in acute stroke patients. Lack of opacification of the ICA and the imaging correlate of the carotid occlusion can be demonstrated

during interpretation of the CT source images as well as with 2D and 3D reconstructions (**Fig. 1.1b**). On the other hand, accurate localization of the carotid occlusion may be difficult with CTA. Ordinarily, CTA is performed in such a way that data acquisition for the CT slices takes place during the first pass of the contrast material through the arterial circulation. In patients with a distal carotid artery occlusion, the more proximal carotid segments are occupied by a blood column that admits contrast material at a very slow rate, if at all. This happens too slowly to be detected during data acquisition for CTA.

Practical Tip

Even if some small distal branch vessels from the ICA are still patent, such as the ophthalmic artery, meningohypophyseal trunk, posterior communicating artery, or anterior choroidal artery, overall blood flow in the ICA is still so diminished that the artery will show a general lack of opacification and appear occluded on CTA. It may be helpful in these cases to carefully reevaluate the noncontrast CT for hyperdense vessel signs or even view the CTA source images with a different window setting to permit a more accurate localization of the occlusion site.

I

Based on the phenomenon of slow blood flow in the ICA described above, CTA may also yield false-positive results. This can easily cause a pseudo-occlusion to be missed. If necessary, a second CTA dataset can be acquired immediately after the first to help localize the occlusion or aid differentiation from a pseudo-occlusion.

As a rule, magnetic resonance imaging (MRI) with MR angiography (MRA) is rarely used in patients with acute stroke. The problems of imprecise localization and differentiation from pseudo-occlusion described above for CT and CTA apply with equal validity to MRI and MRA.

Angiography

The definitive diagnosis and localization of an ICA occlusion can be established by catheter angiography using digital subtraction (DSA) technique (**Fig. 1.1c**). However, the differentiation between occlusion and pseudo-occlusion relies on special techniques that require a cooperative or sedated patient or the use of general anesthesia.

Practical Tip

The diagnostic catheter should be placed just proximal to the presumed ICA occlusion site. This presents no difficulty with extracranial carotid occlusions. The contrast material is then injected at sufficiently high concentration (undiluted if necessary), and the acquisition time of the DSA series should be long enough to detect the slow trickle of contrast material into a blood column, if present, or into the collapsed poststenotic lumen of a pseudo-occlusion. An acquisition time of up to 10–15 seconds at a film rate of 1–0.5 frames/s may be necessary to avoid missing a pseudo-occlusion. Meanwhile, the development of a collateral circulation via extra- or intracranial vessels should be documented to detect, say, retrograde filling of the carotid siphon via the ophthalmic artery (**Fig. 1.2**).

Caution

DSA findings may be misinterpreted in patients with acute distal occlusions of the ICA unless the correct protocol is followed.

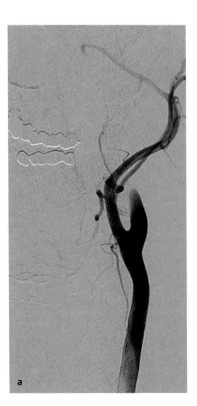
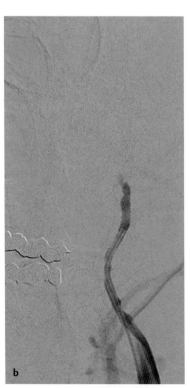

Fig. 1.2a,b   Old occlusion of the cervical carotid artery on DSA.
a Survey image with contrast injection documents an apparent occlusion with pseudotapering at the top of the carotid bulb.
b Selective catheterization of the carotid stump confirms a definitive occlusion in the upper cervical portion of the ICA.

An occlusion of the ICA that also occludes the distal branches (ophthalmic artery, etc.) leads to the stasis of blood throughout the ICA lumen. When the diagnostic catheter is placed into the common carotid artery (CCA) or even the proximal ICA, there will be no distal runoff of injected contrast material and even a very long angiographic series may create the impression of a proximal occlusion. Not infrequently, the injected contrast material may layer along the standing blood column in the extracranial ICA, mimicking the tapered sign or string sign of an extracranial ICA dissection (see the section on Digital Subtraction Angiography, p. 33) (**Fig. 1.2a**). Doubts can be resolved only by a more distal catheterization of the ICA lumen, perhaps advancing the microcatheter past the petrous part of the artery and repeating the angiographic series so that the occlusion site can be accurately located (**Fig. 1.2b**). Sometimes the location and length of an occlusion are clearly appreciated only when endovascular recanalization is performed. By carefully injecting contrast through the microcatheter and advancing the microcatheter and microwire across the occlusion site into the intracranial circulation, the operator can define the entire lumen of the ICA, the occlusion, and the length of the thrombus. Meanwhile the location of the occlusion and whether it can be passed with a catheter can provide clues to the etiopathogenesis of the occlusion.

Pseudo-occlusion of the Internal Carotid Artery

Note

By definition, a pseudo-occlusion of the ICA is present when noninvasive vascular imaging demonstrates a vascular occlusion but invasive catheter angiography documents a high-grade stenosis or partial occlusion.

Three grades of ICA pseudo-occlusion have been described (Kniemeyer et al. 1996):
- *Grade I:* a high-grade stenosis of the ICA in which the original lumen of the carotid artery is preserved (**Fig. 1.3**).
- *Grade II:* a segmental occlusion of the actual carotid lumen, but the distal lumen still carries antegrade flow through vasa vasorum in the carotid wall. Usually the carotid lumen is markedly reduced (**Fig. 1.4**).
- *Grade III:* an actual carotid occlusion in which the ICA stump is perfused by retrograde flow from the external carotid artery (ECA), usually as far as the occlusion site (**Fig. 1.5**).

I

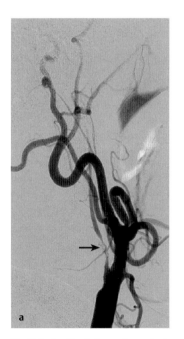 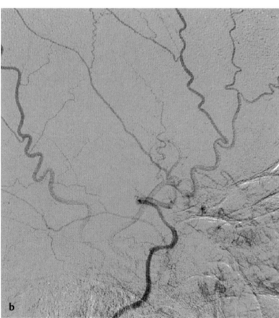

Fig. 1.3a,b Grade I pseudo-occlusion.

a Catheter angiography demonstrates a high-grade proximal stenosis of the ICA (*arrow*). The carotid lumen is preserved but markedly reduced in caliber.

b A long DSA series can still trace the narrowed carotid lumen into the cranial cavity.

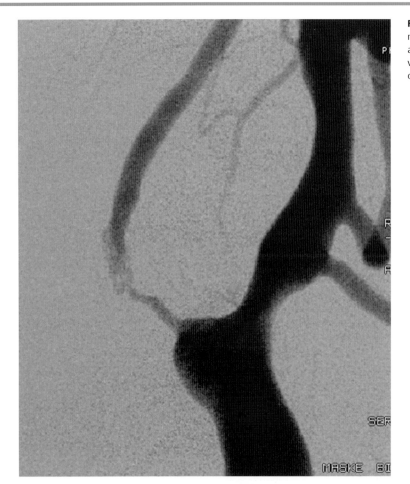

Fig. 1.4   Grade II pseudo-occlusion. Magnified DSA image of the common carotid artery demonstrates the recruitment of vasa vasorum. The original carotid lumen is occluded.

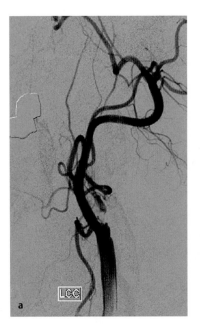

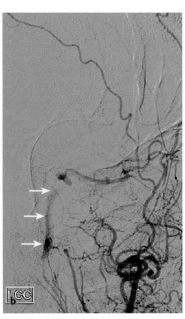

Fig. 1.5a,b   Grade III pseudo-occlusion.
a Survey angiogram shows residual filling of the proximal ICA stump through very small lumina.
b The actual lumen of the cervical and petrous ICA is filled by retrograde flow from ECA collaterals (*arrows*).

Improved imaging by high-resolution ultrasonography and contrast-enhanced MRA has allowed pseudo-occlusions to be detected in a growing number of patients, but definitive diagnosis and staging usually rely on catheter angiography. Pseudo-occlusions of the carotid artery have a relatively high stroke risk of 2–10% per year and therefore constitute an indication for treatment. Grade I pseudo-occlusions are readily accessible to endovascular treatment using a microcatheter technique (Terada et al. 2006). In rare cases even type III pseudo-occlusions are treatable by endovascular recanalization, whereas type II pseudo-occlusions require operative treatment.

Pseudo-occlusions require differentiation from the fairly common spontaneous recanalization of an acute ICA occlusion. In a series of 76 patients with acute ICA occlusions, Szabo et al. (2008) observed spontaneous recanalization in 12 of the cases. Recurrence of cerebral ischemia was noted in 10 of 12 patients during recanalization.

References

Kniemeyer HW, Aulich A, Schlachetzki F, Steinmetz H, Sandmann W. Pseudo- and segmental occlusion of the internal carotid artery: a new classification, surgical treatment and results. Eur J Vasc Endovasc Surg 1996;12(3):310–320

Szabo K, Kern R, Gass A, et al. Early spontaneous recanalization following acute carotid occlusion. J Neuroimaging 2008; 18(2):148–153

Terada T, Tsuura M, Matsumoto H, et al. Endovascular treatment for pseudo-occlusion of the internal carotid artery. Neurosurgery 2006;59(2):301–309, discussion 301–309

I

2 Middle Cerebral Artery Occlusion

C. Riedel

Introduction

The middle cerebral artery (MCA) supplies a large portion of the motor and sensory cortex of the brain. Additionally, the MCA territory of the dominant hemisphere harbors centers for speech reception and production, and the artery supplies other, bilateral centers for higher cognitive functions. Perforating branches from the main trunk of the MCA supply the basal ganglia and the corticospinal tracts.

> **Note**
>
> Occlusions of the MCA trunk are almost always symptomatic because the regions supplied by the MCA are of major functional importance.

The symptoms of an MCA trunk occlusion may be mild in very young patients owing to the presence of extensive collaterals. Generally the symptoms of an ischemic stroke in the MCA territory depend strongly on the site of the occlusion (e.g., proximal or distal main trunk, lenticulostriate arteries, upper and lower groups of the more distal MCA branches).

Segmental Anatomy of the Middle Cerebral Artery

The MCA is the largest branch of the internal carotid artery (ICA). The main trunk of the MCA, called the M1 segment (see also the section on Anatomy, p. 109), runs from the carotid bifurcation along the sylvian fissure between the surfaces of the temporal and frontal lobes to the limen insulae. In its course the main trunk of the MCA runs directly below the anterior perforated substance, a flat area at the base of the brain that is bounded medially by the interhemispheric fissure, laterally by the limen insulae, anteriorly by the division of the olfactory tracts, and posteriorly by the optic tract and temporal lobe. Along the sagittal plane, the perforated substance is subdivided into medial and lateral parts by a line running along the axis of the olfactory tract. This line separates the medial and lateral groups of lenticulostriate arteries, which pass into the perforated substance. Each cerebral hemisphere contains an average of ~10 lenticulostriate vessels (Rosner et al. 1984). Approximately 80% of the branches arise from the posterosuperior wall of the main trunk of the MCA. The other lenticulostriate perforators in the lateral group arise from proximal portions of the M2 branches of

the MCA, mainly from the upper division. The medial lenticulostriate perforators run directly through the perforated substance to the lentiform nucleus, which they supply along with portions of the caudate nucleus and internal capsule.

The lateral lenticulostriate arteries have a slightly larger diameter than those in the medial group. They arch toward the midline before entering the anterior perforated substance. First they wind around the lateral part of the putamen and distribute branches that supply a lateral portion of the anterior commissure, the internal capsule, the posterior part of the head of the caudate nucleus, and the lateral portion of the globus pallidus. More laterally situated structures, the claustrum and capsula extrema, receive their blood supply from insular branches.

Division of the MCA trunk is variable and may follow any of four patterns, some more common than others:
- A single trunk that does not give off equal-sized branches
- Bifurcating pattern
- Trifurcating pattern
- Division into four branches of approximately equal size

In the most common pattern, the MCA bifurcates into upper and lower divisions (64–90% of cases; Gibo et al. 1981). The MCA trifurcates in 12–29% of cases. The other patterns are much less frequent.

> **Note**
>
> The branching pattern of the MCA trunk is of clinical importance in acute ischemic stroke due to differences in the size of territories supplied by the upper and lower divisions. As a result, the clinical manifestations of the occlusion of one of these divisions are highly variable.

The lower group of MCA branches is usually dominant (in ~32% of cases), also supplying most of the cerebral convexity in the MCA territory including the entire temporal lobe and most of the parietal lobe as far as the central region. The upper group of MCA branches is dominant in ~28% of patients. In these cases their territory includes much of the parietal lobe as well as the frontal lobe and may extend to the temporal lobe. In the ~18% of patients with a bifurcating MCA, the upper and lower divisions are approximately equal in size and border each other in continuity with the sylvian fissure.

The 10–12 cortical branches of the MCA, which are variable in different patients, supply a large portion of the cerebral convexity and extend to the territories of the distal branches of the anterior and posterior cerebral arteries (ACA, PCA). These "watershed areas" between territories will shift in response to an acute occlusion of one of the arterial trunks through the recruitment of leptomeningeal collaterals.

Etiology and Clinical Manifestations of Middle Cerebral Artery Occlusion

An occlusion of the main trunk or a proximal branch of the MCA is most often the result of an embolic process or the growth of a mural thrombus located at a more proximal site. In approximately two-thirds of all patients with ischemic stroke, an embolic source can be identified in the heart, ICA, or both (Horowitz et al. 1997). Approximately 50% of emboli originate in the heart, whereas 25% arise from atheromatous plaques in the ICA. Luminal obstruction may also be due to local atheroma formation within the MCA, but this is much rarer in Western countries than in eastern Asia. In rare cases an intracranial dissection may lead to occlusion of the MCA trunk.

Most MCA trunk occlusions start in the proximal part of the vessel. This obstructs the lenticulostriate arteries, causing ischemia in the deep and superficial territories supplied by the MCA. The result is a contralateral sensorimotor deficit, which may be accompanied by aphasia depending on the affected hemisphere. With good collateralization from the ACA and PCA, most ischemic damage occurs to the deep territory of the MCA, resulting in lenticulostriate and capsular infarctions. With more distal occlusions that spare the lenticulostriate territory, the contralateral leg is usually unaffected because the fibers supplying the leg run along the medial wall of the lateral ventricle in the corona radiata, and the corresponding cortical area is supplied by the ACA.

Imaging Studies

Since the introduction of multislice CT scanners, CTA (CT angiography) and CTP (CT perfusion imaging) have become vitally important tools for the evaluation of stroke. A multimodal protocol has been developed for stroke CT analogous to that used in stroke MRI.

> **Note**
>
> For logistic reasons and reasons of patient management, CT is much easier to use than MRI in the evaluation of acute stroke. As a result, CT has become the first-line imaging study at most stroke centers. MRI is more likely to be used in follow-up examinations, chronic stroke patients, and small-vessel diseases than in acute diseases of the larger cervical and intracranial vessels.

This chapter, therefore, will focus on the elements of stroke CT. Details on stroke MRI can be found in specialized textbooks (e.g., Forsting and Jansen 2006; Jansen et al. 2008).

Noncontrast Computed Tomography

At most stroke centers, noncontrast cranial CT is the initial imaging study used for the evaluation of acute ischemic stroke. Besides the exclusion of intracranial hemorrhage and "stroke mimics" (tumor, abscess, subdural hematoma, etc.), noncontrast cranial CT is used mainly to evaluate the extent of early ischemic changes.

Early Ischemic Changes in the Brain Parenchyma

Early ischemic changes (early infarct signs) visible in CT scans of the MCA territory (**Fig. 2.1**) are characterized by hypoattenuation and isoattenuation between the cortical ribbon and white matter and between the basal ganglia and deep white matter (von Kummer et al. 1997). These decreases in CT density are usually attributed to cytotoxic edema in the affected gray and white matter areas. An occlusion of the MCA trunk is usually followed by infarction of the basal ganglia because the lenticulostriate perforators that branch from the main trunk are terminal vessels without collaterals. With good collateralization by an extensive network of leptomeningeal arteries and with early recanalization, the infarction caused by an MCA trunk occlusion may be confined to the basal ganglia. In many cases, however, collateralization from the ACA and PCA cannot adequately supply the MCA territory, and the loss of differentiation in the white matter and basal ganglia, noted above, is accompanied by corticomedullary hypodensities of variable extent. The percentage extent of these early ischemic changes relative to the total size of the MCA territory has been used for over 10 years as a prognostic factor and selection criterion for performing intravenous thrombolysis. For example, an analysis of the data from the European Cooperative Acute Stroke Study (ECASS; Hacke et al. 1995) showed that patients whose early ischemic changes involved less than one-third of the MCA territory derived significantly greater benefit from systemic thrombolysis than comparable patients treated with a placebo. When early ischemic changes involve more than one-third of the MCA territory, treatment outcomes are considerably less favorable and there is a greater risk of hemorrhagic transformation after thrombolysis (von Kummer et al. 1997).

Because evaluating the percentage extent of early ischemic changes relative to the total MCA territory is difficult and prone to errors, the Alberta Stroke Program Early CT (ASPECT) score was developed as an alternative

I

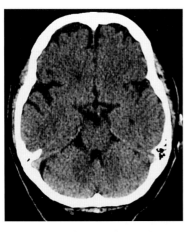 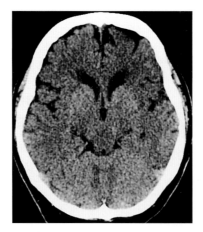 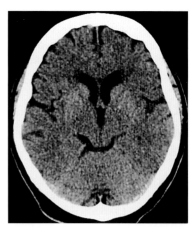

Fig. 2.1   Typical early ischemic changes associated with a thromboembolic occlusion of the main trunk of the left MCA.
Noncontrast cranial CT with a 2.5-mm slice thickness shows loss of gray-white matter differentiation in the area of the left frontal operculum. Also, the lentiform nucleus is obscured relative to the opposite side. CT scans were obtained ~2.5 h after symptom onset marked by global aphasia and predominantly upper limb weakness.

way to define the extent of demarcated infarctions with less interobserver variation. This scoring system (Pexman et al. 2001) subdivides axial CT scans into regions whose involvement by early ischemic changes is described by a 10-point score. The score is calculated from two axial scans, one at the level of the thalamus and basal ganglia and one at the superior border of the caudate nucleus in a plane that just excludes the nucleus from view. Both scans are subdivided into a total of 10 different anatomic regions, and each region is scrutinized for the presence of hypodensities and focal swelling of the brain parenchyma (**Fig. 2.2**). When these early ischemic changes are found in a region, a score of 1 point is assigned to that region.

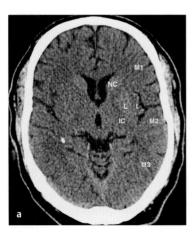 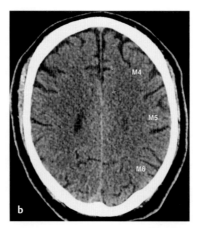

Fig. 2.2a, b   Definition of the ASPECT score for grading the extent of early ischemic changes.
A total of 10 separate regions are defined on two standard axial CT scans of the head. They include the caudate nucleus (NC), lentiform nucleus (L), internal capsule (IC), and insular cortex (I). Additional regions are the anterior MCA cortex (M1), the cortex of the anterior (M2) and posterior temporal lobe (M3), and the MCA cortex above M1 (M4), above M2 (M5), and above M3 (M6). Early ischemic changes in each of these regions cause one point to be deducted from the ASPECT score. Thus a normal-appearing noncontrast cranial CT scan would score 10 points while ischemic changes involving all of the MCA territory would score 0 points. Patients with an ASPECT score ≥ 7 are predicted to have better response to intravenous thrombolysis with recombinant tissue plasminogen activator (rtPA) and a better clinical course after treatment.
a Axial noncontrast CT scan at the level of the thalamus and basal ganglia.
b Axial noncontrast CT scan just above the caudate nucleus.

Early Ischemic Changes in Basal Cerebral Vessels

Besides the changes in the brain parenchyma described above, the early signs of infarction detectable by noncontrast CT also include density changes in the basal cerebral vessels, especially the main trunk of the MCA. Thromboembolic occlusion of the MCA may appear as a focal hyperdensity in the artery when imaged by noncontrast cranial CT. This hyperdense middle cerebral artery (HMCA) sign was described as early as 1983 and validated by DSA studies confirming thromboembolic occlusion of the MCA (Gács et al. 1983). Since then, corresponding focal hyperdensities have been described in the basal cerebral arteries as evidence of vascular occlusion, including the intracranial portion of the ICA (Ozdemir et al. 2008), the proximal PCA (Krings et al. 2006), and the ACA (Jensen et al. 2010). Despite the high specificity of this sign for thrombotic obliteration of the vessel lumen (von Kummer et al. 1994), the HMCA sign has established itself only as one factor for predicting poor response to intravenous thrombolysis (Leys et al. 1992; Moulin et al. 1996; Tomsick et al. 1996).

The prognosis of stroke patients also depends critically on the extent of the occlusion and the length of the obliterated vascular segment (Barber et al. 2001; Somford et al. 2002). Thus, very short occlusions in peripheral branches of the MCA have been identified as focal hyperdensities (MCA dot sign) on noncontrast cranial CT. This sign was found to be associated with a more favorable prognosis than the HMCA sign (Leary et al. 2003). In another study comparing the treatment of stroke patients by mechanical recanalization with intravenous thrombolysis, the interventional treatment was found to achieve better recanalization, especially in patients with a well-defined HMCA sign. To date, however, the hyperdensity sign in a branch of the MCA has not been used in the routine evaluation of acute stroke, either to predict clinical course or to guide the selection of treatment. This is due mainly to the very low sensitivity of the sign. In stroke studies using the HMCA sign as a parameter, its sensitivity for detecting vascular occlusion was found to range from 15% (Qureshi et al. 2006) to 30% (Leys et al. 1992). This low sensitivity is explained by the luminal diameter of the MCA trunk, its predominantly horizontal course, and the slice thicknesses typically used in noncontrast cranial CT. Many studies have employed a slice thickness of 5–10 mm, but the main trunk of the MCA has an average diameter of only ~2.5 mm. With a slice thickness 2–4 times the MCA diameter, the hyperdense intraluminal thrombotic material in one slice is averaged along with an equal or greater quantity of cerebrospinal fluid (CSF) in the adjacent subarachnoid space of the sylvian fissure and also with adjacent brain tissue. This partial-volume effect greatly reduces the likelihood of detecting thrombus in the main trunk of the MCA.

> ### Practical Tip
>
> In one study using thinner CT slices acquired at a considerably higher radiation dose, it was found that hyperdensities caused by thrombi in the proximal MCA were detectable in nearly all cases (Kim et al. 2005). The partial-volume effect described above decreases linearly with the slice thickness, accompanied by a corresponding gain in intraluminal contrast.

The noise level in the image increases only with the square root of the reciprocal of the slice thickness, so the signal-to-noise ratio for thrombus detection rises steadily as the slice thickness is decreased, until the slice thickness is significantly less than the smallest diameter of the thrombus. This principle is illustrated in **Fig. 2.3**, which shows several axial thick-slab maximum intensity projections (MIPs) in a patient with an acute occlusion of the left MCA trunk. The images were reconstructed at various slice thicknesses. As the slice thickness declines, a linear hyperdensity (HMCA sign) becomes increasingly visible in the left sylvian fissure. This correlate of a thrombus in the main trunk of the left MCA is almost totally obscured in images reconstructed with a 5-mm slice thickness, despite its substantial length.

By using thin-slice reconstructions of noncontrast CT scans, it is even possible to make a reliable quantitative assessment of the length of the MCA occlusion based on slice thicknesses of 2.5 mm or less (Riedel et al. 2010). By estimating the thrombus burden in this way, we can predict the likelihood of achieving successful recanalization by systemic thrombolysis. This relationship, and the clinical relevance of the thrombus burden as a prognostic factor for response to systemic thrombolysis, are shown graphically in **Fig. 2.4**, which is based on the results of a current study by the authors. We performed an initial thin-slice reconstruction of noncontrast cranial CT data in patients with acute stroke treated by systemic thrombolysis within the 3-hour therapeutic window. The length of the thrombus was measured and compared with the success of recanalization by thrombolysis (assessed by transcranial Doppler, CTA, or MRA). We also evaluated clinical status at discharge and correlated it with thrombus burden and recanalization rates.

The results of this study suggest that the thrombus burden, when measured as length of occlusion, is not only a good predictor of recanalization by systemic thrombolysis but is also a useful parameter for predicting the initial clinical response to thrombolysis. Prospective treatment studies are still needed to determine whether this parameter can also aid in selecting patients for a mechanical recanalization procedure.

I

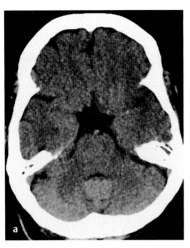 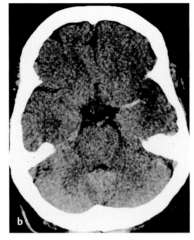 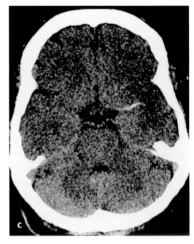

Fig. 2.3a–c   MIPs of basal noncontrast cranial CT scans reconstructed at various slice thicknesses.

a With an axial slice thickness of 5 mm, a definite hyperdense artery sign cannot be identified.

b With a slice thickness of 2.5 mm, image noise is slightly more distinct and a HMCA sign can be seen all along the main trunk of the left MCA.

c With a slice thickness of 0.625 mm, the exact dimensions of the HMCA sign are clearly visible in the very thin-slice reconstruction.

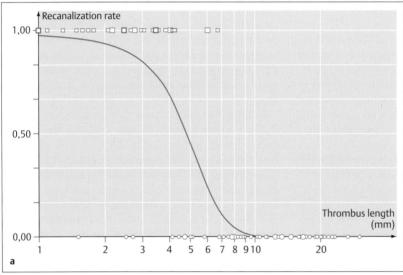

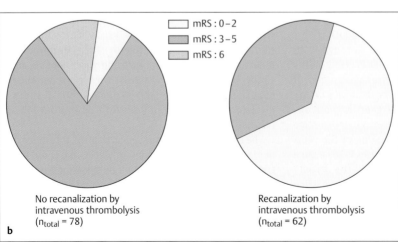

Fig. 2.4a, b   Study on recanalization rates and clinical discharge status after systemic thrombolysis (From Riedel CH, Jensen U, Rohr A, et al. Assessment of thrombus in acute middle cerebral artery occlusion using thin-slice nonenhanced Computed Tomography reconstructions. Stroke 2010;41(8):1659–1664).

a Relationship between recanalization rate by systemic thrombolysis and measurable thrombus length. Each individual patient is represented by a circle (successful recanalization) or a square (no recanalization). A logistic regression shows that almost no recanalization is achieved when thrombus length is > 8 mm.

b The modified Rankin Scale (mRS), which measures patient status at discharge from first hospital admission, indicates a significantly poorer result (average difference of ~2 mRS points) for patients in the failed recanalization group.

CT Perfusion Imaging

Ideally, the inflow dynamics of contrast material through a basal cerebral artery (arterial input function) and its outflow through a large collecting vein (venous output function) should be known in order to determine the above parameters, but older CT scanners with a relatively narrow detector field could typically scan only two or four basal CTP images, thereby missing a large portion of the MCA territory. With the advent of modern multislice CT scanners with a large number of detector rows and a correspondingly wide detector ring, it is now possible to scan almost the entire MCA territory in a single CTP examination. Perfusion imaging with a 64-slice scanner may use a "toggling table" technique (Roberts et al. 2001; Wintermark et al. 2004) in which scans are acquired in an alternating fashion using two different table positions, two scans at each position, to double the effective width of the CT detector. With a detector width of 4 cm, this technique provides an extended craniocaudal coverage of 8 cm, which is sufficient to evaluate a large portion of the supratentorial brain.

Perfusion mapping in stroke patients may reveal hypoperfused territories in which cerebral blood flow is decreased while cerebral blood volume is preserved. Reversible ischemic change is assumed to be present in those areas. Other areas may show decreased cerebral blood flow accompanied by a marked decrease in cerebral blood volume. This pattern represents the "infarcted core" of irreversibly damaged tissue. From the relationship of these territories, one can estimate the volume of brain parenchyma (penumbra, tissue at risk) that is still salvageable by recanalization.

Figure 2.5 illustrates how the toggling table technique can be used to image a large portion of the supratentorial brain. **Figure 2.6** shows infarctions following successful and unsuccessful recanalization by systemic thrombolysis relative to the baseline CTP images.

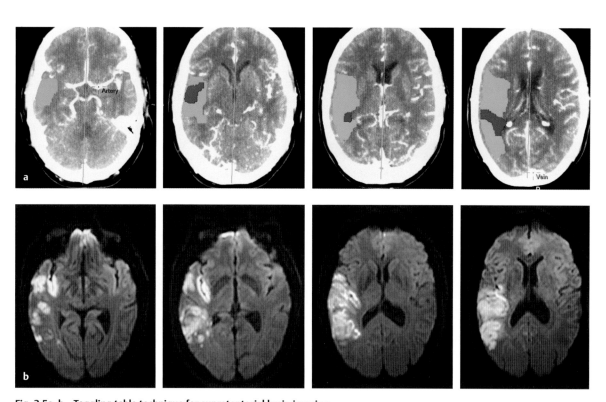

Fig. 2.5a, b   Toggling table technique for supratentorial brain imaging.

a CTP color maps generated from toggling table scans show hypoperfusion of the left MCA territory with areas of decreased cerebral blood flow (*green*) and decreased cerebral blood volume (*red*).

b Diffusion-weighted MR images (DWI) > 24 h after admission document infarction of the hypoperfused brain areas in the CTP maps. CTP fully depicted all of the subsequent infarcted areas.

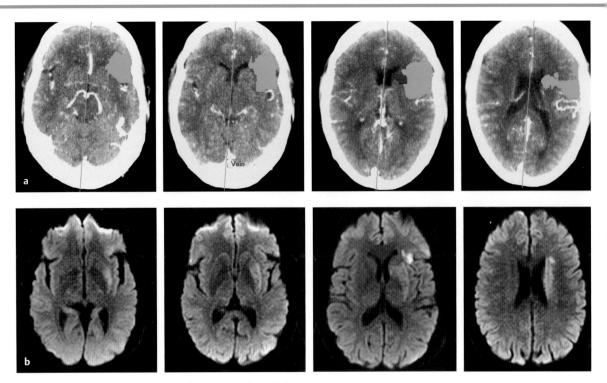

Fig. 2.6a, b   Success of recanalization by systemic thrombolysis.
Parenchyma with decreased cerebral blood volume is found to be infarcted after treatment. The region of hypoperfused brain that showed only a decrease in cerebral blood flow is not infarcted. If recanalization by thrombolytic therapy is unsuccessful, all of the hypoperfused tissue areas in the CTP maps are infarcted.
a CTP before recanalization.
b DWI sequences after successful recanalization of the MCA by systemic thrombolysis.

CT Angiography and Digital Subtraction Angiography

> **Note**
>
> CTA is an important adjunct to noncontrast cranial CT and CTP because it either confirms the site of a thromboembolic occlusion or demonstrates pseudo-occlusion by an embolus that is as yet nonocclusive.

In the case of a long, nonocclusive thrombus in the main trunk of the MCA, it may be appropriate to withhold primary mechanical recanalization or mechanical recanalization after bridging therapy (see section on Bridging Therapy, p. 76), despite the significant thrombus burden. Initial treatment may be limited to intravenous thrombolysis with recombinant tissue plasminogen activator (rtPA, alteplase). In this case the thrombolytic agent does not need to penetrate a long way into the thrombus but can act upon a large surface area of the thrombus. One such scenario is illustrated in **Fig. 2.7**.

Another indication for CTA is to document contrast delivery to thrombus interfaces. This may be limited due to absent or deficient collaterals at the distal end of the arterial occlusion. **Figure 2.8** shows noncontrast cranial CT scans and CTA images from two patients with an acute occlusion of the MCA trunk. In one patient CTA shows contrast material reaching the distal end of the HMCA sign seen on noncontrast cranial CT (see **Fig. 2.8a**), whereas in the second patient CTA shows no luminal opacification distal to the hyperdense MCA segment (see **Fig. 2.8b**), even though the same imaging protocols were used.

If the contrast material does not reach both the proximal and distal ends of the embolus, it is unlikely that there will be adequate delivery of thrombolytic agent to the embolus during systemic thrombolysis. There will also be a risk of appositional thrombus growth at one end of the embolus during treatment if the agent can reach the embolus from one side only. **Figure 2.9** illustrates a special case of poor contrast inflow on CTA and the gain provided by subsequent DSA followed by mechanical recanalization. Noncontrast cranial CT was performed in a 54-year-old woman with left hemispheric symptoms 3.5 h after symptom onset (see **Fig. 2.9a**). The scans excluded intracerebral hemorrhage while showing little evidence of early ischemic changes and only a short hyperdensity in the left bifurcation of the MCA. Subsequent CTA (see **Fig. 2.9b**) demonstrated a cutoff of

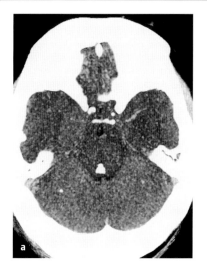

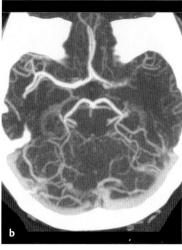

Fig. 2.7a, b Intravenous thrombolysis with rtPA in a 45-year-old woman with fluctuating symptoms of left hemispheric stroke that began 3 h before admission.

a HMCA sign is visible on noncontrast cranial CT.

b MIPs of basal CTA slices in the same patient obtained immediately after noncontrast CT show passage of contrast material along the full extent of the thrombus. After intravenous thrombolysis with rtPA, a hyperdense artery sign was no longer visible in the proximal right MCA and there was no evidence of a demarcated infarction.

vessel opacity at the origin of the main trunk of the left MCA. During subsequent DSA, a microcatheter could be passed into the left MCA trunk without resistance. DSA via the microcatheter (see **Fig. 2.9c**) demonstrated the embolic obstruction of the left MCA bifurcation and the origin of all lenticulostriate perforators arising from the C1 segment of the left ICA. As a result of this normal variant, the blind termination of the vessel lumen was sufficient to decrease flow into the main trunk of the MCA.

Prospective studies are needed to determine whether nonvisualization of the unobliterated vessel lumen close to the occlusion site is useful in predicting response to systemic thrombolysis. In any case, insufficient delivery of contrast material to the distal end of an occlusion is a sure sign of insufficient collateralization. When combined with a decrease in cerebral blood volume, it is an unfavorable prognostic factor for the success of recanalization therapy.

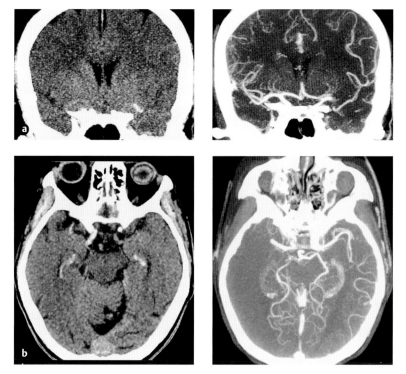

Fig. 2.8a, b Poor contrast delivery to the thrombus due to insufficient collateral vessels.

a Noncontrast cranial CT (*left*) and CTA (*right*). The thrombus in this patient produces an HMCA sign on plain CT and is outlined on both sides by contrast material at CTA.

b In this patient the contrast material reaches the proximal end of the embolus at CTA but does not opacify the distal lumen—most likely a result of insufficient collateral vessels.

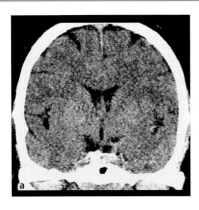
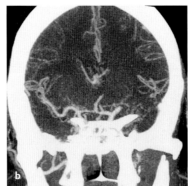
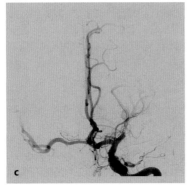
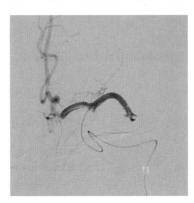

Fig. 2.9a–c   Special case of inadequate contrast material inflow on CTA in a 54-year-old woman with left hemispheric symptoms.

a Noncontrast cranial CT shows a short HMCA sign in the left MCA bifurcation.

b CTA shows cutoff of contrast inflow near the origin of the left MCA trunk from the ICA.

c DSA: Microcatheter series from the freely accessible main trunk of the left MCA demonstrates occlusion of the left MCA bifurcation and the origin of the lenticulostriate perforators from the left ICA as a normal variant, causing the left MCA trunk to appear as an unperfused blind pouch.

References

Barber PA, Demchuk AM, Hudon ME, Pexman JH, Hill MD, Buchan AM. Hyperdense sylvian fissure MCA "dot" sign: A CT marker of acute ischemia. Stroke 2001;32(1):84–88

Demchuk AM, Hill MD, Barber PA, Silver B, Patel SC, Levine SR; NINDS rtPA Stroke Study Group, NIH. Importance of early ischemic computed tomography changes using ASPECTS in NINDS rtPA Stroke Study. Stroke 2005;36(10):2110–2115

Forsting M, Jansen O. MRT des Zentralnervensystems. Stuttgart: Thieme; 2006

Gács G, Fox AJ, Barnett HJ, Vinuela F. CT visualization of intracranial arterial thromboembolism. Stroke 1983;14(5):756–762

Gibo H, Carver CC, Rhoton ALJ Jr, Lenkey C, Mitchell RJ. Microsurgical anatomy of the middle cerebral artery. J Neurosurg 1981;54(2):151–169

Hacke W, Kaste M, Fieschi C, et al; The European Cooperative Acute Stroke Study (ECASS). Intravenous thrombolysis with recombinant tissue plasminogen activator for acute hemispheric stroke. JAMA 1995;274(13):1017–1025

Horowitz DR, Tuhrim S, Weinberger JM, Budd J, Alweiss GS, Goldman ME. Transesophageal echocardiography: diagnostic and clinical applications in the evaluation of the stroke patient. J Stroke Cerebrovasc Dis 1997;6(5):332–336

Jansen O, Forsting M, Sartor K. Neuroradiologie. 4th ed. Stuttgart: Thieme; 2008

Jensen UR, Weiss M, Zimmermann P, Jansen O, Riedel C. The hyperdense anterior cerebral artery sign (HACAS) as a computed tomography marker for acute ischemia in the anterior cerebral artery territory. Cerebrovasc Dis 2010;29(1):62–67

Kim EY, Lee SK, Kim DJ, et al. Detection of thrombus in acute ischemic stroke: value of thin-section noncontrast computed tomography. Stroke 2005; 36 (12): 2745–2747

Krings T, Noelchen D, Mull M, et al. The hyperdense posterior cerebral artery sign: a computed tomography marker of acute ischemia in the posterior cerebral artery territory. Stroke 2006;37(2):399–403

von Kummer R, Meyding-Lamadé U, Forsting M, et al. Sensitivity and prognostic value of early CT in occlusion of the middle cerebral artery trunk. AJNR Am J Neuroradiol 1994;15(1):9–15, discussion 16–18

von Kummer R, Allen KL, Holle R, et al. Acute stroke: usefulness of early CT findings before thrombolytic therapy. Radiology 1997;205(2):327–333

Leary MC, Kidwell CS, Villablanca JP, et al. Validation of computed tomographic middle cerebral artery "dot" sign: an angiographic correlation study. Stroke 2003;34(11):2636–2640

Leys D, Pruvo JP, Godefroy O, Rondepierre P, Leclerc X. Prevalence and significance of hyperdense middle cerebral artery in acute stroke. Stroke 1992;23(3):317–324

Moulin T, Cattin F, Crépin-Leblond T, et al. Early CT signs in acute middle cerebral artery infarction: predictive value for subsequent infarct locations and outcome. Neurology 1996; 47(2):366–375

Ozdemir O, Leung A, Bussière M, Hachinski V, Pelz D. Hyperdense internal carotid artery sign: a CT sign of acute ischemia. Stroke 2008;39(7):2011–2016

Pexman JH, Barber PA, Hill MD, et al. Use of the Alberta Stroke Program Early CT Score (ASPECTS) for assessing CT scans in patients with acute stroke. AJNR Am J Neuroradiol 2001;22(8):1534–1542

Qureshi AI, Ezzeddine MA, Nasar A, et al. Is IV tissue plasminogen activator beneficial in patients with hyperdense artery sign? Neurology 2006;66(8):1171–1174

Riedel CH, Jensen U, Rohr A, et al. Assessment of thrombus in acute middle cerebral artery occlusion using thin-slice nonenhanced Computed Tomography reconstructions. Stroke 2010;41(8):1659–1664

Roberts HC, Roberts TP, Smith WS, Lee TJ, Fischbein NJ, Dillon WP. Multisection dynamic CT perfusion for acute cerebral ischemia: the "toggling-table" technique. AJNR Am J Neuroradiol 2001;22(6):1077–1080

Rosner SS, Rhoton AL Jr, Ono M, Barry M. Microsurgical anatomy of the anterior perforating arteries. J Neurosurg 1984;61(3):468–485

Somford DM, Nederkoorn PJ, Rutgers DR, Kappelle LJ, Mali WP, van der Grond J. Proximal and distal hyperattenuating middle cerebral artery signs at CT: different prognostic implications. Radiology 2002;223(3):667–671

Tomsick T, Brott T, Barsan W, et al. Prognostic value of the hyperdense middle cerebral artery sign and stroke scale score before ultraearly thrombolytic therapy. AJNR Am J Neuroradiol 1996;17(1):79–85

Wintermark M, Smith WS, Ko NU, Quist M, Schnyder P, Dillon WP. Dynamic perfusion CT: optimizing the temporal resolution and contrast volume for calculation of perfusion CT parameters in stroke patients. AJNR Am J Neuroradiol 2004;25(5):720–729

Wintermark M, Sesay M, Barbier E, et al. Comparative overview of brain perfusion imaging techniques. Stroke 2005; 36(9):e83–e99

3 Vertebrobasilar Occlusion

D. Morhard and G. Schulte-Altedorneburg

Introduction

Definition, Etiology, and Incidence

Ischemia in the "posterior" circulation of the brain is caused by atherosclerotic or embolic occlusive processes involving the vertebral arteries, basilar artery, and posterior cerebral arteries. The occlusion of one or more cerebellar arteries (posterior inferior cerebellar artery, anterior inferior cerebellar artery, superior cerebellar artery) is also detectable in many cases (**Fig. 3.1**). Thus, vertebrobasilar occlusions have the same pathogenesis as ischemic infarctions in the anterior circulation. The mortality rate of brainstem strokes is ~3–6% (Glass et al. 2002). These authors found that 21% of 361 patients with brainstem infarction had a poor neurologic outcome (death or severe disability) 30 days after the index event while 28% no longer had a significant neurologic deficit at 1 month (Glass et al. 2002). The largest subset of patients (~50%) retained only minor neurologic deficits.

As in the carotid artery territory, dissections in the vertebrobasilar system are relatively rare with an incidence of 1–1.5 cases per 100 000 population per year. They are an important entity in juvenile stroke, however, which differs from thrombotic and embolic occlusions in its treatment, prognosis, and follow-up (Dittrich et al. 2006).

> **Caution**
>
> Thrombosis of the basilar artery requires differentiation from usually circumscribed lacunar or territorial brainstem and cerebellar infarctions caused by the occlusion of a perforator or cerebellar artery (Pfefferkorn et al. 2006; Schulte-Altedorneburg and Brückmann 2006).

Occlusion of the principal brainstem artery, known in clinical parlance as basilar artery thrombosis, is the most severe form of ischemic stroke—comparable in severity to occlusion of the carotid T (see Chapter 1). When untreated, or when treated with nonthrombolytic agents alone, it has an ~80% mortality rate. The symptoms may be of sudden onset, progressive, or fluctuating. Clinical features depend

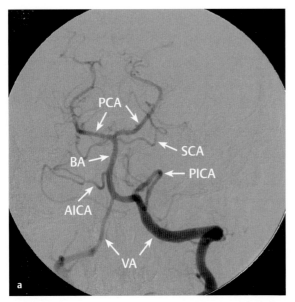
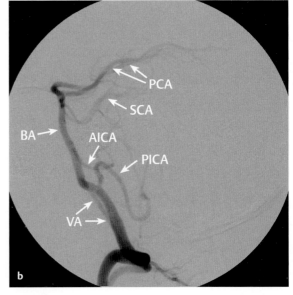

Fig. 3.1a, b DSA after selective contrast injection into the left vertebral artery.

Left side displays typical vascular anatomy with a dominant vertebral artery and large posterior inferior cerebellar artery. Right side shows a variant with a hypoplastic posterior inferior cerebellar artery and a relatively large anterior inferior cerebellar artery.

a Lateral projection.

b PA projection. AICA, anterior inferior cerebellar artery; BA, basilar artery; PCA, posterior cerebral artery; PICA, posterior inferior cerebellar artery; SCA, superior cerebellar artery; VA, vertebral artery.

on the level of the basilar artery occlusion (medulla oblongata, pons, mesencephalon), with or without involvement of the V4 segments of the vertebral artery and P1 segments of the posterior cerebral artery, and thus on the portion of the brainstem predominantly affected by the hypoperfusion (Ferbert et al. 1990). The endovascular treatment of basilar artery thrombosis with thrombolytic agents, first practiced by H. Zeumer in 1982, set the stage for the modern interventional treatment of stroke (Zeumer et al. 1982).

Symptoms of Brainstem and Cerebellar Syndromes

Caution

The combination and severity of brainstem and cerebellar symptoms are highly diverse and, despite typical cardinal signs (vertigo, diplopia, nystagmus, ataxia, dysarthria), may be confused with ischemia in the anterior circulation or with nonneurologic disorders (e.g., blood pressure fluctuations, cardiac arrhythmias, panic attacks, vestibular vertigo, or toxic exposure).

This particularly applies to the cardinal symptom of vertigo. Nonlinear progression or fluctuation of symptoms may also lead to initial misidentification of the syndrome. This pitfall should be considered in the general CT/MRI imaging protocol for strokes (see below). If clinical uncertainty exists, the region of interest should be investigated by (thin-slice) imaging of the entire brainstem, which may even include the cervical spinal cord (Schulte-Altedorneburg and Brückmann 2006).

With a vascular occlusion or "hemodynamically significant" stenosis (defined as > 50% lumen reduction by some authors, > 70% by others), the brainstem syndrome that would be expected in the affected territory will not always develop because the arterial supply and collateral pathways in the vertebrobasilar system can vary greatly in different individuals. This is also true of collaterals to the anterior circulation via external carotid artery (ECA) branches and posterior communicating branches, for example. Accordingly, variants in vascular anatomy (e.g., hypoplasia of an extra- or intracranial vertebral artery segment or a P1 segment of the posterior cerebral arteries) or less than a 50% atherosclerotic stenosis are often a mere coincidence and thus represent incidental findings (Matula et al. 1997; Schulte-Altedorneburg and Clevert 2009).

Macroangiopathic Lesions

This section explores the clinical presentations of common brainstem syndromes as a function of the affected vascular territories.

Vertebral Artery

Sites of predilection for atherosclerotic occlusive disease in the vertebral artery are the ostium (junction of V0 and V1 segments) and the terminal V4 segment. Bilateral high-grade stenoses or occlusions of the vertebral artery may lead to hemodynamically induced transient ischemic attacks with muscular weakness, vertigo, nystagmus, and diplopia. They are a potential source of embolization or autochthonous thrombosis.

A vertebral artery occlusion at the intradural level obstructs the perforators to the lateral medulla oblongata, resulting in a lateral or dorsolateral medulla oblongata syndrome.

Besides vertebral artery occlusion, an occlusion of the posterior inferior cerebellar artery may lead to Wallenberg syndrome, characterized by an ipsilateral Horner triad (ptosis, miosis, hemianhidrosis), contralateral dissociated sensory loss on the trunk and limbs for temperature and pain sensation, vertigo, nausea, hoarseness, dysphagia, and trigeminal neuropathy with pain, burning, and sensory loss on the ipsilateral side of the face. The classic form of Wallenberg syndrome is rarely encountered in everyday practice because pial anastomoses between branches of the anterior inferior cerebellar artery, posterior inferior cerebellar artery, and medulla-supplying perforators from the lower basilar artery can forestall the development of a complete dorsolateral medulla oblongata infarction.

Posterior Inferior Cerebellar Artery

The posterior inferior cerebellar artery is typically a large vessel that supplies more than half of the ipsilateral cerebellar hemisphere. Ischemic infarction produces a typical cerebellar syndrome with vertigo, nausea, vomiting, ipsilateral ataxia, spontaneous rotary nystagmus, dysmetria, rebound phenomenon, and intention tremor.

In many cases the posterior inferior cerebellar artery also helps supply the territory of the anterior inferior cerebellar artery, and its occlusion may give rise to an extensive, potentially malignant cerebellar infarction. This condition presents clinically with decreased level of consciousness, vomiting, hiccups, and abducens paralysis.

Practical Tip

Besides clinical monitoring, close-interval CT follow-ups should be scheduled during the first 4 days to allow for prompt detection and early decompression of incipient obstructive hydrocephalus.

Anterior Inferior Cerebellar Artery

The territory supplied by the anterior inferior cerebellar artery is variable and generally includes rostral portions of the medulla oblongata, the base of the pons, and the cerebellum. Experience has shown that most occlusions are secondary to atherosclerotic changes in the basilar artery or even basilar artery thrombosis. An occlusion leads to cerebellar and pontine deficits marked by vertigo, nausea, nystagmus, ipsilateral ataxia, facial nerve palsy, or even tinnitus.

Superior Cerebellar Artery

Isolated occlusion of the superior cerebellar artery is very rare. It is more common to find (partial) occlusions of the superior cerebellar artery in a setting of basilar tip embolism. Midbrain and/or cerebellar infarctions may occur due to the perimesencephalic course of the vessel. Thus the clinical features may include an ipsilateral Horner triad, astasia, abasia, ataxia, and contralateral dissociated sensory loss.

Posterior Cerebral Artery

Occlusive lesions located in the initial segment of the posterior cerebral artery (proximal to the posterior communicating artery, P1 segment) or just distal to the origin of the posterior communicating artery lead to the obstruction of small paramedian arteries that supply portions of the mesencephalon, thalamus, and geniculate bodies. Thus, an obstruction of these perforators leads to decreased level of consciousness (see also basilar tip embolism, below) with apathy, disorientation, aspontaneity, hemineglect, memory loss, and oculomotor nerve dysfunction.

On the other hand, a more distal occlusion located in the P2 or P3 segment would be expected to produce a cortical syndrome with visual field defects (homonymous hemianopsia to the opposite side, quadrantanopia) due to infarction of the visual cortex.

Basilar Artery

The basilar artery is the central artery supplying the brainstem. Its branches supply all the elementary functional units of the brainstem (e.g., autonomic coordination centers for respiration, circulation and blood pressure; the reticular formation; the center for visual spatial orientation).

The basilar artery is variable in its collateral connections. An intracranial occlusion can be bridged by the circle of Willis, by pial collateralization of the long circumferential arteries, and by the stepladder arrangement of pial collaterals to the short circumferential arteries.

Practical Tip

Symptoms may have an acute onset with immediate loss of consciousness or may be progressive, depending on individual collateral patterns and the location and extent of the basilar artery occlusion.

The vertebrobasilar occlusion may be preceded for a period of hours or weeks by fluctuating prodromal symptoms with vestibular signs (diplopia, vertigo, and nausea), posterior neck pain, or occipital headache. With subsequent appositional thrombosis, these signs will progress to a more severe neurologic syndrome with preservation of consciousness (progressive stroke) or a sudden decrease in consciousness caused by arterioarterial embolism to the basilar artery tip (Ferbert et al. 1990). On the whole, a progressive course is more common than the sudden onset of symptoms (Ferbert et al. 1990).

The following basilar artery syndromes are distinguished according to the level of the occlusion:

- *Caudal vertebrobasilar syndrome:* Predominantly affected brainstem regions are the medulla oblongata and base of the pons. The course is usually progressive, and prodromal symptoms may be present or absent. Lower cranial nerve deficits (nerves IX–XII) present mainly with dysphagia and speech impairment. Ataxia is also present. Pontine base involvement may initially produce hemiparesis, but symmetrical or asymmetrical tetraparesis is more commonly observed.
- *Mid-basilar artery syndrome:* The pons (base and tegmentum) is predominantly affected. Decreased blood flow to the pontine base leads to hemiparesis or, more commonly, symmetrical or asymmetrical tetraparesis. Dysarthria and anarthria are also common. The pontine tegmentum is supplied by perforators arising from the tip or distal bifurcation of the basilar artery. Consciousness becomes impaired if the collateral supply is inadequate or the thrombus spreads farther distally, decreasing blood flow through the perforators at the basilar tip.
- *Basilar tip syndrome:* Predominantly affected brain (stem) regions are the mesencephalon, thalamus, and mesial temporal lobe. Distal embolism causes visual disturbance ranging from field defects to cortical blindness. With occlusion of the basilar tip, the proximal obstruction of both posterior cerebral arteries leads to characteristic "top-of-the-basilar" syndrome. Decreased blood flow to the mesial temporal lobe is characterized by memory loss or altered mental status (agitation and confusion, apathy), in which case consciousness is maintained. With insufficient collateralization of the temporal lobe, the patient also develops cortical blindness with or without anosognosia. Occlusive involvement of the mesodiencephalic perforators may additionally lead to akinetic mutism, pupillary disturbances, and ophthalmoplegia. Consciousness becomes impaired if the thrombus also blocks the paramedian perforators of the mesencephalon arising from the basilar tip and proximal P1 segment.

Locked-in syndrome, which may occur in primary brainstem disorders such as extensive basilar artery thrombosis, brainstem hemorrhage, or brainstem contusions, is characterized by severe tetraparesis or tetraplegia and a loss of all cranial nerve motor functions while perception is preserved. The syndrome is caused by damage to the pontine base while the dorsal portions of the pontine tegmentum are spared. As a result, patients with locked-in syndrome lose all capacity for verbal and motor expression. However, because structures and pathways in the tegmentum (posterior longitudinal bundle and reticular formation) are intact, these patients are awake and conscious and may be able to communicate with their environment through eye movements.

Microangiopathic Lesions

> **Note**
>
> The clinical syndromes described above are rooted in macroangiopathic lesions (territorial infarctions). By contrast, the occlusion of individual perforating arteries (paramedian pontine perforators) gives rise to "lacunar" syndromes that have a microangiopathic cause.

It is common in such cases to observe an isolated sensory and/or motor deficit (contralateral upper limb weakness) and dysarthria not accompanied by neurologic deficits that would indicate a cortical lesion (e.g., aphasia or visual field defects).

Types of Infarction

Infarctions of the vertebrobasilar system are classified as follows:
- Supratentorial infarctions in the territory of the posterior cerebral artery
- Interbrain and midbrain infarctions arising from perforators in the area of the posterior cerebral artery and the top of the basilar artery
- Medulla oblongata infarctions (distal vertebral artery)
- Cerebellar infarctions

Embolic infarctions in the posterior circulation usually stem from vertebrobasilar occlusions but may also be caused by emboli from the anterior circulation (e.g., cases where the posterior cerebral artery arises directly from the internal carotid artery or via large posterior communicating branches). In the case of cerebellar infarctions, the variable vascular supply leads to a less symmetrical pattern of infarction than one would expect in the anterior circulation. The posterior inferior cerebellar artery supplies most of the cerebellar hemispheres (inferior portion with the semilunar and biventer lobules), the cerebellar tonsils, and portions of the cerebellar vermis. Large cerebellar infarcts can produce mass effects leading to malignant infarction with compression of the fourth ventricle and development of hydrocephalus. Infarctions in the territory of the posterior inferior cerebellar artery are the most common of all cerebellar infarctions. Isolated infarctions of the anterior inferior cerebellar artery are rare and most often affect the middle cerebellar peduncle. In variants with a hypoplastic posterior

inferior cerebellar artery, a larger anterior inferior cerebellar artery may be present that can assume the function of supplying the lower cerebellum. The superior cerebellar artery basically supplies the anterior lobe of the cerebellum with the quadrangular lobules, the medullary center (including nuclei), and the superior vermis. Infarctions of the medulla oblongata are most often caused by distal, intradural vertebral artery occlusions. By contrast, pontine and midbrain infarctions, which generally occur at paramedian sites at the level of the pontine base, are caused by the occlusion of perforators from the basilar artery. The angiographic anatomy of the vertebrobasilar system is shown in **Fig. 3.1**.

Imaging Studies

Computed Tomography and CT Angiography

CT is an imaging modality that is available around the clock at most hospitals. Modern stroke CT protocols, while designed mainly for the anterior circulation, are also useful for diagnosing ischemia in the posterior circulation, although there are several key technical and anatomic differences that should be noted with regard to image interpretation.

Noncontrast Cranial CT

Detection of Ischemia

Classic ischemic changes (swelling, loss of corticomedullary differentiation, obscuration of the lentiform nucleus, possible white matter hypodensity) in the supratentorial territory of the posterior cerebral arteries can be detected equally well with older or more recent generations of CT scanners. Early ischemic changes are more difficult to detect, however, in the diencephalon and mesencephalon, in the pons, and in the medulla oblongata. Axial CT scans at the level of the petrous pyramids and skull base consistently show significant beam-hardening artifacts caused by abrupt density changes in the imaged tissues. For example, attenuation changes greater than 1000 Hounsfield units (HU) repeatedly occur at air/bone interfaces in the frontal sinus region and especially around the mastoid air cells. These density changes cause streaky superimposed artifacts that significantly hamper evaluation of the posterior cranial fossa; they can even prevent posterior fossa evaluation with older systems (especially single-slice and two-slice scanners). The diagnostic quality of cranial CT images has risen steadily in recent years, owing to the use of multislice CT systems and special cranial reconstruction algorithms and kernels. As back-projection algorithms have been replaced by computer-intensive iterative algorithms, reconstructions of the posterior fossa can now be generated that are virtually artifact-free. Nevertheless, the generally small infarcted volumes in brainstem ischemia still pose a significant obstacle to early CT detection.

Practical Tip

In most cases, the ability to image infratentorial brain areas without significant artifacts permits an accurate CT evaluation of cerebellar infarctions (**Fig. 3.2**). But although the introduction of multislice CT has significantly reduced artifacts, CT usually cannot reliably exclude ischemic changes in the pons and medulla oblongata during the first 6 h after symptom onset. For this reason, there are certain cases (e.g., uncertain time window) in which diffusion-weighted MRI (DWI) should be added or used as an initial study if it is expected to have therapeutic implications.

In clinical practice, however, a comprehensive review of clinical findings, noncontrast cranial CT, and CT angiography (CTA) images is still an accurate guide for determining whether endovascular treatment is appropriate for a particular patient.

Besides early ischemic changes at the supratentorial level (sulcal effacement and loss of corticomedullary differentiation in the posterior cerebral artery territory), unilateral or bilateral thalamic infarctions, possibly combined with cerebellar infarctions, can provide definite evidence of basilar artery thrombosis on noncontrast cranial CT scans (**Fig. 3.3**). With the normal variant of the posterior cerebral arteries arising directly from the internal carotid arteries on both sides (present in ~20% of patients), long segmental basilar artery thrombosis may exist without causing infarction in the posterior cerebral artery territories. It should be noted in these cases that the vertebrobasilar vessels—especially the top of the basilar artery and the proximal portions of the posterior cerebral arteries (P1 segments)—often have physiologically small caliber, and this should not be mistaken for stenosis on CTA. Isolated unilateral posterior infarctions require correlation with CTA, because the posterior communicating branches often show normal variants that may include an isolated origin of the posterior cerebral arteries from the internal carotid artery, and this configuration could mask a basilar artery thrombosis.

The hyperdense middle cerebral artery (HMCA) sign has been established as a highly specific but not very sensitive sign of arterial occlusion in the anterior circulation. It is only in carefully selected cases that this sign can be applied to the posterior circulation and basilar artery. Puetz et al. (2009) found that the hyperdense basilar artery sign had a sensitivity of 71% and specificity of 98% for detecting basilar artery occlusion in patients with high clinical probability of vertebrobasilar stroke (Goldmakher et al. 2009).

Practical Tip

Earlier studies on the detection of anterior circulation infarcts showed that even experienced (neuro)radiologists and stroke physicians could correctly determine the presence and extent of ischemia in only ~45% of cases based on noncontrast CT scans alone (Wardlaw et al. 1999). This emphasizes the importance of acute and subacute vascular imaging studies (CTA, MR angiography [MRA], duplex, digital subtraction angiography [DSA]) for gaining additional information, especially in patients with suspected vertebrobasilar ischemia.

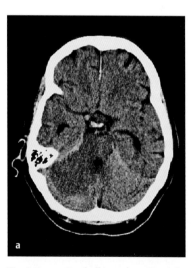 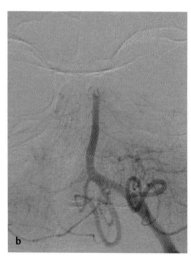 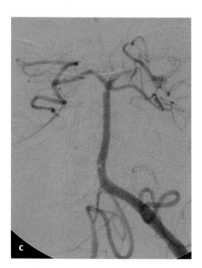

Fig. 3.2a–c   Cerebellar and pontine infarction.
a Noncontrast cranial CT demonstrates a fresh cerebellar and pontine infarction on the right side caused by a basilar tip embolism with occlusion of the superior cerebellar artery and basilar artery perforators.
b DSA findings before intra-arterial recanalization.

c After recanalization, the top of the basilar artery and the left superior cerebellar artery are again visualized by DSA. The right superior cerebellar artery is still occluded. Findings also suggest a small residual thrombus or, less likely, a stenosis just below the basilar tip.

Neuroimaging of Stroke

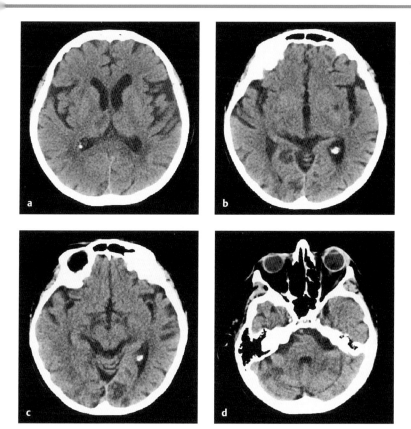

Fig. 3.3 Typical infarction pattern on CT due to basilar artery thrombosis. Small infarctions are demarcated in the right thalamus, precuneus, and left occipital lobe along with bilateral cerebellar infarctions.

Follow-Up Imaging

Cranial CT is also of great value in the subacute imaging of vertebrobasilar ischemia, as malignant cerebellar infarction and parenchymal hemorrhage may develop in patients requiring intensive care after an extensive cerebellar infarction. These cases require a prompt decision on whether to proceed with suboccipital decompressive craniectomy. MRI of ventilated intensive care unit (ICU) patients is an alternative to CT only in selected cases due to the high logistic and technical costs.

CT Angiography

Detection of Ischemia

Angiographic studies play a major role in the diagnosis and etiologic workup of vertebrobasilar ischemia. Besides detecting stenosis, thromboembolism, and thrombosis, angiography is also used to analyze the significance of a circumscribed lesion in relation to overall cerebral hemodynamics. This includes the accurate grading of stenoses and the detection of collateral pathways, asymptomatic vascular pathology, and normal variants.

With older CT systems the size of the scanned region was limited to a few centimeters, but the current standard in stroke CT is to image the entire supra-aortic arterial tree. For this purpose iodinated contrast material is administered through a large-bore IV line, and spiral CTA scans are acquired during the first pass when the contrast material reaches its peak concentration in the arteries. The raw dataset is then used to reconstruct the desired diagnostic images.

Relevant side effects from iodinated contrast material may include contrast-induced nephropathy, anaphylactoid reaction, thyrotoxicosis, and contrast extravasation. In patients with impaired renal function (glomerular filtration rate < 60 mL min^{-1} 1.73 m^{-3} or serum creatinine [rough approximation] > 1.5 mg/dL in men or > 1.2 mg/dL in women), the risk of contrast-induced nephropathy can be reduced by hydrating the patient, injecting a smaller contrast volume, and by giving sodium perchlorate in patients found to have sublatent hyperthyroidism (thyrotropin < 0.4 mU/L). The risk of developing contrast-induced nephropathy depends largely on the injected contrast volume and increases markedly when the iodine dose is ~30 g or higher. Given the extremely low incidence of contrast-induced thyrotoxicosis (estimated < 40 thyroid crises in 5 million contrast injections/year), routine prophylaxis with perchlorate or thiamazole is controversial (van der Molen et al. 2004). Use of the oral antidiabetic agent metformin is a potential concern in diabetic patients, as it may induce life-threatening lactic acidosis in diabetics with impaired renal function who receive iodinated contrast material. For this reason, metformin use should be discontinued for 2 days after the administration of iodinated contrast (Becker 2007).

Besides the placement of a large IV line, preparation of the patient for CTA or CT perfusion imaging (CTP) includes effective immobilization of the head on the examination table. Somnolent patients tend to make gross head movements during contrast injection due to the heat sensation induced by the agent. The resulting motion artifacts may degrade image quality so severely that the examination and contrast injection have to be repeated. High-end scanners offer "high pitch" scan modes that allow supra-aortic CTA to be completed in less than 1 second. One advantage of this feature is that the necessary contrast volume can be reduced to 40–50 mL instead of the 80–100 mL needed in slow scanners. Another advantage is the ability to image the V0 segments of the vertebral arteries (at their origin from the subclavian arteries) without motion artifacts and without the need for complex ECG-gated protocols. The use of a craniocaudal scan direction can also eliminate beam-hardening artifacts in the proximal supra-aortic arteries caused by a highly concentrated contrast bolus in the subclavian vein.

Postprocessing of the CTA raw data should include the generation of thin-slice (1 mm/1 mm thickness/increment) axial multiplanar reconstructions (MPRs), sagittal maximum intensity projections (MIPs) and, if necessary, pseudocoronal (5 mm/5 mm) MIPs.

Caution

Do not interpret CTA based on MIPs alone, as this will probably miss small thrombi located in small-caliber vessels such as the basilar artery.

Bone-removal algorithms and thick-slab MIP reconstructions that resemble MRA images have not proven useful in the posterior circulation (unlike the anterior circulation). This is also true of three-dimensional techniques such as volume rendering and surface reconstructions.

CT Perfusion Imaging

Detection of Ischemia

The third component of a stroke CT protocol is CTP. In this technique CT images are acquired every 1–3 seconds for a designated time period (usually 40–90 seconds) after a contrast bolus injection. This yields a dynamic dataset from which hemodynamic parameters (cerebral blood volume and blood flow) and temporal parameters (MTT, TTP [time to peak], TTD [time to drain], T_{max}) are calculated. These parameters are useful for detecting the infarcted core before it can be seen on noncontrast CT scans. They can also be used to determine the volume of the non-infarcted but hypoperfused penumbra—an area that is potentially salvageable by rapid vascular recanalization (**Fig. 3.4**). This procedure, while well established for the anterior circulation, is of limited usefulness in the posterior circulation. Standard CTP in the anterior circulation maps a brain volume 1–4 cm wide at the level of the basal ganglia. Modern CT scanners can extend the perfusion volume to > 15 cm along the z-axis.

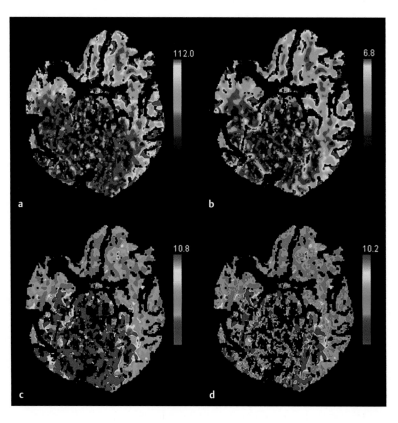

Fig. 3.4a–d   CTP of the posterior cranial fossa with a 128-slice CT scanner. Despite an adjusted (increased) tube current-time product and modern reconstruction techniques, blood flow in the mesencephalon cannot be accurately evaluated. The bilateral cerebellar infarctions are clearly visualized, however.
a Cerebral blood flow.
b Cerebral blood volume
c TTD.
d MTT.

The CTP data are used to evaluate brain perfusion in the basal portions (small perfusion volume) of the territories supplied by the anterior, middle, and posterior cerebral arteries. CTP cannot evaluate di- and mesencephalic blood flow or perfusion in the posterior fossa, however, due to the occurrence of massive beam-hardening artifacts at the skull base and near the petrous pyramids (analogous to non-contrast CT). Image quality can be improved by increasing the tube current–time product (generally by 25%), but this always involves a proportionate increase in dose. It should be noted that in infratentorial CTP, unlike supratentorial CTP, the radiosensitive lens of the eye is consistently exposed to the primary X-ray beam. Even on high-quality CTP images of the posterior fossa, generally it is not possible to evaluate the pons or medulla due to the peculiarities of their blood supply (short and long perforators) and the very small size of the infarcted areas. The perfusion of the cerebellar hemispheres can be evaluated, however (**Fig. 3.5**).

Magnetic Resonance Imaging and MR Angiography

Detection of Ischemia

Stroke MRI can be performed as an alternative to stroke CT in the evaluation of vertebrobasilar ischemia. The main *advantages* of MRI over CT are as follows:
- Excellent soft-tissue contrast
- Accurate evaluation of structures in the posterior fossa (no beam-hardening artifacts as in CT)

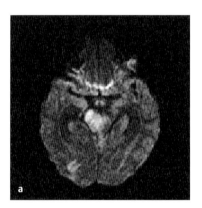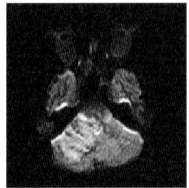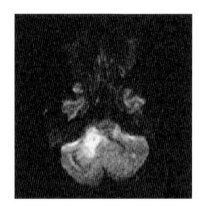

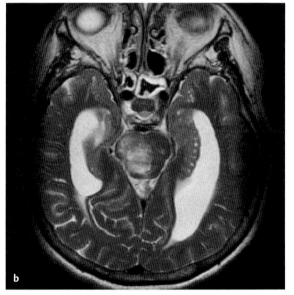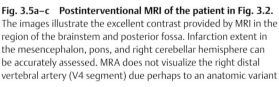
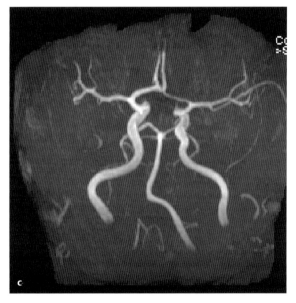

Fig. 3.5a–c   Postinterventional MRI of the patient in Fig. 3.2.
The images illustrate the excellent contrast provided by MRI in the region of the brainstem and posterior fossa. Infarction extent in the mesencephalon, pons, and right cerebellar hemisphere can be accurately assessed. MRA does not visualize the right distal vertebral artery (V4 segment) due perhaps to an anatomic variant or hypoplasia. Perfusion has been fully restored to the larger cerebellar arteries and basilar artery.
a DWI.
b T2w MRI.
c MRA.

- Availability of DWI sequences with excellent visualization of peracute infarctions
- No exposure to ionizing radiation

The main *disadvantages* of MRI relative to CT include:
- Limited availability of equipment and personnel (especially at night and on weekends)
- Numerous contraindications (cardiac pacemaker, MRI-incompatible medical equipment such as spiral-wound ventilation tubes and ECG wires)
- Limited patient monitoring and surveillance capabilities during the MRI examination (~15 min)
- Poor compliance by agitated or somnolent patients
- Relatively high costs

MRI can confidently exclude acute intracranial hemorrhage, but this requires the use of special sequences (DWI, T2*w, and T2w-FLAIR [fluid-attenuated inversion recovery]) and image reading by an experienced radiologist (Wiesmann et al. 2001; Ritter and Schulte-Altedorneburg 2008).

Practical Tip

Stroke MRI protocols for evaluating vertebrobasilar ischemia do not differ from those in the anterior circulation. Key elements are axial DWI, T2*w, and T2w sequences, an optional T2w-FLAIR sequence covering the whole neurocranium, and intracranial time-of-flight (TOF) MRA with complete visualization of the V4 segments and origins of the posterior inferior cerebellar arteries.

Plane selection for parenchymal imaging should provide adequate basal coverage and should include the medulla oblongata. Contrast-enhanced MRA of the cervical arteries is indicated only in cases where intra-arterial recanalization therapy is proposed (and if the examination time does not exceed 3 min).

Practical Tip

T2*w sequences (to exclude hemorrhage) and T2w sequences (mainly to evaluate older ischemic changes) can be omitted in settings where up-to-date noncontrast cranial CT is available. Generally there is no need for additional (e.g., thin-slice) sequences for evaluating the posterior fossa or T1w sequences due to the added time delay.

Analogous to contrast administration in stroke CT, it would be too time-consuming to assess renal function prior to MRI because the likelihood of contrast-induced nephrogenic systemic fibrosis is extremely low—much less than the likelihood of further spread of the infarction due to treatment delay, with potentially catastrophic consequences.

Follow-Up Imaging

MRI also has an important role in the follow-up of patients who do not (or no longer) require intensive care. Since examination time is not a critical concern in these cases, thin-slice DWI and T2w sequences can be obtained for the determination of infarct extent in all areas of the brainstem and cerebellum with considerably greater accuracy than CT. Unenhanced, fat-saturated T1w sequences can detect a subacute arterial wall hematoma (hyperintense crescent) with high sensitivity and specificity. Contrast-enhanced black-blood sequences can even detect inflammatory changes in vessel walls.

Extracranial and Transcranial Doppler and Color Duplex Sonography

Besides the clinical neurologic examination, Doppler and color duplex sonography are the only noninvasive procedures available for the investigation of vertebrobasilar symptoms. With an experienced examiner, the initial ultrasound scan in the emergency department is a fast and rewarding bedside test that can confirm the diagnosis suggested by neurologic examination and can direct the selection of further imaging studies (MRI, MRA, CT, CTA, DSA) and initial therapeutic actions.

Color Duplex Sonography of the Extracranial Cerebral Arteries

Note

Color duplex sonography of the extracranial cerebral arteries differs from other neurovascular studies in that it provides information on extracranial vessel wall morphology and also allows measurements of blood flow velocity and direction in real-time resolution (Schulte-Altedorneburg and Clevert 2009).

Thus, color duplex sonography can yield hemodynamic information (stenoses, occlusions, collaterals) as well as morphologic findings (atherosclerotic plaque, hypoplasia, intimal flap, mural hematoma).

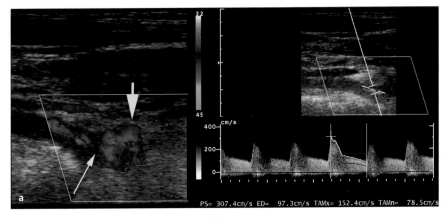
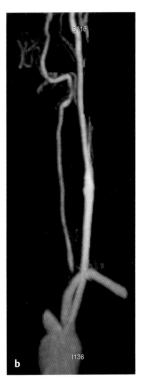

PS= 307.4cm/s ED= 97.3cm/s TAMx= 152.4cm/s TAMn= 78.5cm/s

Fig. 3.6a, b   High-grade proximal stenosis of the vertebral artery.
a Color duplex sonography of the extracranial cerebral arteries.
   Left: intrastenotic constriction of the color band (*thin yellow arrow*), axial view of the subclavian
   artery (*thick arrow*).
   Right: Correlative Doppler spectrum shows a high systolic and end-diastolic flow velocity and
   intrastenotic turbulence (low-frequency flow components).
b Corresponding segmented MIP from contrast-enhanced MRA.

The extracranial segments of the vertebral artery are imaged with a 5- to 10-MHz linear or sector transducer (Schulte-Altedorneburg and Clevert 2009). Kinking, elongation, and anatomic variants (e.g., posteroinferior origin of the vertebral artery from the subclavian artery, vertebral artery arising directly from the aorta in ~5% of cases) may pose an obstacle to continuous extracranial color duplex scanning. (Proximal) stenosis can be recognized by narrowing of the color band and by noting circumscribed flow acceleration and pre- or poststenotic flow changes in the Doppler spectrum (**Fig. 3.6**). Occlusions are characterized by an absence of color flow and by a small, bidirectional occlusion signal. The diameter of the vertebral artery is most easily measured in the V2 artery segment for exclusion of hypoplasia, for example. Dissection-related luminal narrowing in the V1 and V2 segments can often be detected by identifying an intramural hypoechoic hematoma or finding a double lumen along with Doppler spectral changes indicating a steno-occlusive process (Sturzenegger et al. 1993; Dittrich et al. 2006). The sensitivity of ultrasound is only ~85%, however, even when the examination includes transcranial Doppler (Sturzenegger et al. 1993; Dittrich et al. 2006). For this reason, ultrasound should be supplemented by MRI. The presence of low-grade stenoses, very small mural hematomas, and time variations in vessel wall lesions may be a source of false-negative findings.

Color Duplex Sonography of the Transcranial Cerebral Arteries

The V4 segments of the basilar artery are scanned through a transnuchal or transforaminal approach with color duplex sonography (**Fig. 3.7**).

Caution

In many cases the distal third of the basilar artery cannot be adequately evaluated by (noncontrast) color duplex sonography (Schulte-Altedorneburg et al. 2000). This limits the usefulness of this technique for detecting basilar tip embolism.

It may be helpful in these cases to add transtemporal scanning of the initial portions of the posterior cerebral artery and to administer echo contrast agents (Droste et al. 1998; Koga et al. 2002). Occlusions or stenoses of the posterior inferior cerebellar artery or other cerebellar arteries cannot be reliably detected. Contrast-enhanced color duplex sonography has also proven useful for distinguishing distal vertebral artery hypoplasia from occlusion and for detecting stenoses of the distal vertebral artery and basilar artery in cases where it is technically difficult to scan through a transforaminal window (Droste et al. 1998; Koga et al. 2002).

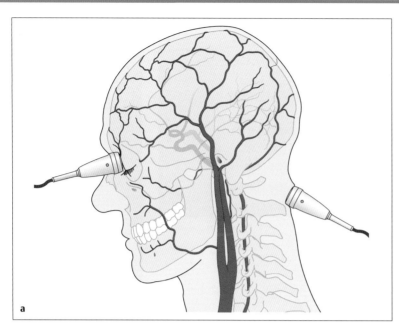

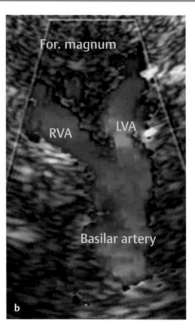

Fig. 3.7a, b   Transcranial color duplex sonography.
a Transcranial approaches (acoustic windows) for scanning the intracranial vertebrobasilar system.
b Transcranial color duplex scan of the V4 segments, the confluence, and proximal two-thirds of the basilar artery. The vertebrobasilar system is pictured upside-down. Normal findings. RVA, right vertebral artery; LVA, left vertebral artery; For. magnum, foramen magnum.

Digital Subtraction Angiography and Patient Selection for Interventional Treatment

Catheter angiography is reserved for cases of vertebrobasilar occlusive disease in which endovascular treatment is already indicated based on the results of (semi) invasive studies. In these cases conventional angiography is the only method that can accurately define the occlusion site, positively distinguish between occlusion and pseudo-occlusion, and define the morphology and hemodynamics of the collateral pathways with high temporal resolution. Semi-invasive techniques cannot quantify a calcified, elongated, symptomatic proximal vertebral artery stenosis with consistent results. In these cases angiography is used to assess the degree of stenosis while stent-protected balloon dilatation is on standby. Given the frequent posterior or posteroinferior origin of the vertebral artery from the subclavian artery, the posteroanterior (PA) projection should be supplemented by oblique views to demonstrate extension of the stenosing plaque from the subclavian artery into the proximal vertebral artery.

The acute treatment of a vertebrobasilar occlusion is indicated whenever there is concomitant involvement of the basilar artery. Isolated occlusions of the vertebral artery, cerebellar arteries, or posterior cerebral arteries are, as a rule, not managed by primary interventional treatment. A high-grade V4 stenosis can be dilated during the treatment of basilar artery thrombosis. Thrombotic material that has migrated into the cerebellar arteries or posterior cerebral arteries is accessible to treatment by thrombolysis or thrombectomy.

Due to significant atherosclerosis and supra-aortic elongation, especially in older patients, catheterization of the vertebral artery may be more difficult than carotid angiography and may pose a higher risk of iatrogenic vessel wall injury. Rare adverse contrast reactions with agitation and transient cortical blindness may be more frequent after vertebral angiography. Thus, patients should be selected carefully for primary selective diagnostic angiography of the vertebrobasilar system after other semi-invasive options have been exhausted.

References

Becker C. Prophylaxis and treatment of side effects due to iodinated contrast media relevant to radiological practice. [Article in German] Radiologe 2007;47(9):768–773

Dittrich R, Dziewas R, Ritter MA, et al. Negative ultrasound findings in patients with cervical artery dissection. Negative ultrasound in CAD. J Neurol 2006;253(4):424–433

Droste DW, Nabavi DG, Kemény V, et al. Echocontrast enhanced transcranial colour-coded duplex offers improved visualization of the vertebrobasilar system. Acta Neurol Scand 1998; 98(3):193–199

Ferbert A, Brückmann H, Drummen R. Clinical features of proven basilar artery occlusion. Stroke 1990;21(8):1135–1142

Glass TA, Hennessey PM, Pazdera L, et al. Outcome at 30 days in the New England Medical Center Posterior Circulation Registry. Arch Neurol 2002;59(3):369–376

Goldmakher GV, Camargo EC, Furie KL, et al. Hyperdense basilar artery sign on unenhanced CT predicts thrombus and outcome in acute posterior circulation stroke. Stroke 2009; 40(1):134–139

Koga M, Kimura K, Minematsu K, Yamaguchi T. Relationship between findings of conventional and contrast-enhanced transcranial color-coded real-time sonography and angiography in patients with basilar artery occlusion. AJNR Am J Neuroradiol 2002;23(4):568–571

Matula C, Trattnig S, Tschabitscher M, Day JD, Koos WT. The course of the prevertebral segment of the vertebral artery: anatomy and clinical significance. Surg Neurol 1997; 48(2):125–131

Pfefferkorn T, Mayer TE, Schulte-Altedorneburg G, Brückmann H, Hamann GF, Dichgans M. Diagnosis and therapy of basilar artery occlusion. [Article in German] Nervenarzt 2006; 77(4):416–422

Puetz V, Sylaja PN, Hill MD, et al. CT angiography source images predict final infarct extent in patients with basilar artery occlusion. AJNR Am J Neuroradiol 2009;30(10): 1877–1883

Ritter MA, Schulte-Altedorneburg G. Imaging of intracerebral haemorrhage—CT, MRI or both? [Article in German] Klin Neurophysiol 2008;39:142–148

Schulte-Altedorneburg G, Droste DW, Popa V, et al. Visualization of the basilar artery by transcranial color-coded duplex sonography: comparison with postmortem results. Stroke 2000;31(5):1123–1127

Schulte-Altedorneburg G, Brückmann H. Imaging techniques in diagnosis of brainstem infarction. [Article in German] Nervenarzt 2006;77(6):731–743, quiz 744

Schulte-Altedorneburg G, Clevert DA. Color duplex sonography of extracranial brain-supplying arteries. [Article in German] Radiologe 2009;49(11):1016–1023

Sturzenegger M, Mattle HP, Rivoir A, Rihs F, Schmid C. Ultrasound findings in spontaneous extracranial vertebral artery dissection. Stroke 1993;24(12):1910–1921

van der Molen AJ, Thomsen HS, Morcos SK; Contrast Media Safety Committee, European Society of Urogenital Radiology (ESUR). Effect of iodinated contrast media on thyroid function in adults. Eur Radiol 2004;14(5):902–907

Wardlaw JM, Dorman PJ, Lewis SC, Sandercock PA. Can stroke physicians and neuroradiologists identify signs of early cerebral infarction on CT? J Neurol Neurosurg Psychiatry 1999;67(5):651–653

Wiesmann M, Mayer TE, Yousry I, Hamann GF, Brückmann H. Detection of hyperacute parenchymal hemorrhage of the brain using echo-planar $T2^*$-weighted and diffusion-weighted MRI. Eur Radiol 2001;11(5):849–853

Zeumer H, Hacke W, Kolmann HL, Poeck K. Local fibrinolysis in basilar artery thrombosis (author's transl). [Article in German] Dtsch Med Wochenschr 1982;107(19):728–731

I

4 Dissections

T. Boeckh-Behrens

Introduction

Arterial dissections, regardless of their location, are defined as intramural hematomas of the artery wall, with or without tearing of the adjacent intima. The hematoma may form primarily in the vessel wall due to rupture of vasa vasorum in the adventitia or media, or it may develop secondarily due to a tear in the intima allowing blood to dissect into deeper wall layers from the artery lumen. A primary intramural hematoma may also spread toward the intima and cause a secondary tear in the intimal wall layers.

Cervical artery dissections are very heterogeneous in terms of their underlying pathogenic mechanism, location, affected individuals, and presenting symptoms.

Note

Dissections in the anterior circulation (internal carotid artery system) should be distinguished from those in the posterior circulation (vertebral artery system) because the location of the dissection determines the clinical presentation. It is also helpful to distinguish secondary dissections caused by trauma or iatrogenic injury from spontaneous dissections that have no discernible cause or result from a trivial injury.

This chapter deals with the diagnosis of dissections in general, regardless of the distinctions noted above. The sections on epidemiology and pathophysiology refer mainly to spontaneous dissections.

Epidemiology

On the whole, spontaneous dissections of the supra-aortic vessels are rare. Several large North American and European studies report an overall incidence between 2.6 and 3 per 100 000 population per year (Giroud et al. 1994; Touzé et al. 2003; Lee et al. 2006; Arnold et al. 2006b). The actual incidence is probably higher when we consider that many oligo- or asymptomatic dissections go unreported. Despite their relatively low incidence, however, dissections are believed to account for up to 25% of all strokes in patients under

50 years of age (Siqueira Neto et al. 1996) and thus represent a significant mortality factor in this population group. The ratio of carotid to vertebral artery dissections is ~3:1 (Lee et al. 2006), although these numbers are becoming more equal as MRI improves our ability to image the posterior circulation. The peak incidence and median age at diagnosis is estimated at 43–46 years, with a large range of variation between 3 and 75 years (Dittrich et al. 2007a).

Pathophysiology

Dissections in the setting of severe blunt or penetrating trauma result from direct injury to the vessel wall. The incidence is ~1–2% of patients who sustain blunt trauma. The risk is higher in patients with severe associated injuries such as facial or basal skull fractures and intracerebral injuries. Severe thoracic trauma has a high association with carotid artery dissections. The vertebral arteries are more commonly affected by cervical fractures and cervical cord injuries.

The mechanism underlying spontaneous arterial dissections is not yet fully understood. Some patients have a history of a minor precipitating event, usually associated with hyperextension, rotation, or sideways bending of the cervical spine (Caso et al. 2005). Dissections have been described after various athletic activities, whiplash injury, vigorous coughing, and even after "visiting the dentist." Given the association between vertebral artery dissections and chiropractic manipulations, it is unclear whether the dissection is a direct result of the manipulation or whether the dissection has caused neck pain that prompts chiropractic visits, implying that there is no direct causal relationship (Haldeman et al. 1999; Dittrich et al. 2007b; Ernst 2007). In several recent studies, MRI has detected an inflammatory process in the vessel wall, often accompanied by evidence of an acute, nonspecific infection (Naggara et al. 2009). The fact that multiple dissections, found in ~13–16% of cases, tend to cluster within the same time frame is consistent with the hypothesis of an inflammatory reaction as an acute trigger mechanism.

But since a precipitating cause often cannot be found, other factors must play a fundamental role. Some authors favor a multifactorial pathogenesis in which a constitutional (perhaps genetic) weakness of the vessel wall combines with exogenous trigger factors such as minor trauma or acute infection to cause acute bleeding into the vessel wall or tearing of the intima (Debette and Leys 2009). This hypothesis is supported by the fact that up to 50% of patients with dissections are found to have associated connective tissue abnormalities in the skin. Patients have also shown an increased incidence of vascular system changes such as impaired vasodilation, increased vessel wall rigidity, aortic arch dilatation, or fibromuscular dysplasia. These changes also appear to have a familial occurrence, which in turn supports a genetic component—as does the association with known genetic connective tissue diseases such as Ehlers–Danlos or Marfan syndrome, although the overall incidence of these diseases is very low.

Clinical Features

As a rule, the symptoms arising from cervical arterial dissections can be positively related to the underlying pathology—that is, an intramural hematoma with or without intimal or adventitial injury at that location.

Initially the intramural hematoma leads to pain, which presents as sudden headache or neck pain with characteristics ranging from "thunderclap" pain of hyperacute onset to a gradual progression of pain symptoms.

Presumably the pain is caused by the activation of pain receptors due to stretching of the vessel wall (Arnold et al. 2006a). Carotid artery dissections may also present with ipsilateral neck pain and tenderness over the course of the vessel (carotidynia).

> **Note**
>
> Overall, pain is the most common initial presenting symptom of a cervical arterial dissection.

The sympathetic nerve plexus for cervical and cranial structures, the carotid plexus, follows the course of the carotid artery and its branches. The mass effect from the intramural hemorrhage may stretch and injure these nerve fibers. The result in 10–30% of cases is an ipsilateral Horner syndrome (miosis, ptosis, enophthalmos). Given the close proximity of the petrous and cavernous portions of the distal internal carotid artery to the lower cranial nerves (especially IX, X, and XII), cranial nerve deficits may arise due to compression at those levels. The most common deficit is hypoglossal nerve palsy, but there may also be involvement of the lingual, facial, and accessory nerves and the chorda tympani. Pulsatile tinnitus occasionally develops. On the whole, cranial nerve deficits are rare, with an incidence of ~7%. Pressure on cervical spinal nerve roots from a vertebral artery hematoma is also very rare.

The purely local symptoms in the initial stage of the disease are followed in more than half of patients by cerebral ischemia or transient ischemic attacks, with symptoms that are typical of the affected vascular territory. Ischemia may occur shortly after the onset of local symptoms or may be delayed by several weeks but almost always develops within one month. Very rarely, ischemic events may occur in the absence of premonitory local symptoms. The pathophysiology of these cases most likely involves tearing of the intima causing release of thrombogenic mediators, and the resulting thrombi later embolize to peripheral vessels. This theory is supported by the observation of territorial embolic distribution patterns in the dependent vascular territories and by the high rate of microembolic signals detectable by transcranial Doppler sonography (Molina et al. 2000; Koch et al. 2004).

Another possible mechanism, though much rarer, relates to hemodynamic infarction patterns in which the intramural hematoma causes such pronounced luminal narrowing that the perfusion pressure in the distal terminal vessels is no longer adequate in patients with insufficient collaterals.

If the mural hematoma spreads into the outer wall layers and involves the adventitia, this may lead to complete rupture of the vessel wall or aneurysmal dilatation, presenting morphologically as a localized pseudoaneurysm or long fusiform expansion (dissecting aneurysm). Because the intracranial portions of the cerebral supply arteries have a thinner media and adventitia and are not covered by an external elastic membrane, the intracranial vascular segments are more susceptible to rupture, leading to subarachnoid hemorrhage (Hart and Easton 1983). It is very rare for subarachnoid hemorrhage to supervene on a cervical artery dissection, however; the incidence in the largest hospital-based study was ~1% (Touzé et al. 2003). On the other hand, asymptomatic dissections appear to be quite common and were detected in ~6% of individuals undergoing routine examinations (Lee et al. 2006).

Imaging Studies

In principle, a cervical artery dissection can be detected by any of the classic imaging modalities—ultrasound, Ct angiography (CTA), digital subtraction angiography (DSA), MRI, and MR angiography (MRA). There are, however, significant differences in the relative merits of these techniques in the diagnosis of dissections.

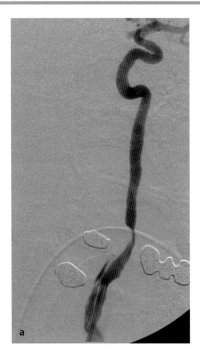

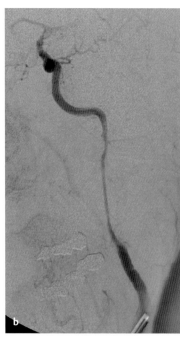

Neuroimaging of Stroke

Fig. 4.1a, b   Appearance of internal carotid artery dissections on DSA.
a Proximal, catheter-induced dissection of the internal carotid artery with high-grade luminal narrowing and a visible intimal flap.
b Long-segment dissection of the internal carotid artery with a string sign and peripheral embolic M1 occlusion.

Digital Subtraction Angiography

Caution

DSA, once the gold standard for diagnosing dissections before the large-scale introduction of sectional imaging modalities, is no longer recommended today for the diagnosis of this disease.

The reasons for this include invasiveness, ionizing radiation exposure, and the inability to image the hematoma itself, with the result that DSA may miss dissections that do not cause significant luminal narrowing or wall irregularity. Catheter angiography may even cause intimal injury in rare cases (**Fig. 4.1a**).

DSA may be considered as an adjunct only in isolated equivocal cases and in the setting of proposed interventional treatments for hemodynamically significant stenosis or peripheral emboli treatable by mechanical recanalization (**Fig. 4.1b**). Morphologically, a dissection may appear on DSA as a sharply tapered, frequently long vascular segment with luminal narrowing ("string sign," see **Fig. 4.1b**) or as a complete occlusion. An intimal flap dissected from the vessel wall may occasionally appear as a linear filling defect (see **Fig. 4.1a**).

CT Angiography

CTA can no longer be recommended as a standard routine test (Diener and Putzki 2008). In addition to concerns about radiation exposure, CTA is inferior to MRI in the detection of mural hematoma. CTA is useful, however, for evaluating the classic signs of caliber irregularities in the affected artery, high-grade stenoses, long-segment stenoses, and possible pseudoaneurysmal dilatation or segmental changes (**Fig. 4.2**). Also, it is equivalent to MRI during the early phase (< 2 days) when the morphology of the mural hematoma is not yet clearly visible by MRI. Its high availability and shorter examination time are additional reasons why CTA will continue to play an important and perhaps essential role during the acute phase.

Ultrasound

With its speed and widespread availability, (color-coded) Doppler and duplex sonography has become perhaps the most widely used initial imaging study in clinical practice. There are several reasons, however, why ultrasound cannot be recommended as a stand-alone test.

Ultrasound is very sensitive for detecting proximal cervical artery dissections in both the anterior and posterior circulations (> 90% of cases), but it is much less sensitive to dissections near the skull base and within the

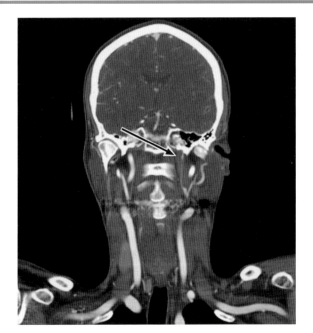

Fig. 4.2 Long segmental dissection of the left internal carotid artery with a string sign on CTA. The arrow indicates the string sign in the left internal carotid artery (coronal image).

transverse foramina. Thus in the case of vertebral artery dissections, ultrasound cannot adequately evaluate the most common site of occurrence, the V3 segment before the artery enters the foramen magnum. Sensitivity is also low for carotid artery dissections that are causing only local symptoms with pain and Horner triad; ultrasound findings may be normal in more than 30% of these cases (Arnold et al. 2008). This is probably because significant luminal narrowing is rare in cases of this kind, and so the hemodynamic effects of a relatively high-grade mural hematoma are not detectable by Doppler scanning.

Practical Tip

For these reasons, ultrasound is recommended only as a screening tool in patients with a suspected dissection. Negative Doppler findings in clinically suspicious cases should warrant further investigation by MRI or CTA. Even if Doppler findings are positive, additional imaging should be done to confirm the diagnosis. Once a dissection has been established, however, ultrasound is an effective follow-up tool, especially for evaluating the success of recanalization.

The mural hematoma in both carotid and vertebral artery dissections appears morphologically and functionally as a hypoechoic wall structure with adjacent luminal irregularity or an abrupt caliber change. The dissected flap appears as an intraluminal membrane with or without

active blood flow into a second, false lumen. Aneurysmal dilatation of the vessel lumen or a pseudoaneurysm may also be detectable in some cases.

Besides these specific, direct morphologic signs, ultrasound may also show indirect hemodynamic changes that provide nonspecific evidence of a vascular stenosis, such as flow acceleration or a bidirectional flow pattern with or without signs of occlusion.

Magnetic Resonance Imaging and MR Angiography

MRI examination with MRA has become the new gold standard for the diagnosis of cervical artery dissections. This modality can demonstrate the morphologic vascular changes noted above (sharply tapered long-segment stenosis or occlusion without other atherosclerotic wall changes at a typical location, intraluminal flaps, pseudo-aneurysms, or long-segment ectasia). Additionally, MRI can visualize the mural hematoma and may even show intracerebral diffusion abnormalities relating to a previous embolic or hemodynamic event.

Note

MRI can detect all characteristic changes that may occur in the setting of an arterial dissection.

Thus, an optimum MRI protocol for a suspected cervical dissection should include an intracerebral diffusion-weighted imaging (DWI) sequence to detect ischemic events, an unenhanced T1w sequence with fat suppression, preferably in axial and coronal planes to detect the mural hematoma (**Fig. 4.3**), and contrast-enhanced MRA (more sensitive than time-of-flight [TOF] MRA) for the detection of caliber irregularities, occlusions, and pseudo-aneurysms (**Figs. 4.4** and **4.5**).

It should be noted that in the early acute phase (< 48 h after the intramural hemorrhage), the mural hematoma may still appear isointense in T1w sequences if sufficient extracellular methemoglobin has not yet formed in the hematoma. CT scans are just as sensitive during this phase; a perivascular soft-tissue mass with adjacent luminal narrowing can provide indirect evidence of the hematoma and dissection.

Caution

A mural hematoma in the acute phase (first or second day) may not yet be hyperintense on MRI and may elude detection. Greater attention should be given to indirect signs (wall irregularity, diffusion abnormalities, flow changes, etc.) during this phase.

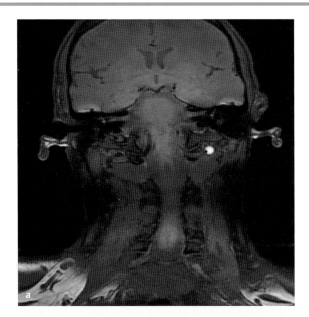

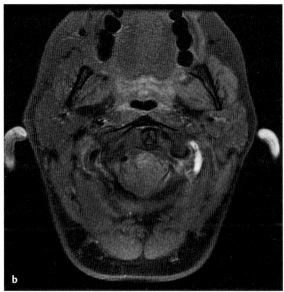

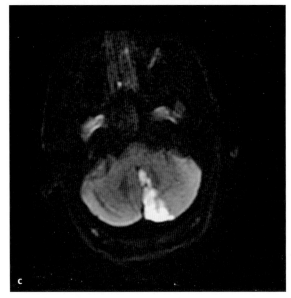

Fig. 4.3a–c   Left vertebral artery dissection in the atlas loop with hyperintense mural hematoma and associated (partial) infarction of the posterior inferior cerebellar artery.

a Typical hyperintense mural hematoma in a coronal fat-suppressed T1w sequence caused by a vertebral artery dissection in the atlas loop (site of predilection for vertebral artery dissections).

b Residual lumen in high-grade stenosis appears as a faint linear hypointensity at the center of the vessel (axial image).

c MRA shows associated (partial) infarction of the left posterior inferior cerebellar artery, most likely due to embolism caused by spread of the dissection to the origin of the posterior inferior cerebellar artery, occluding the vessel.

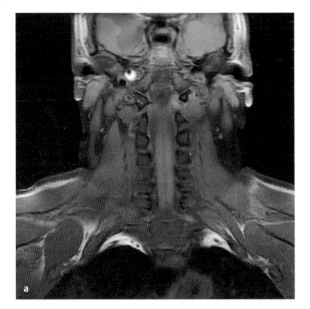

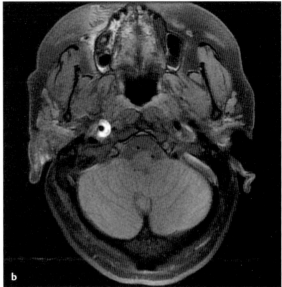

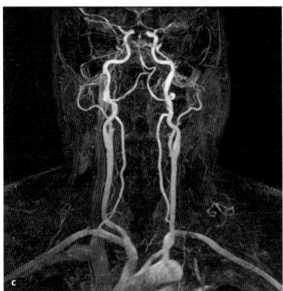

Fig. 4.4a–c   Right carotid artery dissection just below the skull base, with a hyperintense mural hematoma and pseudoaneurysmal dilatation of the internal carotid artery on MRA.

a Coronal T1w sequence with fat suppression displays the mural hematoma as a hyperintense mass. Blood flow in the slightly narrowed residual lumen appears hypointense at the edge of the hematoma.

b Axial T1w sequence with fat suppression.

c MRA shows the dissection as a distinct contour irregularity with low-grade stenosis. Tapering gives way to abrupt luminal expansion (pseudoaneurysm) at the distal end of the dissection.

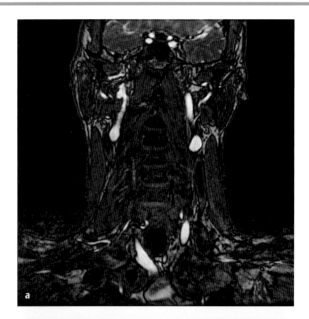

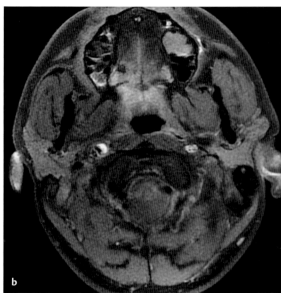

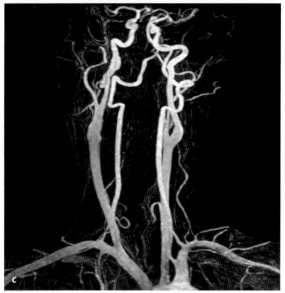

Fig. 4.5a–c   Right carotid artery dissection just below the skull base, with a hyperintense mural hematoma and marked pseudoaneurysmal dilatation of the internal carotid artery on MRA.

a Coronal T1w sequence with fat suppression.
b Axial T1w sequence with fat suppression.
c MRA shows sharp tapering of the dissected lumen with a typical pseudoaneurysm appearance.

Table 4.1 Radiologic signs of a cervical artery dissection

Modality	Imaging signs	Diagnostic role
DSA	• Sharply tapered, irregular, long-segment luminal narrowing (string sign) • Possible tapered occlusion • Linear filling defect caused by intimal flap • Possible distal embolic branch occlusion	Rarely indicated for diagnosis of cervical artery dissection Possible indications: planning therapeutic interventions (stenting, mechanical recanalization) or cases with equivocal findings
CTA	• Long-segment stenosis, luminal irregularity • Mural hematoma may appear as perivascular structure of soft-tissue density	Very useful in acute settings because it is fast and widely available Mural hematoma is not yet clearly definable by MRI in the acute phase

Ultrasound	• Direct morphologic criteria:
	  - Stenosis
	  - Hypoechoic mural hematoma
	  - Intimal flap, two lumina
	• Indirect hemodynamic criteria:
	  - Flow acceleration
	  - Bidirectional flow, "slosh phenomenon"
	  - Occlusion
		Useful only for screening or follow-up due to low sensitivity at skull base and for dissections with scant luminal narrowing
		Caution: very examiner dependent!
		Fast and widely available

MRI	• Mural hematoma is hyperintense in fat-saturated T1w sequences • Contrast-enhanced MRA can detect wall irregularity and stenosis • Possible pseudoaneurysm, wall ectasia • Possible intracerebral diffusion abnormalities due to secondary emboli	Current gold standard This modality can demonstrate all typical signs

Summary

The radiologic signs of a cervical artery dissection are reviewed in **Table 4.1**.

References

Arnold M, Cumurciuc R, Stapf C, Favrole P, Berthet K, Bousser MG. Pain as the only symptom of cervical artery dissection. J Neurol Neurosurg Psychiatry 2006a;77(9):1021–1024

Arnold M, Kappeler L, Georgiadis D, et al. Gender differences in spontaneous cervical artery dissection. Neurology 2006b;67(6):1050–1052

Arnold M, Baumgartner RW, Stapf C, et al. Ultrasound diagnosis of spontaneous carotid dissection with isolated Horner syndrome. Stroke 2008;39(1):82–86

Caso V, Paciaroni M, Bogousslavsky J. Environmental factors and cervical artery dissection. Front Neurol Neurosci 2005;20:44–53

Debette S, Leys D. Cervical-artery dissections: predisposing factors, diagnosis, and outcome. Lancet Neurol 2009;8(7):668–678

Diener HC, Putzki N, Eds. Leitlinien für Diagnostik und Therapie in der Neurologie. 4th ed. Stuttgart: Thieme; 2008

Dittrich R, Nassenstein I, Bachmann R, et al. Polyarterial clustered recurrence of cervical artery dissection seems to be the rule. Neurology 2007a;69(2):180–186

Dittrich R, Rohsbach D, Heidbreder A, et al. Mild mechanical traumas are possible risk factors for cervical artery dissection. Cerebrovasc Dis 2007b;23(4):275–281

Ernst E. Adverse effects of spinal manipulation: a systematic review. J R Soc Med 2007;100(7):330–338

Giroud M, Fayolle H, André N, et al. Incidence of internal carotid artery dissection in the community of Dijon. J Neurol Neurosurg Psychiatry 1994;57(11):1443

Haldeman S, Kohlbeck FJ, McGregor M. Risk factors and precipitating neck movements causing vertebrobasilar artery dissection after cervical trauma and spinal manipulation. Spine 1999;24(8):785–794

Hart RG, Easton JD. Dissections of cervical and cerebral arteries. Neurol Clin 1983;1(1):155–182

Koch S, Rabinstein AA, Romano JG, Forteza A. Diffusion-weighted magnetic resonance imaging in internal carotid artery dissection. Arch Neurol 2004;61(4):510–512

Lee VH, Brown RD Jr, Mandrekar JN, Mokri B. Incidence and outcome of cervical artery dissection: a population-based study. Neurology 2006;67(10):1809–1812

Molina CA, Alvarez-Sabín J, Schonewille W, et al. Cerebral microembolism in acute spontaneous internal carotid artery dissection. Neurology 2000;55(11):1738–1740

Naggara O, Touzé E, Marsico R, et al. High-resolution MR imaging of periarterial edema associated with biological inflammation in spontaneous carotid dissection. Eur Radiol 2009;19(9):2255–2260

Siqueira Neto JI, Santos AC, Fabio SR, Sakamoto AC. Cerebral infarction in patients aged 15 to 40 years. Stroke 1996;27(11):2016–2019

Touzé E, Gauvrit JY, Moulin T, Meder JF, Bracard S, Mas JL; Multicenter Survey on Natural History of Cervical Artery Dissection. Risk of stroke and recurrent dissection after a cervical artery dissection: a multicenter study. Neurology 2003;61(10):1347–1351

5 Cerebral Venous and Sinus Thrombosis

J. Linn

Introduction

Epidemiology

Cerebral venous and sinus thrombosis (CVST) is a relatively rare but important cause of stroke. It accounts for less than 1% of all strokes in Europe. The estimated annual incidence of CVST is ~3–4 cases per 1 million in adults, and ~7 cases per 1 million in newborns, infants, and children. The disease may occur in all age groups and in both sexes, although young and middle-aged women (< 40 years) are most commonly affected (Stam 2005).

Risk Factors

To date, a wide variety of predisposing factors as well as several important direct causes for CVST are known. The most important risk factors and causes of CVST are acquired or congenital coagulation disorders; oral contraceptive use; pregnancy; lactation; and ear, nose, and throat infections. Over 40% of patients are found to have two or more predisposing factors, but 15–20% of all patients have no identifiable risk factors (Ferro et al. 2009).

Subtypes

Three subtypes of CVST are distinguished according to the location of the thrombosis—that is, the venous structures affected. This distinction is clinically relevant because the subtypes differ in their symptoms and prognosis. Also, the value of different imaging sequences differs considerably depending on the site of the thrombosis (Linn and Brückmann 2010).

- *Sinus thrombosis:* This refers to the thrombotic occlusion of one or more of the dural venous sinuses. Sinus thrombosis is by far the most common form of CVST. The superior sagittal sinus is most often affected, followed by the transverse sinus (Ferro et al. 2009; **Figs. 5.1** and **5.2**).
- *Deep cerebral venous thrombosis:* This refers to thrombosis of the internal cerebral veins, vein of Galen, and/or the basal veins of Rosenthal and their tributaries. Most authors also include the straight sinus with the deep cerebral veins. Involvement of the deep cerebral

veins is present in ~10% of all patients with CVST. It is usually accompanied by sinus thrombosis. Isolated thrombosis of the deep cerebral veins is much less common (Ferro et al. 2004; **Fig. 5.3**).
- *Cortical vein thrombosis:* Thrombosis of the cortical veins refers to a thrombosis of the superficial veins of the cerebral convexities including the vein of Labbé. Like deep cerebral vein thrombosis, cortical vein thrombosis occurs most often in combination with sinus thrombosis. In these cases, the superior sagittal sinus is most often involved. Cortical vein thrombosis often develops secondary to superior sagittal sinus thrombosis due to retrograde spread of thrombotic material from the sinus into the cerebral veins draining into the sinus (**Fig. 5.4**). This process most commonly affects the frontal cortical veins, followed by the parietal veins (Linn et al. 2010). Isolated thrombosis of one or more cortical veins is very rare and has been described only in isolated case reports and small case series.

Evaluation of the cortical veins poses a special diagnostic challenge to the radiologist. This is mainly because the cortical veins, unlike the dural sinuses and deep cerebral veins, show striking intra- and interindividual variations in number, diameter, and anatomic location. These hamper the interpretation of angiographic studies. Therefore, these techniques are of limited used for the evaluation of the cortical veins and cannot serve as gold standard technique. More recently, T2*-weighted gradient-echo sequences have proven very effective for this application (see below and **Fig. 5.4**). Consequently, the number of reported cases has risen sharply in recent years. Today many authors believe that cortical vein involvement is much more common than previously described. It is also reasonable to assume that isolated cortical vein thrombosis is not as rare as previously thought but simply went undetected in earlier studies.

Clinical Signs and Symptoms

In contrast to arterial strokes, the symptoms of CVST usually have a subacute onset. The clinical presentation is nonspecific, and heterogeneous. The most common initial, very unspecific symptom is severe headache, which occurs in 75–90% of all patients. In addition to headache, patients often develop other signs of increased

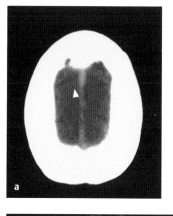

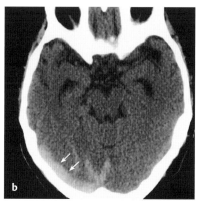

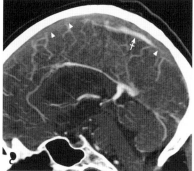

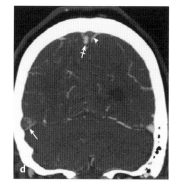

Fig. 5.1a–d Sinus thrombosis on non-contrast CT and CTA. A 70-year-old woman who suffered from predominantly right-sided headaches for several days due to thrombosis of the superior sagittal sinus (*arrowheads* in **a**, **c**, and **d**) and right transverse sinus (*arrows* in **b** and **d**).

a, b Noncontrast CT scans (**a, b**) show a hyperdense vessel sign (cord sign) in the affected sinuses (*arrows* and *arrowheads* in **a** and **b**, respectively) as a direct sign of thrombosis.

c, d CT angiography. Sagittal and coronal multiplanar reconstruction from MPRs (**c** and **d**) demonstrate the thrombosis as a filling defect in the affected vessels (*arrows* and *arrowheads* in **c** and **d**, respectively). The *crossed arrows* in **c** and **d** indicate a prominent cortical vein that drains into the thrombosed superior sagittal sinus.

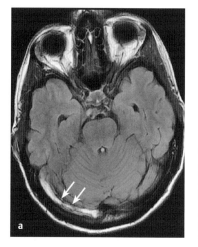

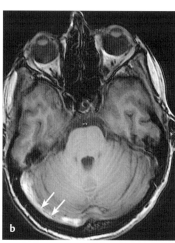

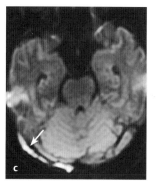

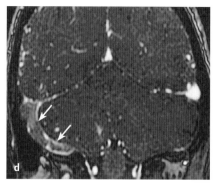

Fig. 5.2a–d Direct MR signs of subacute right transverse sinus thrombosis (*arrows* in **a–d**) in a 32-year-old man who had been symptomatic (headaches and nausea) for 10 days, consistent with a subacute phase of thrombosis.

a FLAIR sequence. The thrombotic material in the right transverse sinus (*arrows*) appears hyperintense.

b T1w sequence. Again, the thrombotic material in the right transverse sinus (*arrows*) appears hyperintense.

c The thrombotic material also has high signal intensity on diffusion-weighted MRI (*arrow*).

d Coronal reconstruction of contrast-enhanced MRA shows no contrast filling of the affected sinus (*arrows*).

I

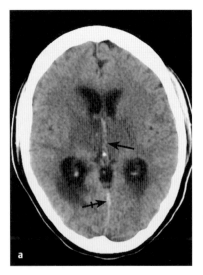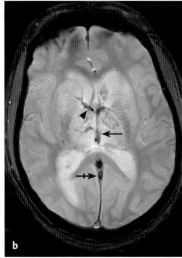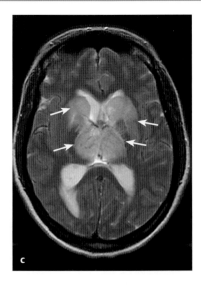

Fig. 5.3a–c   Direct and indirect signs of deep cerebral vein thrombosis
in a 32-year-old woman with thrombosis of the deep cerebral
veins (*arrows* in **a** and **b**), thalamostriate veins (*arrowhead* in **b**),
and straight sinus (*crossed arrows* in **a** and **b**) causing bilateral
edema in the thalamus and basal ganglia (*arrows* in **c**).

a The thrombotic material shows high attenuation on noncontrast
CT (dense vein sign, *arrow*).

b The thrombotic material has low signal intensity on T2*w MRI
(*arrow, arrowhead, crossed arrow*).

c T2-weighted sequence vividly defines the extent of associated
venous edema (*arrows*).

intracranial pressure such as dizziness, nausea, and visual
disturbances. Other symptoms of CVST depend basically
on the location and extent of the thrombosis (Ameri
and Bousser 1992; Stam 2005). Other important factors
that determine clinical presentation are patient age, the
presence of concomitant parenchymal changes, and the
interval from symptom onset to diagnosis. Focal neurologic deficits can occur, depending on the site of the
venous occlusion, and may include cranial nerve deficits
and focal seizures.

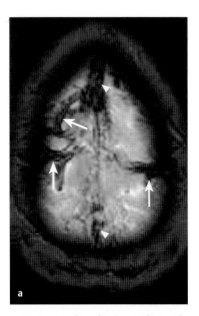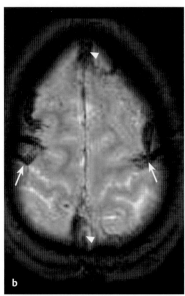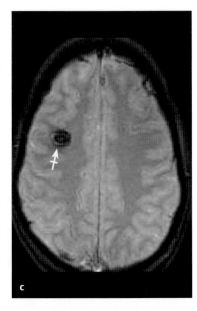

Fig. 5.4a–c   Value of T2*w gradient-echo MRI for detecting cortical vein thrombosis.
A 45-year-old woman with thrombosis of the superior sagittal
sinus (*arrowheads* in **a** and **b**) and bilateral frontal cortical veins
(*arrows* in **a** and **b**). Right frontal hemorrhage due to venous stasis
(*crossed arrow* in **c**) is present as an indirect sign of thrombosis.

Cortical vein involvement is clearly appreciated only in the T2*w
sequence where the affected veins appear as very hypointense
tubular structures. The other MR sequences (*not shown*) showed
direct signs of thrombosis only in the superior sagittal sinus.

Involvement of the deep cerebral veins or cortical veins significantly affects the clinical presentation. Patients with deep cerebral vein thrombosis present with a decreased level of consciousness in over 70% of cases (Pfefferkorn et al. 2009). Cortical vein thrombosis is often characterized by focal or generalized seizures, hemiparesis, aphasia, hemianopsia, or other focal neurologic deficits. Symptoms of increased intracranial pressure may be absent, especially when thrombosis is limited to the cortical veins (Jacobs et al. 1996).

Laboratory Findings

Normal D-dimer levels have a high negative predictive value for suspected CVST. Nevertheless, D-dimer levels may be normal in up to 25% of cases, especially in patients with isolated thrombosis of the deep cerebral veins. False-negative results in these cases are presumably due to the relatively small thrombus volume (Pfefferkorn et al. 2009).

Prognosis and Outcome

The outcome of CVST has improved significantly in recent decades. This is due largely to improvements in imaging modalities and effective treatment methods using intravenous or subcutaneous low-molecular-weight heparin. Today CVST has a very good prognosis when diagnosed early, with complete recovery achieved in 80% of patients (Diener and Putzki 2008). It should be added, however, that the interval from symptom onset to definitive diagnosis still averages 7 days, despite modern imaging modalities (Stam 2005). This interval may be considerably longer in patients with deep cerebral vein thrombosis, in males, and in patients who present only with signs of increased intracranial pressure. This is due mainly to the very unspecific and variable symptoms of the disease and its delayed or subacute clinical onset, especially in the small subset of patients who have normal D-dimer levels.

This delay accounts for the poorer outcomes in ~10–15% of patients with CVST. Besides a delay in diagnosis, there are other risk factors that are associated with a poor outcome:

advanced age, male gender, parenchymal hemorrhage secondary to venous congestion, involvement of the deep cerebral veins or right transverse sinus, and the presence of CNS infection or an intracerebral tumor as a precipitating cause (Ferro et al. 2004). Although involvement of the deep venous system is a risk factor for a poor or even fatal course, a recent study found that even this condition has a better outcome today than in earlier studies. It was shown that 75% of patients improved significantly when treated with intravenous or subcutaneous low-molecular-weight heparin, achieving a modified Rankin Score (mRS) of 2 or higher, signifying little or no functional disability. The remaining 25% of patients deteriorated with progressing coma, even though most of them received endovascular recanalization therapy (Pfefferkorn et al. 2009).

Imaging Studies

Direct and Indirect Signs of Cerebral Venous and Sinus Thrombosis

Imaging studies can reveal both direct and indirect signs of CVST, regardless of the site of the venous occlusion. Direct signs are signal or density changes caused by the thrombotic material itself; indirect signs are associated signal abnormalities in the brain parenchyma.

- *Direct signs:* "Positive" visualization of the thrombus in an affected vein or sinus by noncontrast CT or MRI, or "negative" visualization of the thrombus as a filling defect in digital subtraction angiography (DSA), CT angiography (CTA), or other contrast-enhanced images, as well as absence of a flow signal in flow-sensitive venous time-of-flight MR angiography (TOF MRA).
- *Indirect signs:* The following parenchymal changes can be found as indirect signs of CVST on CT and MR images: venous edema or venous infarction, subarachnoid hemorrhage, and parenchymal hemorrhage due to venous congestion. In contrast to arterial strokes, the edema in CVST typically does not conform to arterial territories but crosses territory boundaries. Most often a vasogenic edema is found, while acute ischemic arterial infarctions typically present with a cytotoxic edema. In the case of dural sinus or cortical vein thrombosis, the edema typically affects the cortex and/or the adjacent subcortical white matter. By contrast, deep cerebral vein thrombosis is typically associated with unilateral or most often bilateral edema or venous infarction in the thalamus and basal ganglia (Linn and Brückmann 2010; see **Fig. 5.3**). If parenchymal hemorrhage is detected at the time of diagnosis, it correlates with more severe initial symptoms and a poorer outcome (Ferro et al. 2004).

I

Digital Subtraction Angiography

Long considered the diagnostic gold standard for CVST, DSA no longer has a significant role in the diagnosis of this disease, having been largely replaced by CTA and MRI.

> **Note**
>
> Today DSA is no longer a standard tool for suspected CVST but is reserved for cases being considered for interventional treatment such as local thrombolysis or mechanical recanalization (Diener and Putzki 2008).

However, DSA is still superior to MRI and CTA in its spatial and temporal resolution and can provide very precise dynamic information, especially on collateral venous drainage pathways. This capability can yield important additional information in selected cases.

For the cortical veins, a few authors still claim that DSA can provide higher sensitivity than other modalities, although no systematic data have been published to support this hypothesis. In patients with isolated thrombosis of one or more cortical veins, DSA may show an "absent" cortical vein and/or a partially opacified vein with an abrupt cutoff. Dilated cortical veins functioning as collaterals may be visible in the surrounding area. The value of this sign is limited, however, by the large intra- and interindividual variations of the number and anatomic location the cortical veins as described above. As a result, the direct signs of thrombosis on DSA are of limited value and the diagnosis of cortical vein thrombosis by DSA is based mainly on the following *indirect signs:*

- Detection of a focal delay in venous drainage
- Signs of venous congestion in parenchyma drained by the occluded vein
- Detection of cortical collaterals, also known as "corkscrew vessels"

> **Caution**
>
> The above limitations of DSA for evaluating the cortical veins also apply to other angiographic techniques including CTA and the various MRA techniques.

Magnetic Resonance Imaging

Today MRI is regarded as the gold standard for the diagnosis of CVST (Stam 2005), although CTA is increasingly found to be equivalent to MRA alone (see below; Diener and Putzki 2008).

Direct Signs of CVST on MRI

Cerebral venous thrombosis shows rather complex signal characteristics on MRI depending on the age of the thrombus (acute, subacute, or chronic stage) and on the type of MRI sequence used. In contrast, the location of the thrombus does not influence its imaging appearance—that is, the signal characteristics of the thrombotic material are the same regardless of whether the dural sinuses, deep cerebral veins, or cortical veins are affected (Linn and Brückmann 2010).

> **Note**
>
> A detailed knowledge of the complex, time-dependent signal characteristics of the venous thrombus is essential for the correct interpretation of MR images in CVST.

Spin-Echo Sequences

During the acute phase of thrombosis (days 0–5 from symptom onset), the thrombus typically has low signal intensity in T2-weighted (T2w) spin-echo sequences and is isointense in T1w spin-echo sequences. Because of these signal characteristics, the thrombus itself may be difficult to distinguish from normal flow signal in the venous vessels. This considerably limits the sensitivity of these sequences, especially during the days immediately after symptom onset. In the subacute phase (days 6–15), the venous clot becomes increasingly hyperintense in both T2- and T1w sequences (Teasdale 2000; **Fig. 5.2**). On FLAIR and proton-density-weighted sequences, the thrombus signal characteristics are very similar to those in T2w spin-echo sequences (Linn et al. 2010). Although these signal patterns are found in the majority of cases, there are isolated cases in which the signal characteristics may show considerable variations (**Table 5.1**).

Due to the complexity of the clot signal characteristics, the interpretation of MRI in CVST requires a great deal of experience to avoid diagnostic and also technical pitfalls. As an example of potential technical pitfalls, a hyperintense signal from normal venous flow can mimic a thrombus in T1w sequences acquired without adequate flow compensation (**Fig. 5.5**). These pitfalls represent a disadvantage of MRI compared with CTA, which is easier to interpret in CVST (Teasdale 2000; Linn and Brückmann 2010).

Diffusion-Weighted MRI

In some cases the venous thrombus shows restricted diffusion in diffusion-weighted MRI with a hyperintense signal in B1000 images and a decreased apparent

Tab. 5.1 Dependence of thrombus signal intensity in T1- and T2-weighted spin-echo sequences on the delay after symptom onset

MRI sequence	Signal intensity of thrombus	Percentage of patients affected (%)		
		Acute phase (days 0–5)[a]	Subacute phase (days 6–15)[a]	Chronic phase (> 15 days)[a]
T1w	Hyperintense	30	**71**	39
	Isointense	**68**	29	**54**
	Hypointense	2	0	7
T2w[b]	Hyperintense	25	**52**	**43**
	Isointense	10	32	**45**
	Hypointense	**65**	16	12

[a] Days refer to delay after symptom onset.
[b] The signal intensities described for T2-weighted sequences also apply to FLAIR and proton-density sequences.
The signal intensities most commonly found in a particular phase are boldfaced for emphasis.

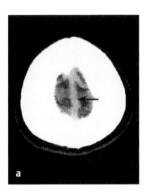
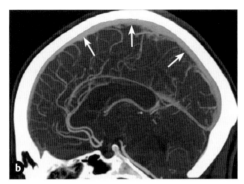
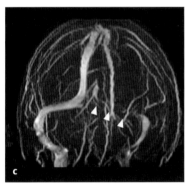
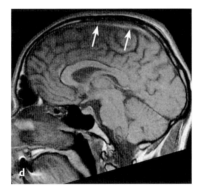
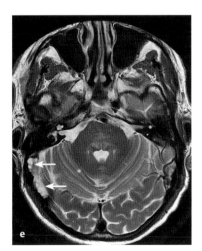
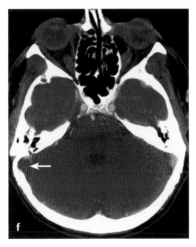

Fig. 5.5a–f Potential pitfalls in the imaging of CVST.

a Unenhanced CT. False-positive cord sign in the superior sagittal sinus (*arrow*) of a 42-year-old man with headaches.

b CT angiography (sagittal reconstruction). Same patient as shown in **a**. CTA shows normal contrast filling of the superior sagittal sinus (*arrows*), excluding thrombosis.

c TOF MRA in a healthy 30-year-old subject. Hypoplasia of the left transverse sinus (*arrowheads*) is common and should not be mistaken for thrombosis.

d Sagittal T1w sequence without flow compensation, performed in another healthy volunteer. Normal blood flow in the superior sagittal sinus appears hyperintense due to lack of flow compensation (*arrows*). This, too, may be mistaken for thrombosis.

e Prominent pacchionian granulations are easily identified as such in the T2w image (*arrows*).

f The prominent pacchionian granulations in **e** produce a filling defect on CTA (*arrow*). They are respectively isointense to CSF in all modalities and sequences, which aids in their positive identification.

I

diffusion coefficient in the ADC map. The diagnostic value of this finding is limited by the fact that it occurs mainly in the subacute phase of thrombosis when a hyperintense thrombus signal is seen on FLAIR and T2w and T1w images. At this stage, it is relatively easy to make a diagnosis based on these sequences even without additional information (see **Fig. 5.2**). Furthermore, the sensitivity of this sign is rather low, ranging from ~4% to 40% in different studies (Lövblad et al. 2001; Linn et al. 2010). There is, however, initial evidence that the detection of a hyperintense clot on diffusion-weighted MRI might be a useful prognostic factor in predicting the likelihood of spontaneous recanalization. In an initial study, the presence of restricted diffusion in the clot was associated with low recanalization rates (Favrole et al. 2004).

T2*-Weighted Gradient-Echo Sequence

Recent findings have shown that the T2*w gradient-echo sequence is excellent for the diagnosis of CVST. This is particularly true in the acute phase of the disease, when the thrombus is still isointense in T1w sequences. T2*w imaging, even soon after symptom onset, displays the thrombus as a homogeneous, markedly hypointense tubular structure with an associated "blooming" effect. Published reports consistently document the value of this sequence in the acute phase of thrombosis (Selim et al. 2002; Idbaih et al. 2006; Leach et al. 2007). The findings at later stages are somewhat less consistent. Some authors have described a relatively strong time-dependence of the hypointense signal, which they observed in 90% of cases during the first week but only in 9–32% of cases by the subacute or chronic phase (Leach et al. 2007). Other authors found that the hypointensities persisted for up to 1 year after symptom onset and were present in more than 30% of cases at 4-month follow-up (Idbaih et al. 2006).

The T2*w sequence is particularly rewarding in patients with suspected cortical vein thrombosis (see **Fig. 5.4**). It has proven far superior to all other MRI sequences and CTA for evaluating the cortical veins. Hence this sequence is currently considered to be the gold standard for the diagnosis of isolated or combined cortical vein thrombosis and for the exclusion of cortical vein involvement by dural sinus thrombosis (Boukobza et al. 2009; Linn et al. 2010).

Note

The T2*w sequence should be implemented as a standard sequence for the routine diagnosis or exclusion of CVST, as it is the only technique that can accurately evaluate the cortical veins.

Practical Tip

To avoid a false-positive interpretation of a T2*w sequence, a linear hypointense signal should be taken as a direct sign of venous thrombosis only if:

- it is prominent—it produces a blooming effect that extends past the normal vascular diameter
- it shows a round cross-section in slices perpendicular to the course of the signal
- it conforms to the anatomic course of a vessel.

A chronic subarachnoid hemorrhage or focal superficial siderosis, defined as a hypointense linear signal within the superficial layers of the cerebral cortex, should not be misinterpreted as a hypointense venous thrombus. Superficial siderosis is typically found in patients with cerebral amyloid angiopathy or in patients with vasculitis (Linn et al. 2009).

Susceptibility-weighted sequences are a recent addition to the MRI sequence repertoire. They are even more sensitive than conventional T2*w sequences for detecting susceptibility changes, and provide an excellent tool for the detailed visualization of cerebral venous anatomy. Various acquisition and postprocessing methods can be used to produce susceptibility-weighted images. The sequence is known by the acronyms SWI (susceptibility-weighted imaging) and SWAN (susceptibility-weighted angiography). To date, these sequences have been used only in selected patients with CVST (Kawabori et al. 2009; Linn and Brückmann 2010). These isolated cases have yielded very promising results, although it should be noted that even normally perfused veins appear hypointense in these sequences, which can hamper interpretation as venous thrombus would also appear as hypointense signal. Systematic prospective studies are needed to determine the value of SWI for the diagnosis of CVST.

Venous MRA Techniques

Various MRA techniques can be used for imaging the cerebral venous vessels. Venous TOF MRA is the most widely used method for routine clinical imaging. It is a flow-sensitive sequence in which the thrombus can be directly identified as a flow void in the affected vascular segment. The following potential pitfalls and artifacts should be considered in interpreting this sequence, however (Ayanzen et al. 2000):

- Slow blood flow or blood flow in the acquisition plane can mimic the absence of flow.
- The presence of a hypoplastic or aplastic transverse sinus (usually the left) may be mistaken for a thrombus when MRA is used alone (see **Fig. 5.5**). In a significant proportion of healthy control subjects, no venous flow signal is detected in one transverse sinus, due to hypoplasia

of this respective sinus (typically the left one), which should not be misinterpreted as a thrombotic occlusion.
- A thrombus in the subacute stage, which is very hyperintense on T1w images, can mimic a normal flow signal in TOF MRA.

Practical Tip

To reduce misinterpretations in TOF MRA, it is strongly recommended that the source images also be reviewed. Image analysis should not be based on three-dimensional maximum-intensity projection reconstructions (MIPs) alone.

MRA is subject to the same limitations as DSA and CTA for imaging the cortical veins due to the marked anatomic variations in these vessels (see above).

Besides TOF MRA, phase-contrast techniques as well as contrast-enhanced venous MRA (see **Fig. 5.2**) and contrast-enhanced MPRAGE (magnetization-prepared rapid acquisition gradient echo) sequences can also be used to evaluate CVST.

Additionally there are promising new MRA techniques such as time-resolved MRA, which may become important in the future for evaluating the cerebral veins and dural sinuses. It has been shown, for example, that the combination of dynamic and static three-dimensional MRA, known as combined four-dimensional MR venography, is superior to TOF MRA for the assessment of venous structures (Meckel et al. 2010). Further studies are needed to evaluate the diagnostic yield of these sequences and the effect of higher field strengths with regard to the diagnosis of CVST.

Indirect Signs of CVST in MRI

MRI is the most sensitive modality for detecting secondary parenchymal changes as indirect signs of venous thrombosis. T2-, proton-density-, and FLAIR-weighted sequences are best suited for detecting venous edema and venous infarction (see **Fig. 5.3**), while the T2*w gradient echo sequence is best for detecting hemorrhagic imbibition and hemorrhage due to venous congestion (see **Fig. 5.4**).

Diffusion-weighted MRI in CVST shows highly variable or heterogeneous findings in the brain parenchyma. It may reveal cytotoxic or vasogenic edema or a mixed pattern. Studies in patients as well as in animal models have shown evidence that cytotoxic edema precedes vasogenic edema in CVST. This is manifested by a decrease of the ADC in the very early stage of thrombosis, followed later by a normalization or increase in the ADC (Ducreux et al. 2001; Srivastava et al. 2009).

Computed Tomography

Noncontrast CT

At most clinical institutions, noncontrast CT is still the method of first choice for the emergency evaluation of suspected neurologic disease. This is due mainly to wide availability of the method, its cost effectiveness, and short examination time.

On noncontrast CT, a fresh thrombus produces a homogeneous hyperdense signal in the affected sinuses. This direct sign of thrombosis is called the cord sign or dense vein sign (Linn et al. 2009; see **Figs. 5.1** and **5.3**). Both terms are applied rather inconsistently in the literature to veins as well as sinuses. Here we use the term "cord sign" for the dural sinuses and "dense vein sign" for the cerebral veins. This direct sign of thrombosis, marked by high attenuation of the thrombotic material itself, is most apparent during the first week of the disease, and thus during the acute phase. Over a period of 7–14 days the thrombus first becomes isodense and later hypodense. It has been shown that the cord sign in the dural sinuses has a relatively low sensitivity and specificity of 25–65% (Virapongse et al. 1987; Linn et al. 2009; see **Fig. 5.5**). For a thrombosis of the cortical veins, the dense vein sign has a sensitivity of only 25% (Linn et al. 2010).

Caution

Noncontrast CT alone cannot reliably detect or exclude thrombosis of the dural sinuses or cortical veins.

Although noncontrast CT is of limited value for sinus and cortical vein imaging, it is much better suited for detecting thrombosis of the deep cerebral veins. Studies have shown that the dense vein sign has a sensitivity of 100% and a specificity > 99% for the presence of isolated or combined deep cerebral vein thrombosis (see **Fig. 5.3**). This applies both to the overall diagnosis of this disease and to the determination of the extent of thrombosis and the involvement of the individual deep cerebral veins (Linn et al. 2009).

Note

Noncontrast CT is a valuable tool for the diagnosis of suspected deep cerebral vein thrombosis. Its rapid availability and cost effectiveness make it excellent for this application.

Potential pitfalls in noncontrast CT that may lead to false-positive or false-negative findings regarding the presence of a cord sign or dense vein sign are as follows:
- *Partial-volume effects:* These effects, caused by adjacent bony structures and especially the calvarium,

may give rise to false-positive hyperdense areas. This particularly applies to the dural sinuses and cortical veins, which are in close proximity to the calvarium. Evaluation of the deep cerebral veins is not hampered by this effect owing to the deep location of the vessels.

- *Normal venous blood flow:* Normally flowing venous blood may appear slightly hyperdense on noncontrast CT, especially when the hematocrit is high (see **Fig. 5.5**).
- *Delayed initial imaging:* Noncontrast CT may be false-negative for sinus thrombosis, showing absence of a hyperdense vessel sign, in patients with mild clinical symptoms (e.g., thrombosis limited to one sinus) causing initial imaging to be delayed. The thrombus may then appear isodense again on noncontrast CT, yielding a false-negative result.

Although MRI is superior to noncontrast CT for detecting associated parenchymal changes as indirect signs of thrombosis, noncontrast CT is also very sensitive and specific in detecting these secondary effects of thrombosis (Linn et al. 2007; see **Fig. 5.3**).

Contrast-Enhanced Computed Tomography

The "empty delta sign" in contrast-enhanced CT has been described as a direct sign of CVST. It is best detected on slices perpendicular to the affected sinus axis and refers to a triangular-shaped hypodense center (corresponding to the thrombosed sinus lumen) bordered by a "empty" triangular-shaped enhancing rim. The sign is typically found in the superior sagittal sinus (Virapongse et al. 1987). It occurs because the walls of the affected sinus show contrast uptake (causing peripheral enhancement) while the thrombus within the sinus does not (causing central absence of enhancement). Today, however, contrast-enhanced CT and the empty delta sign have become less important in the diagnosis of CVST owing to the wide availability of CTA.

CT Angiography

Note

According to the latest statement of the American Heart Association and the American Stroke Association on the diagnosis and management of cerebral venous thrombosis, venous CTA is at least equivalent to venous MRA alone in the diagnosis of CVST (Saposnik et al. 2011).

The cerebral veins and dural sinuses can be imaged and evaluated at high spatial resolution with multislice CTA. This method enables high-quality multiplanar reconstructions and three-dimensional MIPs that can further facilitate the evaluation of the cerebral venous system. With regard to the visualization of small cerebral veins, the inferior sagittal sinus, and the nondominant transverse sinus, there is growing evidence that CTA may be superior to venous TOF MRA. A major advantage of CTA over flow-sensitive TOF MRA is that CTA is not susceptible to flow artifacts. This is particularly important in the presence of a hypoplastic vessel such as the left transverse sinus. The short examination time and the ability to simultaneously visualize the arterial and venous cerebrovascular system by using a suitable scan delay can further increase the value of CTA, especially in the acute setting (Klingebiel et al. 2001).

CTA displays the thrombus as a filling defect in the affected vessel (see **Fig. 5.1**). One study comparing multislice CTA with the gold standard of MRI found that CTA had a sensitivity and specificity of 100% for the diagnosis of sinus thrombosis (Linn et al. 2007). Although CTA delineates the small cerebral vessels very accurately, no systematic studies have been done on the value of CTA in diagnosing deep cerebral vein thrombosis, to date.

Caution

As for the cortical veins, CTA has been found to have very low sensitivity in the detection of cortical vein thrombosis and is not considered suitable for this application (Linn et al. 2010).

The following factors could be responsible for misinterpretations (mostly false-negative) in CTA:

- *Cord sign and dense vein sign:* In the acute phase of thrombosis, a very hyperdense thrombus on CTA (cord sign, dense vein sign) can mimic normal contrast filling of the affected vessel, leading to a false-negative result. This error can be avoided by also obtaining a noncontrast CT scan that shows the thrombus as a dense vein sign. This could be particularly important for evaluating the deep cerebral veins on CTA.
- *Chronic organized thrombus:* Instead of causing a filling defect, this type of thrombus may show enhancement on CTA, leading to a false-negative interpretation.
- *Partial-volume effects:* Partial-volume effects from the enhancing walls of small veins could obscure a filling defect at the center of the vessel. This limitation is especially true for small-caliber veins such as the cortical veins.
- *Pacchionian granulations:* Prominent pacchionian granulations are a theoretical source of false-positive findings (see **Fig. 5.5**). In practice, however, it has been shown that arachnoid granulations can regularly be

distinguished from thrombosis by their typical round or oval shape, smooth margins, and isodensity to cerebrospinal fluid (CSF) (Linn et al. 2007).

Radiation exposure is only a minor disadvantage of CTA. The effective dose from a multislice CTA examination at 120 kV is < 1 mSv, which is even less than the mean effective dose from noncontrast CT.

Summary

MRI with a multisequence protocol including venous MRA and T2*w imaging is currently considered the gold standard for the diagnosis of CVST. However, the interpretation of MRI in venous thrombosis requires a detailed knowledge of the time- and sequence-dependent signal characteristics of thrombi, and this may be a disadvantage of MRI relative to CTA in routine examinations. Multislice CTA is a very fast, widely available, and cost-effective technique that is regarded as equivalent to MRA in suspected sinus thrombosis.

Noncontrast CT alone cannot reliably exclude sinus thrombosis or cortical vein thrombosis, but it is very sensitive for the detection of deep cerebral vein thrombosis. Accordingly, special attention should be given to possible hyperdensity of the deep cerebral veins during the interpretation of noncontrast CT.

T2*w MRI is essential in patients with suspected involvement of the cortical veins or isolated cortical vein thrombosis because other imaging techniques have very low sensitivity for this application.

References

Ameri A, Bousser MG. Cerebral venous thrombosis. Neurol Clin 1992;10(1):87–111

Ayanzen RH, Bird CR, Keller PJ, McCully FJ, Theobald MR, Heiserman JE. Cerebral MR venography: normal anatomy and potential diagnostic pitfalls. AJNR Am J Neuroradiol 2000;21(1):74–78

Boukobza M, Crassard I, Bousser MG, Chabriat H. MR imaging features of isolated cortical vein thrombosis: diagnosis and follow-up. AJNR Am J Neuroradiol 2009;30(2):344–348

Diener HC, Putzki N, Eds. Leitlinien für Diagnostik und Therapie in der Neurologie. 4th ed. Stuttgart: Thieme; 2008

Ducreux D, Oppenheim C, Vandamme X, et al. Diffusion-weighted imaging patterns of brain damage associated with cerebral venous thrombosis. AJNR Am J Neuroradiol 2001;22(2):261–268

Favrole P, Guichard JP, Crassard I, Bousser MG, Chabriat H. Diffusion-weighted imaging of intravascular clots in cerebral venous thrombosis. Stroke 2004;35(1):99–103

Ferro JM, Canhão P, Stam J, Bousser MG, Barinagarrementeria F; ISCVT Investigators. Prognosis of cerebral vein and dural sinus thrombosis: results of the International Study on Cerebral Vein and Dural Sinus Thrombosis (ISCVT). Stroke 2004;35(3):664–670

Ferro JM, Bacelar-Nicolau H, Rodrigues T, et al; ISCVT and VENOPORT investigators. Risk score to predict the outcome of patients with cerebral vein and dural sinus thrombosis. Cerebrovasc Dis 2009;28(1):39–44

Idbaih A, Boukobza M, Crassard I, Porcher R, Bousser MG, Chabriat H. MRI of clot in cerebral venous thrombosis: high diagnostic value of susceptibility-weighted images. Stroke 2006;37(4):991–995

Jacobs K, Moulin T, Bogousslavsky J, et al. The stroke syndrome of cortical vein thrombosis. Neurology 1996;47(2):376–382

Kawabori M, Kuroda S, Kudo K, et al. Susceptibility-weighted magnetic resonance imaging detects impaired cerebral hemodynamics in the superior sagittal sinus thrombosis—case report. Neurol Med Chir (Tokyo) 2009;49(6):248–251

Klingebiel R, Zimmer C, Rogalla P, et al. Assessment of the arteriovenous cerebrovascular system by multi-slice CT. A single-bolus, monophasic protocol. Acta Radiol 2001;42(6):560–562

Leach JL, Strub WM, Gaskill-Shipley MF. Cerebral venous thrombus signal intensity and susceptibility effects on gradient recalled-echo MR imaging. AJNR Am J Neuroradiol 2007;28(5):940–945

Linn J, Ertl-Wagner B, Seelos KC, et al. Diagnostic value of multidetector-row CT angiography in the evaluation of thrombosis of the cerebral venous sinuses. AJNR Am J Neuroradiol 2007;28(5):946–952

Linn J, Pfefferkorn T, Ivanicova K, et al. Noncontrast CT in deep cerebral venous thrombosis and sinus thrombosis: comparison of its diagnostic value for both entities. AJNR Am J Neuroradiol 2009;30(4):728–735

Linn J, Brückmann H. Cerebral venous and dural sinus thrombosis: state-of-the-art imaging. Clin Neuroradiol 2010;20:25–37

Linn J, Michl S, Katja B, et al. Cortical vein thrombosis: the diagnostic value of different imaging modalities. Neuroradiology 2010;52(10):899–911

Lövblad KO, Bassetti C, Schneider J, et al. Diffusion-weighted mr in cerebral venous thrombosis. Cerebrovasc Dis 2001;11(3):169–176

Meckel S, Reisinger C, Bremerich J, et al. Cerebral venous thrombosis: diagnostic accuracy of combined, dynamic and static, contrast-enhanced 4D MR venography. AJNR Am J Neuroradiol 2010;31(3):527–535

Pfefferkorn T, Crassard I, Linn J, Dichgans M, Boukobza M, Bousser MG. Clinical features, course and outcome in deep cerebral venous system thrombosis: an analysis of 32 cases. J Neurol 2009;256(11):1839–1845

Saposnik G, Barinagarrementeria F, Brown RD Jr, et al; American Heart Association Stroke Council and the Council on Epidemiology and Prevention. Diagnosis and management of cerebral venous thrombosis: a statement for healthcare

I

professionals from the American Heart Association/American Stroke Association. Stroke 2011;42(4):1158–1192

Selim M, Fink J, Linfante I, Kumar S, Schlaug G, Caplan LR. Diagnosis of cerebral venous thrombosis with echo-planar T2*-weighted magnetic resonance imaging. Arch Neurol 2002;59(6):1021–1026

Stam J. Thrombosis of the cerebral veins and sinuses. N Engl J Med 2005;352(17):1791–1798

Srivastava AK, Kalita J, Haris M, Gupta RK, Misra UK. Radiological and histological changes following cerebral venous sinus thrombosis in a rat model. Neurosci Res 2009;65(4):343–346

Teasdale E. Cerebral venous thrombosis: making the most of imaging. J R Soc Med 2000;93(5):234–237

Virapongse C, Cazenave C, Quisling R, Sarwar M, Hunter S. The empty delta sign: frequency and significance in 76 cases of dural sinus thrombosis. Radiology 1987;162(3):779–785

Summary and Recommendations Part I

O. Jansen and H. Brueckmann

Imaging studies are essential in the evaluation of stroke patients. When it comes to strokes, however, "time is brain" and available options such as CT and MRI should be applied with maximum efficiency to save time. Moreover, there is a growing need to establish a network structure between smaller hospitals or hospitals with no capacity for interventional therapies and neurovascular centers that offer all therapeutic options to expedite patient selection based on imaging studies. The main goals of this selection process are to determine the pathogenesis of the stroke and define possible treatments and therapeutic windows for individual patients. In the future, then, telemedical and teleradiologic networks will function more efficiently to ensure that, after their initial imaging workup, stroke patients are placed on the most appropriate treatment paths. This process requires active and effective communication between central and peripheral stroke facilities.

For at least a decade, the capabilities and protocols of "stroke MRI" have advanced our knowledge of the pathophysiology of stroke, especially ischemic stroke. Today, however, CT with its options of CTA and CTP (whole-brain perfusion imaging) has become the primary diagnostic tool in most patients. This particularly applies to ischemic strokes in the anterior circulation. Large studies on intravenous thrombolysis (ECASS: see pp. 9 and 57; NINDS: see p. 56) still based patient selection entirely on noncontrast CT, mainly to differentiate between ischemic and hemorrhagic stroke. During the course of these studies on intravenous thrombolysis, early ischemic changes became increasingly important in defining exclusion criteria for intravenous thrombolysis (one-third MCA rule). Today, however, further advances in CT technology and the widespread availability of multislice scanners with a large number of detector rows have made it possible to perform almost a complete vascular and parenchymal workup in stroke patients on a broad scale within a very short time. The practice of combining noncontrast CT with CTA and/or CTP (known as "CT+") has increasingly become the centerpiece of early diagnosis in patients who are candidates for active stroke therapy based on the severity of the stroke and the available time window. On the other hand, the interpretation of stroke CT should not be limited to the evaluation of reconstructions or perfusion maps but should include information from the source images. The analysis and interpretation of these data will provide at least an experienced diagnostician with comprehensive information on the current and individual status of ischemic stroke patients. But as we saw in Chapter 2, multislice CT can do more than supply functional information; it can also provide additional information on the location of the occlusion and the pathogenesis of the ischemia.

The ability to detect and define the thrombus causing the occlusion based solely on the skilled interpretation of thin-slice noncontrast CT scans apparently enables us to predict whether a given patient will benefit from intravenous or intra-arterial recanalization therapy (see Chapter 6). The use of thin-slice reconstructions from noncontrast cranial CT lets us accurately determine the length of the occlusion of the middle cerebral artery or internal carotid artery, provided the slice thickness of the individual scans does not exceed 2.5 mm. This technique makes it possible to determine the individual thrombus burden, which in turn correlates with the success rate of recanalization by systemic thrombolysis. Studies show that intravenous thrombolysis is extremely unlikely to dissolve thrombi more than 6 mm long, and presumably these patients would benefit more from an intra-arterial recanalization procedure (e.g., thrombectomy). CTP, on the other hand, makes it possible to estimate the volume of potentially salvageable tissue (penumbra) as a basis for selecting patients who will benefit from active recanalization therapy.

The situation is somewhat different for ischemic strokes in the posterior circulation. These tend to be smaller infarctions that, while detectable by CTP, are missed more frequently than in the anterior circulation. CTA can detect thrombus and occlusion in the basilar artery, but noncontrast CT usually cannot determine whether the brainstem has already sustained damage, due to the difficulty of appreciating early ischemic changes in that region. MRI is much more sensitive for this application and is better for deciding whether or not recanalization is still appropriate for a particular patient. Thus, there are cases in which MRI with diffusion-weighted imaging should be used as an adjunct to emergent CT or even as an initial study if it is expected to have therapeutic implications. In cases where vertebrobasilar thrombosis is detected or strongly suspected, there should be little hesitation in proceeding with catheter angiography, which can provide a fast and confident diagnosis in this type of stroke. Overall, vertebrobasilar thrombosis is the most severe type of stroke with the highest mortality risk, and this often justifies an aggressive diagnostic approach. As a rule, however, vertebrobasilar thrombosis can be diagnosed by sectional imaging studies, and diagnostic catheter angiography is used in cases where it will be followed by interventional recanalization therapy.

In summary, the diagnostic workup of acute ischemic stroke should proceed swiftly but, for optimum treatment selection, should continue until it has answered pivotal questions relating to acute cerebral ischemia:

1. Has the patient suffered an ischemic stroke?
2. Is the vessel still occluded?
3. Where is the occlusion located and how long is the thrombus?
4. How large is the infarcted core?
5. Is there is significant volume of tissue at risk?

These questions should be addressed quickly and specifically in all severe strokes using available imaging modalities, most notably CT. The addition of MRI may be advisable in the posterior circulation.

The diagnostic workup of patients with vessel wall dissections is usually done in the subacute phase, when the positive detection of a mural hematoma has a greater impact on long-term management (anticoagulant medication?) than treatment during the acute phase. While dissections in the anterior extracranial vessels can be diagnosed with reasonable accuracy in the subacute phase (i.e., after 2–3 days) by active detection of the mural hematoma, it is occasionally difficult to detect dissections in the posterior circulation, especially at the level where the vertebral artery pierces the dura. The initial imaging study of choice in both the anterior and posterior circulations is MRI with MRA. Careful scrutiny with thin-slice imaging is necessary to detect or exclude a mural hematoma in a vertebral artery dissection. In equivocal cases, it is occasionally necessary to repeat the examination later in the methemoglobin stage when the mural hematoma will be easier to detect. If vertebral artery status is unclear, it may be appropriate to proceed with catheter angiography to establish a definitive diagnosis.

CVST is also frequently diagnosed in the subacute phase of the disease, and repeated examinations are occasionally necessary to establish the diagnosis. While dural sinus occlusions can generally be diagnosed by applying the proper technique (see Chapter 5), the main diagnostic challenge is to detect or exclude the thrombosis of small vessels, i.e., the cortical veins or basal sinuses (e.g., cavernous sinus). As in the diagnosis of dissections, a meticulous technique and possible repeat examinations may be needed to establish the presence or absence of small-vessel thrombosis. The diagnostic repertoire has been particularly enriched by the use of new and expanded MRI techniques (with susceptibility weighting, DWI, or T2*w). Contrast-enhanced TOF angiography with data acquisition during the contrast bolus phase has also raised the diagnostic level, and it should always be possible to detect even small venous thromboses when a targeted search is made. The key factor in diagnosing these thromboses is to consider them in the differential diagnosis in the first place, and then tailor the diagnostic strategy accordingly. It is clear that noncontrast CT is no longer suitable for detecting or excluding CVST. The ability to generate very thin-slice CT angiograms using multislice scanners and an optimized venous bolus phase has significantly increased the diagnostic value of this modality.

Treatment of Acute Ischemic Stroke

6 Thrombolysis

Intravenous Thrombolysis

G. F. Hamann

Introduction

Most strokes occur when a clot occludes an artery that supplies the brain. This underlies the rationale of administering a clot-dissolving (thrombolytic) agent that can reduce the damage from ischemic infarction by restoring blood flow. This is most likely to be successful when blood flow is re-established shortly after the occlusion. The danger of this therapy is that it may lead to hemorrhage in brain areas that have been softened due to ischemia. As of 1992, ~700 patients had been treated by intravenous thrombolysis in six randomized studies. A Cochrane Review published in 2003 covered 5727 patients treated with thrombolytic agents (Wardlaw et al. 2003), and the most recent Cochrane Review (Wardlaw et al. 2009) covered 7152 patients. Most patients had been treated within 6 h from the onset of their stroke. The most widely used agent, approved for use in the United States, Canada, and most European countries, was rtPA (alteplase).

Basic Principles of Coagulation Physiology

Coagulation

The thrombotic occlusion of a cerebral artery may be embolic or may result from local thrombosis due to endothelial damage, platelet activation and aggregation, and thrombin formation. The complex coagulation system has four main components:
- Endothelium
- Soluble and cellular components of the coagulation and fibrinolytic system
- Cellular blood constituents, especially platelets
- Blood flow

These four components interact in an tight-knit fashion to regulate coagulation (Preissner 2004). The role of the endothelium is to shield potentially thrombogenic vascular contents from the environment, so its basic function is to prevent coagulation and maintain unrestricted flow. Activated platelets can bind only to endothelium that is not fully intact. **Figure 6.1** shows the processes that are associated with intact and damaged endothelium. Important properties of the endothelium that can initiate and reinforce clotting are the formation and secretion of

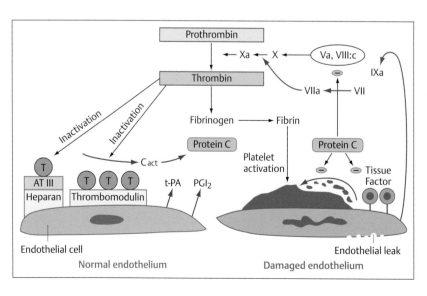

Fig. 6.1 Graphic representation of coagulation cascades in the case of intact endothelium (*left*) and damaged endothelium (*right*; after Hamann).
AT III, antithrombin III; C_{act}, protein C activator; T, thrombin; tPA, tissue-type plasminogen activator; PGL_2, prostacyclin; Va, VII, VIIa, VIII:c, IXa, X, Xa, and protein C, coagulation factors.

plasminogen activator inhibitor-1 (PAI-1), initiation of the endothelial factor VII–tissue factor complex, the formation of von Willebrand factor, and platelet adhesion. Conversely, endothelium in an intact state has considerably more *antithrombotic* properties such as thrombomodulin formation, protein C activation, antithrombin binding, and the formation and secretion of prostacyclin, which inhibits platelet aggregation.

The factors of the coagulation and fibrinolytic system may lead to plasmatic coagulation or clot dissolution. The end result of plasmatic coagulation is the platelet-induced transformation of soluble fibrinogen into fibrin and the formation of insoluble, stable fibrin polymers. The proteins involved in this process consist mainly of serine proteases (coagulation factors II, VII, IX, X, XI, XII, and protein C inhibitor). Serine proteases can exert their full effect at the site of an endothelial lesion only by forming a complex with cofactors, calcium, phospholipids, and their substrates. In understanding coagulation, it is helpful to distinguish between an exogenous system and an endogenous system

- *Exogenous system:* This is the system by which platelets aggregate at the site of an endothelial defect and form a thrombus (clot). Extravascular tissue factor from subendothelial cells forms a calcium-dependent complex with factor VII or VIIa, which activates factor VII as well as factors IX and X. The factors Xa and Va can form a calcium-dependent complex that activates factor II to IIa—that is, converts prothrombin to thrombin. This step is called initiation. The activation of factor IX by the tissue factor VIIa complex is an amplification mechanism that serves to increase thrombin formation (the "Josso loop"). The resulting thrombin can now activate factor XI to XIa, which creates another mechanism, called propagation, that can increase thrombin generation. Thrombin activates factors V, VIII, and XIII and is also a potent platelet activator. It converts fibrinogen to fibrin, splitting off the fibrin peptides A and B. Even small amounts of thrombin can convert very large amounts of fibrinogen to fibrin.
- *Endogenous system:* This is an in-vitro phenomenon. Nevertheless, it is useful to recognize the endogenous system because one of the most widely used clinical tests, the activated partial thromboplastin time (aPTT) test, covers this part of the coagulation system and exploits the fact that factor XII can be activated by contact with nonphysiologic foreign surfaces (Hamann 2010).

Fibrinolysis

Fibrin formation is accompanied by a simultaneous activation of the fibrinolytic cascade. The endothelial cells mainly secrete tissue-type plasminogen activator (tPA), which binds to fibrin and forms a fibrin–tPA–plasminogen complex. One result of this process is the formation of plasmin from plasminogen. Plasmin splits fibrin and dissolves temporary clots. The resulting cleavage products lead to an increased interaction between plasminogen and tPA, stimulating the formation of Lys-plasminogen, which is more fibrin-specific. Plasmin also initiates the formation of the activated two-chain form of tPA. Dissolution of the clot destroys the platelets contained in the clot, causing them to release PAI-1. Extracellular fibrinolysis stimulates neoangiogenesis and tissue remodeling (Hamann 2010).

Endogenous Plasminogen Activators

- *tPA:* tPA is a single-chain glycosylated serine protease with a molecular mass of 70 kDa. The molecule has four different domains: a finger (F) domain, an epidermal growth factor (E) domain, a two-kringle domain (K1 and K2), and the serine protease domain. The C-terminal serine protease domain has an active site where plasminogen cleavage can occur. The two-kringle domain of tPA resembles the plasminogen domain. The finger domain and K2 domain are responsible for binding to fibrin. Single-chain tPA can be converted by plasmin cleavage to a double-chain form, which is also active. The plasma half-life of the single- and double-chain forms of tPA is ~3–8 min, averaging 3.5 ± 1.4 min. tPA is naturally released by endothelial cells, neurons, astrocytes, and microglia. It is broken down in the liver. tPA is classified as a "fibrin-specific" thrombolytic because it activates plasminogen most effectively when it is bound to fibrin. Desmopressin can raise the blood levels of tPA, while heparin and heparan sulfate can increase its activity. Today a single-chain form of tPA is produced by recombinant technology and is marketed under the generic name alteplase.
- *Urokinase:* Urokinase is a plasminogen activator whose precursor prourokinase is formed in renal endothelial cells and by malignant cells. Single-chain prourokinase binds fibrin-selective plasminogen. Prourokinase can be produced by recombinant technology. The cleavage of prourokinase yields a heavy double-chain urokinase molecule with a molecular mass of 54 kDa, which is split further into a low-molecular-weight (31 kDa) urokinase activator. Both the high- and low-molecular forms are enzymatically active and convert plasminogen to plasmin. Their plasma half-life is ~9–12 min, similar to that of rtPA.

Exogenous Plasminogen Activators

These compounds are typically derived from nonhuman tissues or cells.

- *Streptokinase:* The best-known exogenous plasminogen activator, streptokinase is a single-chain polypeptide derived from β-hemolytic streptococci. It binds plasminogen and activates circulating plasminogen to plasmin. In the process, it is transformed into a streptokinase–plasmin complex. This complex can then be inactivated by α-2-antiplasmin. Previous streptococcal infections may have stimulated the formation of antibodies that can neutralize streptokinase and reduce its efficacy. Streptokinase has a plasma half-life of 4 min, and its complex has a second half-life of 30 min.

- *Anisoylated plasminogen–streptokinase activator complex (APSAC):* This agent consists of plasminogen non-covalently bound to streptokinase. APSAC has a half-life of 70 min, which is longer than that of tPA. It has been used in the treatment of myocardial infarction.
- *Desmoteplase:* This agent is a recombinant plasminogen activator produced from the saliva of the vampire bat (*Desmodus rotundus*). Its α form is even more fibrin-selective than tPA. It has a longer half-life and appears to be the most potent plasminogen activator now available.
- *Staphylokinase:* This enzyme is derived from *Staphylococcus aureus*. Its fibrin specificity is low.
- *Tenecteplase:* This is the primary thrombolytic agent now used in the treatment of myocardial infarction and pulmonary embolism. It is a mutant of tPA with a longer half-life of ~17 ± 7 min, higher fibrin specificity, higher resistance to PAI-1, and greater lytic activity on clots.

Direct Thrombolytic Agents

Microplasmin is a new thrombolytic agent that has a special role because it consists only of the active portion of the plasmin molecule. This enables it to dissolve blood clots directly rather than by plasminogen activation. Its efficacy therefore does not depend on the local abundance of plasminogen.

Experimental Studies of Thrombolysis in Acute Stroke

There are significant differences in the coagulation physiology of different animal species, and between animals and humans. As a result, we must be very careful when applying the results of animal studies to clinical medicine.

As early as 1963, Meyer et al. used cats and monkeys as experimental models for investigating the intravenous or intra-arterial administration of bovine or human plasmin in stroke (Meyer et al. 1963). These agents dissolved blood clots with a high rate of intracerebral hemorrhage. In 1985, Zivin et al. showed that tPA could improve neurologic outcomes following embolization with artificially produced clots (Zivin et al. 1985). In the following year, del Zoppo et al. found that 3 h after reversible balloon compression of the MCA in baboons, the intracarotid infusion of urokinase improved neurologic outcome and reduced infarct size without evidence of significant

intracerebral hemorrhage (del Zoppo et al. 1986). In 1987, Slivka and Pulsinelli observed that both tPA and streptokinase, when administered 24 h after experimentally induced stroke in rabbits, increased the rate of intracerebral hemorrhage (Slivka and Pulsinelli 1987). They also found that administering the agent early after the occlusion did not increase the risk of hemorrhage. On the other hand, a 1989 study by Lyden et al. showed that rtPA did not increase the incidence of cerebral hemorrhage in rabbits, regardless of when it was administered (10 min, 8 h, or 24 h after cerebral embolism; Lyden et al. 1989). Lyden et al. later compared different thrombolytic agents—tPA, streptokinase, and saline as a control—in the rabbit embolic model (Lyden et al. 1990). They found that streptokinase, but not rtPA, caused a significant increase in the rate and size of intracerebral hemorrhages. rtPA was administered at 90 min in three doses (3, 5, and 10 mg/kg body weight) whereas streptokinase was administered in a dose of 30 000 U/kg at 5, 90, and 300 min. No clear dose dependence was observed, but results varied with the agent used: streptokinase was significantly less effective than rtPA. Interestingly, these investigators already noted the fact that when tPA did dissolve the clot, it resulted in an incidence of cerebral hemorrhage twice high as the placebo. This finding led to the conclusion that reperfusion was responsible for the higher rate of hemorrhagic transformation. In 1991, Clark et al. showed that aspirin and tPA acted synergistically to cause intracerebral hemorrhage in a rabbit embolism model (Clark et al. 1991). It was later found that tPA in a rat model caused microvascular damage at high doses (comparable to human use) but caused significantly less damage at lower doses (Burggraf et al. 2003). Tenecteplase appears to be associated with higher hemorrhage rates in animal studies, whereas microplasmin appears to be better tolerated when used in neural tissue (Burggraf et al. 2010).

> **Note**
>
> In summary, experimental studies found that tPA had a better safety profile than other thrombolytic agents, especially streptokinase. It was safe when administered early after the occlusion. Cerebral hemorrhage was most strongly associated with recanalization and later administration.

Clinical Studies of Thrombolysis in Acute Stroke

First Efficacy Studies

The initial results of attempts to introduce thrombolysis as a treatment option for acute stroke were extremely discouraging. This applies particularly to studies that were done in the pre-CT era. Besides suffering from a lack of imaging options to exclude intracerebral hemorrhage, these studies also employed a significantly longer time window. In 1965, Meyer et al. conducted a study in 73 patients with acute progressive strokes (Meyer et al. 1965). The treatment group received streptokinase + heparin, whereas the control group received heparin only. There were significantly more deaths in the treatment group, and the control group had better outcomes. In 1976, Fletcher et al. studied 31 patients with acute stroke who received three different doses of intravenous urokinase or a placebo (Fletcher et al. 1976). The time window for these cases was 36 h. The study showed that urokinase could be administered without causing serious deficits. The number of patients was very small; the mortality rate was 16%.

In the wake of these two studies by Meyer et al. and Fletcher et al., thrombolysis was considered unsuitable for the treatment of strokes. Once the safety and efficacy of tPA had been documented in animal models, del Zoppo et al. conducted a study in 193 patients with acute ischemic stroke who received different doses of rtPA 8 h after the onset of stroke symptoms (del Zoppo et al. 1992). Angiography documented the occlusion of an extra- or intracranial cerebral artery in all patients. Exclusion criteria were a minor deficit, transient ischemic attacks, severe stroke with hemiplegia, decreased level of consciousness, gaze deviation, blood pressures higher than 200/120 mmHg, and CT evidence of hemorrhage or mass effect with a midline shift. Patients with early CT changes were not excluded from the study. The primary end point was the angiographic detection of recanalization and/or intracerebral hemorrhage with neurologic deterioration. This landmark study documented the clinical possibilities of thrombolysis. Approximately 40% of all patients achieved recanalization of the occluded artery. There was no relationship between dose and recanalization. Patients with smaller clots (i.e., distal vascular occlusions) showed the best recanalization rates. The incidence of all possible hemorrhagic changes was 30.8%. Symptomatic hemorrhages occurred in 9.6% of the patients, and the mortality rate was 12.5%. Hemorrhagic transformation did not increase at the dose that had been used for coronary thrombolysis. This led the authors to conclude that the dose of rtPA used for coronary thrombolysis was also the perfect dose for the treatment of acute stroke.

The first NINDS study was published in 1992 (Brott et al. 1992). In a dose-escalation study design, 74 patients with acute ischemic stroke were treated with incremental doses of rtPA (0.35–1.08 mg/kg body weight) within 90 min of symptom onset. Intracerebral hemorrhage did not occur in any of the 58 patients treated with ≤ 0.85 mg/kg rtPA. Intracranial hemorrhage occurred only at higher doses. Hemorrhage with neurologic deterioration (symptomatic hemorrhage) occurred only in patients treated with rtPA at doses ≥ 0.95 mg/kg. Significant neurologic improvement occurred in 30% of the patients at 2 h from the start of treatment and in 46% at 24 h. Clinical neurologic improvement was not found to be dose-dependent. The investigators concluded that the highest possible safe dose of rtPA was probably < 0.95 mg/kg. However, this conclusion was ultimately based on just three symptomatic hemorrhages that occurred in a total of 74 patients, so it was possible that a higher dose could be both safe and more effective.

In the same year, Haley et al. (1992) conducted another dose-escalation study in 20 patients with acute ischemic stroke who received rtPA between 91 and 180 min after symptom onset. The risk of symptomatic intracerebral hemorrhage was stated as 10% overall and 17% in the two higher-dose groups. Three different doses were used: 0.6, 0.85, and 0.95 mg/kg body weight. Three patients had improved by at least 4 points at 24 h.

That same year, Mori et al. (1992) did a study to determine whether rtPA was safe when administered intravenously at a dose of 6 or 12 million units within 6 h after symptom onset. Angiograms were obtained before and after thrombolytic therapy. These Japanese researchers confirmed that rtPA improved recanalization rates. The functional outcome (Barthel score) also showed significant improvement. This study, like the study by del Zoppo et al. (1992), confirmed the capability of rtPA to open occluded vessels.

The Bridging Trial was published in 1993. Haley et al. investigated 27 patients who had received 0.85 mg/kg intravenous rtPA or a placebo within 3 h after stroke onset (Haley et al. 1993). The study was a randomized, double-blind, placebo-controlled trial. Despite its small size, the study showed that patients treated within 90 min from symptom onset did show neurologic improvement at 24 h. Six of 10 patients treated with rtPA within 90 min improved by 4 or more points on the NIHSS at 24 h, compared with just one patient in the placebo group. In the groups that were treated at 91–180 min after onset, two patients in the rtPA group improved at 24 h, and two improved in the placebo group.

Large Randomized Multicenter Placebo-Controlled Studies

ECASS I Study

Published in 1995, the European Cooperative Acute Stroke Study (ECASS I) study included 620 patients treated with 1.1 mg/kg body weight of intravenous rtPA or placebo within 6 h from stroke onset (Hacke et al. 1995). This study found no significant efficacy of intravenous thrombolysis in an intention-to-treat analysis. The 109 patients with protocol violations (17.4% of all patients) were excluded, leaving a target population of 511 patients. The protocol violations consisted mainly of including patients with major strokes (> ⅓ hypodensity of MCA territory on CT) who were taking anticoagulants or hemodilutants, missed

Treatment of Acute Ischemic Stroke

II

hemorrhages on initial CT, uncontrolled hypertension, and lack of follow-up. The target population showed a significant point difference in the mRS scale between the two treatment groups, with no difference in rates of intracerebral hemorrhage but with a higher rate of large parenchymal hemorrhages in the rtPA-treated patients. More hemorrhagic infarcts were documented in the placebo group. The mortality rates at 30 days were the same. The ECASS study also showed a significant difference when the NINDS global end point was applied. This was a post-hoc analysis, however, and the overall results of the study do not support a recommendation for routine intravenous thrombolysis in acute ischemic stroke patients.

NINDS Study

Also published in 1995 (National Institute of Neurological Disorders and Stroke rtPA Stroke Study Group 1995), the NINDS study was the first randomized, placebo-controlled multicenter study that showed the efficacy of rtPA in the treatment of acute stroke when administered within 3 h of symptom onset. The NINDS study differed from the ECASS study in several respects: perhaps the major difference was that the rtPA dose in the NINDS study was only 0.9 mg/kg. Moreover, the NINDS study was strictly controlled for blood pressure, which had to be less than 185/95 mmHg. The NINDS study had two parts with an identical protocol but different end points. Part 1 tested whether rtPA had clinical activity as indicated by an improvement of 4 points on the NIHSS or a complete resolution of neurologic deficits by 24 h. Part 2 assessed clinical outcome at 3 months according to scores on the Barthel index, mRS, Glasgow outcome scale, and NIHSS. The numbers of patients enrolled were 291 in Part 1 (144 in the rtPA group, 147 in the placebo group) and 333 in Part 2 (168 in the tPA group and 165 in the placebo group). In Part 1, 67 patients (47%) improved in the tPA group and 57 patients (39%) improved in the placebo group. This difference was not statistically significant ($p < 0.21$). In Part 2 of the study, assessing clinical outcome, it was found that the number of patients with good outcomes was higher in the tPA group than in the placebo group. The probability of having little or no disability at 3 months was 30–50% higher in the rtPA group. Specifically, the percentage of patients with a mRS of 0 or 1 at 3 months was 39% in the rtPA group vs. only 26% in the placebo group. This was a statistically significant difference in favor of rtPA. Symptomatic hemorrhage occurred in 6.4% of the rtPA-treated patients compared with only 0.6% of the placebo-treated patients. The mortality rate at 3 months was essentially the same in both groups (17% in the rtPA group vs. 21% in the placebo group). This means that, despite an increased risk of hemorrhage, treatment with rtPA did not affect mortality. Treatment with rtPA resulted in a more favorable prognosis. Interestingly, this effect did not depend on the subtype of stroke and

applied equally to micro- and macroangiopathic strokes and cardioembolic strokes. Factors that were particularly associated with an increased risk of hemorrhage after rtPA treatment were a severe stroke, pronounced brain edema, or a midline shift. It was also found that patients treated with rtPA had at least a 30% greater likelihood of living independently at 1 year than patients treated with placebo. This improved outcome was not associated with increased disability or mortality. The rates of recurrent strokes at 1 year were the same in the tPA and placebo groups (Kwiatkowski et al. 1999).

> **Note**
>
> The NINDS study opened the window for the widespread use of rtPA in humans with acute ischemic stroke within 3 h after symptom onset.

ECASS II Study

The ECASS II study (Hacke et al. 1998), like ECASS I, was a multicenter, double-blind randomized trial. It investigated 800 patients with acute stroke treated with 0.9 mg/kg of rtPA or a placebo within 6 h of stroke onset. The exclusion criteria were similar to the NINDS criteria but also included early infarct signs on CT involving more than one-third of the MCA territory, decreased level of consciousness, or hemiplegia with fixed deviation of gaze (conjugate deviation). Patients who had received anticoagulants or antithrombotic therapy during the first 24 h were also excluded. There were no significant differences in the rate of patients who had a good prognosis (mRS = 0–1 on day 90): 40.3% in the rtPA group and 36.6% in the placebo group. The rate of intracerebral hemorrhage was significantly higher in the rtPA group (8.8%) than in the placebo group (3.4%).

Streptokinase Studies

Three studies investigated the use of streptokinase in acute stroke patients: the MAST-E, MAST-I, and ASK studies.

MAST-E (Multicenter Acute Stroke Trial—Europe Study Group 1996) was a double-blind, placebo-controlled randomized study. Patients were treated with 1.5 million units of intravenous streptokinase or placebo within 6 h. No difference was found in the primary outcome parameters (death or severe disability). More patients died in the streptokinase group, which also showed an increased incidence of symptomatic intracerebral hemorrhage. Approximately 60% of the streptokinase patients and 75% of the placebo patients also received heparin, and 20% in each group received aspirin. Assessment at 6 months showed a small, not statistically significant proportion of deaths in the streptokinase group plus a trend toward less disability in that group.

MAST-I (Multicentre Acute Stroke Trial—Italy (MAST-I) Group 1995) was a randomized controlled study with a four-arm design in which patients were treated with intravenous streptokinase, streptokinase plus aspirin, aspirin alone, or a placebo. No other anticoagulants were given. No benefits were found for any particular subgroups. A statistically significant increase in early mortality was documented in the aspirin group and the streptokinase group.

In the ASK study (Australian Streptokinase Study; Donnan et al. 1996), 340 patients randomized from various centers were treated with intravenous streptokinase or a placebo within 4h of stroke onset. The study was terminated early due to the poorer outcomes in the streptokinase-treated patients. Intracerebral hemorrhage occurred in 9.6% of the patients in the streptokinase group and none of the patients in the placebo group. The streptokinase patients had a higher incidence of hypotension and a significantly higher mortality rate.

> **Note**
>
> All three studies supported the conclusion that streptokinase is not indicated in the treatment of acute stroke.

ATLANTIS Study

The ATLANTIS study (Alteplase ThromboLysis for Acute Noninterventional Therapy in Ischemic Stroke; Clark et al. 1999) was a double-blind randomized study that tested the safety and efficacy of 0.9 mg/kg body weight intravenous rtPA in patients within 6 h of symptom onset. The time window was later shortened to 5 h. The study was terminated early when an interim analysis showed that it was unlikely that any benefit would be derived from rtPA. There was no difference in the primary end point. As expected, the rate of symptomatic intracerebral hemorrhages was higher in the rtPA-treated group. A post-analysis of patients treated with rtPA within 3 h of stroke onset showed that those patients were more likely to have a favorable outcome (60.9% in the rtPA group vs. 26.3% in the placebo group). This difference was statistically significant, but it was based on a post-hoc analysis. Symptomatic intracerebral hemorrhage occurred in 13% of the rtPA-treated patients and none of the placebo-treated patients.

ECASS III Study

The ECASS III study (Hacke et al. 2008b) tested the efficacy and safety of alteplase in the treatment of acute stroke within a 3- to 4.5-h time window after symptom onset. A total of 821 patients were enrolled in the double-blind study and were randomly assigned to receive intravenous alteplase (0.9 mg/kg body weight) or a placebo.

The primary end point of the study was a good treatment outcome defined as an mRS of 0 or 1, in contrast to a poor outcome (mRS = 2–6). The secondary end point was a global outcome analysis of four neurologic and disability scores. Safety end points included death and symptomatic intracerebral hemorrhage. Of the 821 stroke patients studied, 418 were assigned to the alteplase group and 403 to the placebo group. The median time to alteplase administration was 3 h 59 min. Approximately 10% of the patients were treated in the time window from ≥ 3 to ≤ 3.5h, 46% from > 3.5 to < 4h, and 40% from > 4 to ≤ 4.5h. Significantly more patients treated with alteplase had a good outcome at 90 days (mRS = 0 or 1; 54% vs. 45.2%; OR 1.34; 95% CI 1.02–1.76; $p = 0.04$). A global outcome analysis also showed a benefit of alteplase therapy (OR 1.28; 95% CI 1.00–1.65; $p < 0.05$). The incidence of any intracerebral hemorrhage and symptomatic intracerebral hemorrhage was significantly higher in the alteplase group (any intracerebral hemorrhage: 27.0% vs. 17.6%; $p = 0.001$; symptomatic intracerebral hemorrhage: 2.4% vs. 0.2%; $p = 0.008$). The mortality rates were the same in both groups (7.7% vs. 8.4%; $p = 0.68$).

The ECASS III study (Bluhmki et al. 2009) joins the NINDS study of 1995 as the second large, randomized multicenter study to document the efficacy of rtPA in the treatment of acute stroke. Nevertheless, it should be noted that the treatment benefit achieved in the 3- to 4.5-h time window is moderate. The likelihood of a good treatment outcome not requiring help with daily activities increases by 28%, and the number of treatments necessary to achieve an mRS of 0 or 1 is 14. The overall risk of symptomatic intracerebral hemorrhage, while low and within expected limits (2.4% vs. 0.2%), was still significantly increased. On the positive side, the ECASS III study was a "true" 3- to 4.5-h study: 87% of the patients were treated within a time window of 3.5–4.5 h. Thus, the crucial question of efficacy in the latter part of the 3- to 4.5-h time window—a question not answered in the SITS registry (Safe Implementation of Treatments in Stroke)—has now been positively confirmed. Analysis by subgroups (patients grouped by age, sex, stroke severity, time to treatment, diabetes, hypertension, atrial fibrillation, smoking, or use of platelet inhibitors) showed no benefit differences in any of the subgroups (Bluhmki et al. 2009). It remains unclear why the 45% rate of good outcomes in the placebo group in ECASS III was ~6% higher than in the old NINDS study of 1995. Is this a stroke-unit effect or just a coincidence?

> **Note**
>
> Even in an expanded time window of 3–4.5 h, thrombolysis has been shown to be safe and effective. This does not mean, however, that we can take our time in treating patients for stroke. The cardinal rule still applies: Time is brain!

Japanese Studies Using a Lower rtPA Dose

In an initial multicenter open-label single-arm study (Yamaguchi et al. 2006), 103 patients in Japan received intravenous rtPA at a dose of 0.6 mg/kg body weight; 38% of the patients had a very good outcome with mRS = 0 or 1, and 6 symptomatic intracerebral hemorrhages occurred. The authors theorized that the lower dose of rtPA may be just as safe and effective in Japanese patients as the approved dose of 0.9 mg/kg. The J-ACT II study (Mori et al. 2010) investigated the efficacy and safety of 0.6 mg/kg body weight of rtPA administered within 3 h after onset of ischemic stroke symptoms in patients with an MCA occlusion confirmed by MRA. In the 58 patients studied, a recanalization rate of 52% was achieved by 6 h and 69% by 24 h. In all, 46.6% of the patients had a good clinical outcome (mRS = 0 or 1) after thrombolytic therapy, and no hemorrhages occurred. Recanalization at 6 h was an independent predictor of favorable outcome. No difference was found relative to treatment with 0.9 mg/kg of rtPA. No information is currently available on the follow-up of low-dose intravenous thrombolysis, and corresponding action recommendations cannot be made.

Microplasmin Study

Thijs et al. (2009) published the results of an intravenous microplasmin phase II study that had a double-blind, randomized, placebo-controlled design. The 40 patients in the study had been admitted between 3 and 12 h after an ischemic stroke: 10 of them received a placebo, 6 received microplasmin at a dose of 2 mg/kg body weight, 12 received 3 mg/kg, and 12 received 4 mg/kg. The therapy was well tolerated; only one fatal hemorrhage occurred. Microplasmin leads to the neutralization of α-2-antiplasmin in the serum. Clinical parameters were not significantly altered given the small case numbers, and currently there are no plans to conduct larger randomized efficacy studies with this agent.

Desmoteplase Studies

A desire for higher recanalization rates and lower rates of symptomatic intracerebral hemorrhage in an expanded time window beyond 3 h has prompted efforts to develop new thrombolytic agents. Desmoteplase is a fibrin-specific plasmin activator found to have an acceptable safety profile in earlier phase II studies—DIAS (Hacke et al. 2005 and DEDAS (Furlan et al. 2006)—also showing a trend toward higher reperfusion rates relative to placebo and greater clinical efficacy in a time window of 3–9 h.

The DIAS II study (Hacke et al. 2009) was a phase III study aimed at confirming the results of DIAS and DEDAS, documenting safety and efficacy in patients with acute stroke, and detecting the presence of tissue at risk by diffusion- and perfusion-weighted MRI and CT perfusion (CTP). In a randomized, placebo-controlled, double-blind double-dose study, patients were randomly assigned to a group treated with 90 or 125 μg/kg of desmoteplase or placebo. One inclusion criterion was the presence of a 20% mismatch, i.e., visual estimation of a perfusion abnormality (penumbra) 20% larger than the diffusion abnormality.

The primary end point was clinical improvement of ≥ 8 points on the NIHSS score or an NIHSS score of ≤ 1 point at 90 days, an mRS of 0–2 points, and a Barthel index of 75–100 points. Secondary end points were change in lesion volume between baseline and day 30, rate of symptomatic intracerebral hemorrhage, and mortality rate. In this study 193 patients were randomized, and 186 were treated: 57 received 90 μg/kg desmoteplase, 66 received 125 μg/kg, and 63 received placebo. The median baseline NIHSS score was 9 points, and 30% (53 of 179) of the patients had a vascular occlusion detectable by MRA. The core lesion and mismatch volumes were small (median initial infarct volume was 10 cm^3, mismatch volume was 52 cm^3). The clinical response rates did not differ significantly among the different groups. The changes in lesion volume over time were also similar. The rates of symptomatic intracerebral hemorrhage were higher in the treatment groups (3.5% and 4.5% vs. 0% for placebo). The mortality rate in the 125-μg group, at 21%, was markedly higher than in the low-dose and placebo groups. One-third of the patients were treated in the 3- to 6-h time window and two-thirds in the 6- to 9-h time window.

The results of the DIAS II study are disappointing. It is interesting to analyze the study, however, because it suggests which patients may benefit from thrombolysis over an expanded time window of up to 9 h based on MRI or CT findings:

- Patients with a large mismatch volume, i.e., a small diffusion abnormality and a large perfusion abnormality
- Patients with a proximal vascular occlusion (M1 or M2 segment)
- Patients who have had a mild stroke (NIHSS ≥ 14 with a proximal vascular occlusion)
- Patients who recanalize

These patients were in the minority in the DIAS II study. Only 30% of the patients had a vascular occlusion that was detectable by MR angiography (MRA) or CT angiography (CTA). The mismatch volume was ~80 cm^3, meaning that only a small tissue volume was salvageable by recanalization. Another reason for the disappointing result was the MR and CT criteria. A mismatch volume of 20% of the tissue area with abnormal perfusion is too small and mainly encompasses oligemic tissue. Given this baseline condition, there was no reason to expect a significant benefit from reperfusion therapy. Criteria for effective thrombolysis in the expanded time window are a high recanalization rate and low rate of intracerebral hemorrhage. Desmoteplase was unable to meet these criteria in the DIAS II study.

Tenecteplase Study

A clinical phase IIb study with tenecteplase was designed to define the optimum dose while demonstrating safety and efficacy in comparison with rtPA. The study in question was a multicenter, double-blind, randomized trial using tenecteplase doses of 0.1, 0.25, and 0.4 mg/kg body weight, which were compared with 0.9 mg/kg of rtPA. After the best dose was found, it was supposed to be used in treating 100 pairs of patients with tenecteplase and rtPA. The study was terminated due to slow recruitment and could not establish the effective dose (Haley et al. 2010). The high tenecteplase dose was associated with the highest bleeding rate, which was not unexpected on the basis of experimental data (Burggraf et al. 2010). It remains to be seen whether further studies on the agent will be forthcoming.

MRI-Based Thrombolysis

"Mismatch" is the difference between the size and extent of the DWI lesion (diffusion abnormality) relative to the larger PWI lesion (perfusion abnormality). The DWI/PWI mismatch is useful for defining tissue at risk, i.e., tissue that is at risk for infarction but is still potentially salvageable by treatment. In a German multicenter study of 174 MRI-selected patients (Thomalla et al. 2006), 62% of the patients were treated with tPA within 3 h and 38% within 3–6 h on the basis of MRI mismatch findings. The outcome data were compared with pooled data from the ATLANTIS, ECASS, and NINDS trials. A good outcome was achieved in 48% of the MRI-selected tPA patients compared with 33% of pooled placebo patients and 40% of pooled tPA-treated patients. This indicates a slight superiority of MRI-based therapy. Safety was dramatically improved, however. The rate of symptomatic intracerebral hemorrhage was only 3% in the MRI-selected patients, compared with 8% in the pooled tPA group and 2% in the pooled placebo group.

The Australian EPITHET study (De Silva et al. 2010) is an important study that investigated the efficacy of intravenous thrombolysis in stroke administered within a 3- to 6-h time window after symptom onset. Besides delayed thrombolysis, this study indirectly investigated the mismatch concept. While this concept seems logical and sound from a pathophysiologic standpoint, it has not been prospectively evaluated in selecting patients for thrombolytic therapy. In the EPITHET study, patients were selected by cranial CT. Afterward they were randomly assigned to rtPA or placebo groups, and then diffusion-weighted MRI was performed. Lesion size on baseline MRI was later compared with T2w MRI performed at 90 days. The primary end point was increase in lesion size between the two MRIs. Unfortunately, the primary end point was not significantly different between the two examinations, resulting in a negative study. While all the results tended to support the efficacy of thrombolysis, the benefit was not statistically significant. It is noteworthy that only a slight improvement was achieved in tPA patients with good outcomes (mRS = 0–3) (22% vs. 20% for all patients; 19% vs. 17% for mismatch patients). On the other hand, thrombolysis was associated with a nonsignificant but notable increase in the incidence of death or severe disability (18% vs. 9% for all patients; 15% vs. 8% for mismatch patients). A meta-analysis of MRI-based intravenous thrombolysis (Mishra et al. 2010) calls for more rigorous evaluation of the mismatch concept and a large, randomized confirmation study.

> **Note**
>
> Patient selection based on DWI/PWI mismatch by MRI allows for successful thrombolysis at 4.5 h, but further prospective studies are needed to investigate and confirm this concept.

Meta-analysis

A meta-analysis (Lees et al. 2010) analyzed the individual data for rtPA-treated patients and placebo patients from clinical studies to determine the efficacy of this agent over time. This meta-analysis added the 821 ECASS III patients and the 100 EPITHET patients to the 2775 patients that had previously been pooled in the meta-analysis. The analysis included patients treated up to 6 h after stroke onset, yielding a total of 1850 rtPA-treated patients and 1820 placebo-treated patients. The earlier the patients were treated, the higher the percentage of patients with an mRS of 0 or 1 at 3 months. A benefit of intravenous thrombolysis was no longer seen by 270 min (4.5 h) after stroke onset (**Fig. 6.2**). Patients treated at 0–90 min had an OR of 2.55 (95% CI 1.44–4.52) for a favorable outcome at 3 months. Patients treated at 91–180 min had an OR of 1.64 (95% CI 1.12–2.40), and patients treated

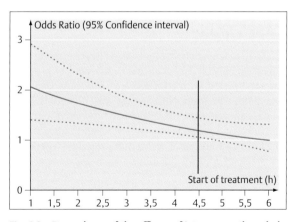

Fig. 6.2 Dependence of the efficacy of intravenous thrombolysis on time to treatment. Thrombolysis is effective when started up to 4.5 hours after symptom onset (*black bar*). Odds ratio refers to the group with an mRS of 0—1 (after Lees et al. 2010).

at 181–270 min had an OR of 1.34 (95% CI 1.06–1.68). These differences were significant. The OR at 270 min was 1.22 (95% CI 0.92–1.61), which was not statistically significant. Large symptomatic hemorrhages occurred in 96 of the alteplase-treated patients and 18 of the placebo patients. Mortality rates increased significantly with time from stroke onset to start of treatment (mean 95% CI 0.78 [0.41–1.48] for 0–90 min; mean 95% CI 1.13 [0.70–1.82] for 90–180 min; mean 95% CI 1.22 [0.87–1.71] for 180–270 min; mean 95% CI 1.49 [1.00–2.21] for 271–360 min). The authors concluded that the meta-analysis supported the efficacy of intravenous thrombolysis within a time window of 4.5 h, but that every effort should be made to shorten the delay in initiating treatment.

> **Note**
>
> Intravenous thrombolysis is effective when started up to 4.5 h from the onset of acute stroke. Individual patients should be treated as soon as possible.

Everyday Practice of Intravenous Thrombolysis in Acute Stroke

In June 1996, the U.S. Food and Drug Administration (FDA) approved the use of intravenous rtPA at a dose of 0.9 mg/kg body weight when administered within 3 h after onset of an acute stroke. This regimen was approved in Europe in April 2002. Since then, there have been numerous observational studies documenting the use of thrombolysis in routine treatment settings. There is no need to review all of this research, but here we take a closer look at two of the larger studies: CASES and SITS-MOST.

CASES Study

CASES (Canadian Activase for Stroke Effectiveness Study), published in 2005 (Hill et al. 2005), analyzed 1135 stroke patients treated with rtPA between February 1999 and June 2001. The mean NIHSS score was 15. Follow-up at 90 days showed that 30% of the patients had minimal or no neurologic sequelae and that 46% were independent. The rate of intracerebral hemorrhage was 4.6%. There was a 15% rate of protocol violations.

SITS-MOST Study

The SITS-MOST registry (Safe Implementation of Thrombolysis in Stroke—Monitoring Study) compiled data from over 11 000 stroke patients treated by thrombolysis at

more than 700 stroke units in 35 countries (Wahlgren et al. 2007). The registry, mandated by the European Medicines Evaluation Agency (EMEA) to provide more data on the safety and efficacy of thrombolysis within the 3-h time window, has become an important database for the everyday practice of thrombolysis. The SITS registry has not only confirmed the efficacy of thrombolysis but has shown a lower rate of intracerebral hemorrhages outside of study conditions (1.7% vs. 5.1%).

Another important aspect revealed by the comparison of participating centers is the enormous gap between door-to-imaging times and door-to-needle times. Door-to-imaging times ranged from 9 to 90 min (averaging 28 min for all centers), while the door-to-needle times ranged from 20 to 139 min (average of 73 min). Short door-to-needle times are an important quality indicator, and ~30 min is a reasonable time goal with proper organization.

One study used the SITS registry to assess the efficacy and safety of thrombolysis within the expanded time window of 3–4.5 h (Wahlgren et al. 2008). A total of 664 ischemic stroke patients that received thrombolysis from 3 to 4.5 h after stroke onset (average 195 min) were compared with 11 865 patients treated within 3 h (average 140 min). Study end points were the occurrence of symptomatic intracerebral hemorrhage detected by cranial CT, clinical deterioration by NIHSS $\geq$ 4 within 24 h, mortality at 3 months, and favorable outcome at 3 months defined as a score of 0–2 on the mRS.

The 3- to 4.5-h group was 3 years younger on average, had less severe strokes (NIHSS = 11 vs. 12), and had lower rates of hypertension and hyperlipidemia. The mean treatment times differed by 55 min between the two groups (140 vs. 195 min), and 50% of the 3- to 4.5-h group were treated within 15 min past the 3-h time window. None of the end points differed significantly between the two treatment groups: the rate of symptomatic intracerebral hemorrhage was 2.2% vs. 1.6%, mortality rate was 12.7% vs. 12.2%, and favorable treatment outcome was 58% vs. 56.3%.

It is beyond the scope of this chapter to review the ~50 publications dealing with single-center or pooled experience on the routine use of rtPA.

> **Note**
>
> Intravenous rtPA can be used in everyday practice with the same safety and efficacy as in large studies. It is reasonable to conclude that intravenous thrombolysis with rtPA in the 3-h and even 4.5-h time window can reduce deaths and severe disability by ~30%.

Guidelines

Different guidelines offer different recommendations on intravenous thrombolysis. The guidelines stated below are the ones that are currently followed by the

American Heart Association (Adams et al. 2007; del Zoppo et al. 2009):

- The intravenous administration of rtPA is recommended within a 4.5-h time window for the treatment of ischemic stroke at centers experienced with this therapy (0.9 mg/kg body weight, maximum dose 90 mg, 10% of total dose given as initial bolus, the remaining 90% by infusion over 60 min).
- Blood pressure should be less than 185/110 mmHg before and during thrombolytic therapy.

Thrombolysis is generally contraindicated in patients with major strokes (NIHSS > 25) and extensive early ischemic changes, due to the risk of secondary cerebral hemorrhage. Thrombolysis cannot be recommended in patients with uncontrolled hypertension (blood pressure > 185/110 mmHg despite multiple treatment attempts).

Guidelines in the United States (Adams et al. 2007) recommend intravenous thrombolysis with rtPA administered at 0.9 mg/kg body weight (maximum of 90 mg) over a 60-min period, with the initial 10% given by bolus injection within 3 h after symptom onset. Besides intracerebral hemorrhage, the risk of airway swelling and obstruction is noted as a potential serious side effect (Adams et al. 2007). Patients with epileptic seizures may receive thrombolysis if the treating physician believes that the residual symptoms are due to ischemia rather than Todd's (postictal) paralysis.

According to German approval criteria, the treatment may be administered only by a physician trained and experienced in critical care neurology. Other approval restrictions in Germany pertain to patients with a history of stroke and coexisting diabetes and a blood glucose level < 50 mg/dL or > 400 mg/dL. These restrictions are not adequately supported by study data, however. Labeling also cautions against treating patients > 80 years of age with intravenous rtPA, although several observational studies have shown that intravenous thrombolysis is also safe and effective in older patients.

Practical Recommendations

According to the Ad Hoc Committee representing the National Stroke Foundation and Stroke Society of Australasia (2009) and the American Heart Association (AHA) Statement on expanding the time window (del Zoppo et al. 2009), the following criteria should be applied in selecting patients for intravenous thrombolysis:

- Treatment is initiated within 4.5 h from the onset of clinical symptoms.
- A measurable, clinically significant neurologic deficit is present (NIHSS > 0).
- Cranial CT shows no hemorrhage or other cause for the clinical symptoms.
- The patient is over 18 years of age.

Absolute contraindications to thrombolysis are as follows:
- Unknown time of onset
- Coma
- Complete hemiplegia with fixed deviation of gaze
- Rapid resolution of symptoms
- Seizure at symptom onset
- Blood pressure > 185 mmHg systolic and/or > 110 mmHg diastolic in repeated measurements despite therapy
- Clinical suspicion of subarachnoid hemorrhage, even with negative cranial CT
- Presumed septic embolism
- Known bleeding diathesis, heparin administration in prior 48 h with increased partial thromboplastin time
- Prothrombin time > 1.7
- Platelets < 100 000/μL
- Blood glucose < 50 or > 400 mg/dL

The following are relative contraindications that still allow for thrombolysis but only after detailed consideration and informed consent:
- NIHSS > 22
- Age > 80 years
- Hypodensities in cranial CT > ⅓ of MCA territory
- Stroke or head trauma in prior 3 months
- Major surgical procedure in prior 2 weeks
- Earlier subarachnoid hemorrhage, intracerebral hemorrhage due to angioma or other bleeding source
- Myocardial infarction in prior 30 days
- Needle biopsy of hollow viscus during prior 30 days with risk of uncontrolled bleeding
- Trauma with internal injuries in prior 30 days
- Gastrointestinal or other bleeding in prior 30 days
- Arterial puncture in prior 7 days
- Severe, untreatable comorbid condition that may jeopardize the success of thrombolysis (e.g., terminal cancer)

The following factors predict a favorable outcome of intravenous thrombolysis, listed in order of descending importance (Demchuk et al. 2001):
- Mild clinical severity
- Absence of diabetes mellitus
- Normal cranial CT
- Normal blood pressure before treatment

> **Note**
>
> Always look for reasons to proceed with thrombolysis in stroke patients, not for reasons to withhold it.

II

Special Cases

Systemic Thrombolysis in Basilar Artery Thrombosis

The treatment of the most severe form of stroke, basilar artery thrombosis, continues to be based on personal experience, case series, and nonrandomized studies (see the section on Basilar Artery Thrombosis, p. 116). The main reason for this is the fortunately low incidence of basilar artery thrombosis. At most centers with facilities for interventional neuroradiologic treatment, patients with basilar artery stroke are managed by intra-arterial thrombolysis, which may be combined in varying degrees with mechanical recanalization techniques.

The registry data of the Basilar Artery International Cooperation Study (BASICS; Schonewille et al. 2009) attempt to expand the evidence base for basilar artery thrombosis. A total of 619 patients were entered in the registry from 2002 to 2007, but 27 patients were excluded from analysis because their outcomes could not be determined due to lack of follow-up data. Of the remaining 592 patients, 183 were treated with antithrombotic therapy only (generally intravenous heparin) and 121 received intravenous thrombolysis analogous to the NINDS study. The largest group of patients ($n = 288$) were treated by intra-arterial thrombolysis. No significant differences were found among the different treatment modalities. Patients with moderately severe clinical deficits after basilar artery thrombosis could not benefit from more aggressive therapy such as intra-arterial thrombolysis. Patients with severe symptoms were more likely to be harmed by antithrombotic therapy alone, but no differences were found between intra-arterial and intravenous thrombolysis. It is very clear that registry data are of limited analytical value, but it is equally clear that these data show no evidence that patients with basilar artery thrombosis benefit more from intra-arterial thrombolysis than from intravenous thrombolysis.

> **Note**
>
> Following diagnosis, intravenous thrombolysis should be initiated according to the NINDS protocol. The patient should then be transferred to a center with facilities for interventional neuroradiologic treatment. Based on current information, facilities should definitely be available for mechanical recanalization.

Sonothrombolysis

Indirect mechanical clot dissolution with transcranial ultrasound is an interesting approach to augmenting thrombolytic therapy. This is desirable because the recanalization rates after systemic thrombolysis range only from 30 to 50% in different studies. The concept of sonothrombolysis has been pursued for several years.

Smaller studies using ultrasound energies higher than the standard 2 MHz showed that transcranial ultrasonography may lead to increased rates of symptomatic intracerebral hemorrhage and were discontinued for that reason (Daffertshofer et al. 2005). In the CLOTBUST trial, the recanalization rate in the ultrasound group was increased from 30 to 49% with no associated increase in the rate of symptomatic intracerebral hemorrhage (Alexandrov et al. 2004). On the other hand, the study, which was not designed to prove clinical efficacy, did not show any significant clinical improvement. A calculation on a efficacy study revealed ~600 patients per treatment arm.

The effect of sonothrombolysis can be increased by using an ultrasound contrast agent consisting of gas-filled microspheres. The microspheres absorb ultrasound energy and begin to oscillate, transferring mechanical energy to the environment. This creates small defects in the thrombus, forming sites that are more receptive to attack by rtPA. The new ultrasound contrast agent with C3F8-μS (perflutren C3F8 liquid microspheres) has better stability than older agents, and this should result in greater efficacy. Molina et al. (2009) applied this principle in a prospective randomized clinical study. They investigated safety aspects and recanalization rates with a combined regimen consisting of rtPA, transcranial ultrasound (2 MHz), and C3F8-μS. The study included acute stroke patients who were treated within the 3-h time window and had an abnormal MCA waveform on transcranial ultrasound (12 patients in the tPA + ultrasound + C3F8-μS treatment arm, and 3 patients in the tPA + ultrasound control arm). None of the patients developed a symptomatic intracerebral hemorrhage (primary end point of this safety study); however, four patients did have an asymptomatic intracerebral hemorrhage (three in the group with ultrasound + C3F8-μS and one in the control group). In 75% of the treated patients, C3F8-μS could be detected past the site of the MCA occlusion, with transcranial Doppler showing an improved MCA flow rate in 83% of cases. Comparison of the tPA + ultrasound + C3F8-μS treatment arm with the control arm in the multicenter CLOTBUST trial (tPA only; $n = 63$) with identical inclusion criteria showed significantly higher complete and partial recanalization rates at 2 h with a nonsignificant improvement in neurologic outcomes (NIHSS). The authors conclude that combination therapy consisting of tPA, ultrasound, and C3F8-μS is safe and leads to improved flow rates in the MCA after vascular occlusion.

> **Note**
>
> Sonothrombolysis appears to be effective, and it is time for a randomized controlled study with sufficiently large case numbers to evaluate efficacy and rate of symptomatic intracerebral hemorrhages (Tsivgoulis et al. 2010).

Thrombolysis in Pregnancy and the Puerperium

The treatment of acute stroke in pregnant women poses a special problem. Pregnancy and the puerperium were recognized as exclusion criteria in large studies on thrombolysis, and this caveat is noted in technical information and labeling. Besides the risk of teratogenesis, there is the serious danger of excessive bleeding, especially in the puerperium. Cronin et al. (2008) recently reviewed several case series relating to this problem. In 172 pregnant patients who received thrombolysis, 8% experienced severe bleeding complications. Ultimately, the use of thrombolysis in pregnant women with acute stroke must be decided on a case-by-case basis. It is possible, but requires very careful consideration and disclosure (Cronin et al. 2008).

Thrombolysis in Stroke Due to Arterial Dissection

Many neurologists feel that it is dangerous to use thrombolysis in patients with an arterial dissection (see the section on Cervical Artery Dissections, p.124). Intracranial dissections in particular are believed to have a high association with an increased hemorrhage risk. A Swiss group (Engelter et al. 2009) has shown, however, that thrombolysis can be used in patients with cervical dissections and is reasonably safe. In the Swiss database on thrombolysis, 55 of 1061 patients (5.2%) had a dissection of the cervical vessels. Thrombolysis in this group was not as successful as in the non-dissection group (36% vs. 44% of patients with good clinical status at 3 months). The rates of cerebral hemorrhage and death were the same in both groups, however. Consequently there is no reason to exclude these patients from thrombolytic therapy.

Thrombolysis in Patients with Microangiopathy

The severity of cerebral microangiopathy is considered a risk factor for cerebral hemorrhage in response to thrombolysis. Ariës et al. (2010) found that patients with leukoaraiosis were at greater risk for cerebral hemorrhage than control patients and had a poorer prognosis than controls. Another study showed, however, that patients with small artery occlusions had an even better functional outcome after thrombolysis than other patients. They had a lower incidence of intracerebral hemorrhage and disability (Fluri et al. 2010). An analysis of the NINDS data (Demchuk et al. 2008) showed that microangiopathy detectable by cranial CT did not adversely affect the outcome of thrombolysis. Similar results were reported by the Canadian thrombolysis group and the CASES registry (Palumbo et al. 2007).

> **Practical Tip**
>
> At present, there is no reason to withhold intravenous thrombolysis from patients with microangiopathy.

Age, Sex, and Thrombolysis

Effect of Patient Age

Regulatory approval in some countries stipulates an upper age limit of 80 years for intravenous thrombolysis, but there is little scientific evidence to support this restriction. Numerous studies have shown that even older patients can be treated with similar efficacy and safety. Toni et al. (2008) compared 41 patients over 80 years old with 207 patients < 80 years treated by intravenous thrombolysis and found that the rates of intracerebral hemorrhage were similar in both groups. The older patients had a significantly higher mortality rate (34%) than the younger group (10.6%). The rates of favorable clinical outcomes were 44% and 58.5%, respectively. Berrouschot et al. (2005) reported similar results based on an analysis of German data: 38 of 228 patients in this series were > 80 years old. A good clinical outcome was achieved in 26.3% of the > 80-year-olds and in 46.8% of the younger patients. The rates of intracerebral hemorrhage were the same. Both groups of authors conclude that intravenous thrombolysis can be performed in elderly patients with increased mortality. A Finnish group (Meretoja et al. 2010) studied 159 patients over 80 years old in a total population of almost 1000 patients. Age predicted a poor prognosis with an OR of 2.18 (95% CI 1.27–3.73).

> **Caution**
>
> Age alone is not an absolute contraindication, but intravenous thrombolysis in patients > 80 years old is associated with higher mortality and a poorer prognosis.

Younger patients have a good prognosis after thrombolysis. Putaala et al. (2009) found a significantly better prognosis in 48 patients 16–49 years of age than in older patients: 27% of the younger patients had a complete recovery, vs. only 10% of older patients. Canadian authors report similar results: in 99 of 1120 patients, thrombolysis was performed at < 50 years of age. Mortality was significantly lower in these younger thrombolysis patients than in the older group, but both groups had a similar prognosis (Poppe et al. 2009a).

> **Note**
>
> Patients < 50 years of age with acute stroke appear to have a better prognosis with intravenous thrombolysis than older patients.

Influence of Patient Sex

Sex differences in the results of thrombolysis are not significant, as a French study has shown (Meseguer et al. 2009). On the other hand, it appears that women are less likely to receive thrombolysis than men under otherwise equal conditions (Reeves et al. 2009).

> **Note**
>
> There are no differences between men and women in the efficacy of intravenous thrombolysis.

Off-Label Thrombolysis

Treatment outside of approved restrictions is a major practical problem. Meretoja et al. (2010) found that, based on the experience of the Finnish group, the treatment of 51% of patients had violated one or more eligibility conditions for intravenous thrombolysis. Some patients were too old, the NIHSS was < 5, intravenous antihypertensives had been used, symptom-to-needle time was > 3 h, blood pressure at thrombolysis was > 185/110 mmHg, or patients were on oral anticoagulants. Except for age (see above), all the other off-label uses had no prognostic significance and did not lead to an increased rate of intracerebral hemorrhage.

> **Caution**
>
> Off-label thrombolysis should be avoided but does not necessarily lead to increased hemorrhage or other complications.

Prior Illnesses and Treatments

Platelet Aggregation Inhibitors

Several studies address the problem of prior treatment with platelet inhibitors. In some countries rtPA approval recognized prior treatment with platelet aggregation inhibitors as an exclusion criterion. The most important study is based on the SITS-MOST registry (Diedler et al. 2010). Of 11 865 patients in the registry who received intravenous thrombolysis, 3782 had been premedicated with platelet inhibitors. The mortality rates were the same in both groups. Symptomatic intracerebral hemorrhage occurred in 1.1% of patients not on antiplatelet therapy, 2.5% of patients on platelet inhibitors, 1.7% on clopidogrel, 2.3% on aspirin and dipyridamole, and 4.1% on aspirin plus clopidogrel. Only the combination of aspirin and clopidogrel was associated with a significantly increased rate of intracerebral hemorrhage. Despite the higher incidence of hemorrhage, another group of authors (Uyttenboogaart et al. 2008) reported a greater net benefit of intravenous thrombolysis in patients taking antiplatelet drugs.

> **Note**
>
> Prior treatment with platelet aggregation inhibitors is not an absolute contraindication to intravenous thrombolysis. Caution should be exercised in patients taking aspirin plus clopidogrel. These patients may receive thrombolysis but should be explicitly informed of the up to fourfold increase in intracerebral hemorrhage risk.

Atrial Fibrillation

Atrial fibrillation appears to be an important independent risk factor for a poorer prognosis after intravenous thrombolysis (Kimura et al. 2009a; Sanák et al. 2010). In one study, patients with atrial fibrillation were found to have an average mRS of 2.5 at 90 days compared with a score of 1.0 in patients without atrial fibrillation (Sanák et al. 2010). One reason may be that patients with atrial fibrillation tend to have more severe stroke and more frequent occlusions of large cerebral vessels.

Persistent Foramen Ovale

On the other hand, a persistent foramen ovale appears to be a favorable prognostic factor for thrombolytic outcome. The only significant independent factor that could be identified in 22 patients with a dramatic improvement of thrombolysis was the presence of a right-to-left shunt, with an OR of 5.9 (95% CI 1.1–27.3; Kimura et al. 2009b).

Metabolic Syndrome

There is evidence that a metabolic syndrome can reduce the efficacy of intravenous thrombolysis. The biochemical and molecular changes in metabolic syndrome appear to create a resistance to clot lysis, especially in women (OR 17.5 for unsuccessful recanalization; 95% CI 1.9–163; Arenillas et al. 2009).

Diabetes Mellitus

Several studies have shown that diabetes reduces the efficacy of thrombolysis while increasing the risk of intracerebral hemorrhage and other complications. For example, the Canadian CASES study (Poppe et al. 2009b) showed that 18% of nondiabetics and 70% of diabetics were in a hyperglycemic state during intravenous thrombolysis. This was an independent predictor of death, cerebral hemorrhage, and severe disability.

Elevated Body Temperature

Norwegian results indicate that an elevated body temperature, which is otherwise a poor prognostic factor in stroke, can improve response to thrombolysis. This may result from the reaction rate–temperature rule, in which a higher temperature correlates with higher enzymatic thrombolytic activity (Naess et al. 2010).

Mild Symptoms and Thrombolysis

It has often been asked whether thrombolysis is appropriate for patients with relatively mild clinical symptoms or patients with resolving symptoms. In a series of 32 patients with predominantly isolated aphasia who received intravenous thrombolysis, 94% had a good outcome and 46% had complete regression of symptoms with only one reported asymptomatic hemorrhage (Köhrmann et al. 2009). In another study, however, 27% of too-good-to-treat patients suffered severe disability or death (Smith et al. 2005).

> **Caution**
>
> Isolated clinical syndromes such as aphasia, or resolving symptoms, do not mean that thrombolysis should be withheld. These patients often have an unfavorable prognosis without thrombolysis, whereas thrombolysis is safe.

Stroke Mimics

For a long time it was feared that patients misdiagnosed with ischemic stroke would be harmed by intravenous thrombolysis. A detailed history, complete neurologic examination, baseline imaging, and laboratory tests will help avoid diagnostic errors. In the acute setting, however, there will always be patients who receive systemic thrombolysis in the mistaken belief that they have had a stroke. This is especially likely in cases where a history is not given by the patient or a third party—a common situation in patients who are aphasic, comatose, or demented. But a small study has provided at least partial reassurance for these cases, showing that intravenous thrombolysis did not harm patients who had been misdiagnosed with a stroke. In this Swiss study, 7 of 250 patients (2.8%) who received thrombolysis were classified as stroke mimics. The most commonly missed diagnosis was epileptic seizure with Todd's paralysis. Stroke mimics were often characterized by global aphasia without hemiparesis (42.9% vs. 3.3%). An allergic reaction or a symptomatic or asymptomatic intracranial hemorrhage was not observed in stroke mimics. As expected, a favorable course was noted in 85% of the stroke mimics compared with just 35.4% of the stroke patients. The authors concluded that improper treatment with rtPA is rare and that there is little risk that patients will be harmed by this therapy (Winkler et al. 2009).

> **Practical Tip**
>
> Inadvertent thrombolysis for a stroke mimic is harmless. Better to have too much thrombolysis than too little!

Side Effects and Hemorrhages

The principal side effects of intravenous thrombolysis are angioneurotic edema causing potentially life-threatening airway obstruction, intracerebral hemorrhage, and recurrent stroke.

Angioneurotic edema appears to occur at a rate of ~1% and is five times more common in patients previously treated with angiotensin converting enzyme (ACE) inhibitors (Engelter et al. 2005). It is managed by immediate intubation to provide oxygenation and establish a secure airway.

> **Practical Tip**
>
> It is important to consider the rare but life-threatening complication of angioneurotic edema in patients who develop acute respiratory distress during or after thrombolysis.

The problem of intracerebral hemorrhage is an inherent problem of thrombolytic therapy. The rate of intracerebral hemorrhage in the NINDS study was 6.4% (vs. 0.6% with a placebo). Unfortunately, it is difficult to bring this problem into focus due to different definitions and classifications of both clinical and radiologic criteria; different rates may be a result of different definitions.

In principle, the rate of symptomatic intracerebral hemorrhages in stroke patients not treated by thrombolysis is low (0–0.6%). It is increased up to 10-fold by thrombolytic therapy. Predictors of cerebral hemorrhage may be early ischemic changes on cranial CT and protocol violations (Martí-Fábregas et al. 2007). A special relationship exists between high blood pressure and bleeding complications. Thus, a blood pressure > 185/110 mmHg is significantly associated with a 2.59-fold increase in risk for cerebral hemorrhage (95% CI 1.07–6.25) (Tsivgoulis et al. 2009).

II

Besides blood pressure, a hyperglycemic metabolic state plays a similar negative role. A blood glucose level < 110 mg% on admission was found to be associated with a 2.1% rate of intracerebral hemorrhage in patients who received thrombolysis. This rate was 3.6% at levels of 110–150 mg%, and 6.4% at levels > 150 mg% (Paciaroni et al. 2009).

Caution

Intravenous thrombolysis for acute stroke is inevitably associated with an increased incidence of intracerebral hemorrhage. It is important to consider blood pressure and blood sugar limits to keep the risk of hemorrhage as low as possible.

Best Practice

Following the aphorism that "time is brain," it is essential to optimize the prehospital and in-hospital phases of thrombolysis. A Canadian study showed that the selective referral of patients with suspected acute stroke to hospitals with a stroke unit could significantly increase the tPA treatment rates for ischemic stroke (Gladstone et al. 2009). All patients with clinical suspicion of acute stroke were referred to a regional stroke center; acute referral to local hospitals without a stroke unit was not allowed. The emergency medical team followed a strict ambulance destination decision rule, and the care team at the stroke unit was directly notified by telephone in advance. This protocol doubled the number of patients with acute stroke arriving at the stroke center within a 2.5-h time window, and it more than doubled the thrombolysis rate from 9.5% to 23.4% ($p = 0.01$). Fifty percent of patients with ischemic stroke arriving within 2.5 h received rtPA thrombolysis. This study shows that a coordinated prehospital phase provides an immediate increase in thrombolysis rates resulting in improved acute causal therapy. Another point that should not be underestimated is the importance of educating the general public. Despite repeated, vigorous information campaigns, there seems to be little public awareness of stroke warning signs and available treatments. In one survey conducted in the United States, 4724 people were asked whether they knew about the possibilities of acute stroke treatment with rtPA. Only 32.2% of those surveyed knew that strokes could be treated acutely with a thrombolytic drug. Of that percentage, only half knew that the time window for that therapy was limited (at that time) to 3 h (Anderson et al. 2009).

In-hospital procedures should also be optimally organized. Every effort should be made to achieve door-to-needle times of ~30 min.

Outlook

Various ideas have been proposed for combining thrombolysis with neuroprotective drugs to make the treatment safer and more effective in the future. Unfortunately, combination therapies have failed in the past because individual neuroprotective agents were not shown to be effective. Several approaches are currently being discussed: endogenous uric acid (Amaro et al. 2007) to prevent lipid oxygenation; combining caffeine and hypothermia with thrombolysis (Martin-Schild et al. 2009); and, very recently, combining a proteosome inhibitor with thrombolysis, which has yielded excellent results in an experimental setting (Zhang et al. 2010). The point is that we should not view intravenous thrombolysis as being independent of other stroke treatments but should, whenever possible, integrate thrombolysis into the protocol of the stroke unit (Pérez de la Ossa et al. 2009).

For the present, expanding the time window for thrombolysis beyond 4.5 h can be recommended only in clinical studies that employ MRI criteria and other imaging techniques, but perhaps in the future it will become a part of routine clinical care (Mishra et al. 2010).

Within a broad framework of future developments, leading international experts in acute stroke emphasize the importance of stroke centers as an essential component in the process of improving the safety and efficacy of intravenous thrombolysis (Hachinski et al. 2010).

Intra-arterial Thrombolysis
B. Eckert

Introduction

The introduction of local intra-arterial thrombolysis by Hermann Zeumer in 1981 marked a milestone in the treatment of acute stroke (Zeumer et al. 1982). For the first time, local intra-arterial thrombolysis provided a causal therapeutic approach that could eliminate the offending vascular occlusion, and this was the only recanalization therapy available for many years. Technological advances and initial study results in subsequent years contributed greatly to the design of studies on intravenous thrombolysis performed in the 1990s (see p. 52). Following the success of the randomized placebo-controlled NINDS studies (National Institute of Neurological Disorders and Stroke rtPA Stroke Study Group 1995) and the ECASS II study (Hacke et al. 2008a), intravenous thrombolysis became the only approved treatment for acute stroke up to 4.5 h after symptom onset. As for local intra-arterial thrombolysis, to date there has been only one successful randomized placebo-controlled study in patients with an MCA occlusion (Furlan et al. 1999). Local intra-arterial thrombolysis is considered the treatment of choice for proximal, clinically severe vascular occlusions, especially in a delayed time window. Today a variety of mechanical thrombectomy systems and special intracranial stents have significantly expanded endovascular treatment options. The results of available pilot studies suggest that these techniques can provide faster and more effective recanalization than local intra-arterial thrombolysis alone. Nevertheless, local intra-arterial thrombolysis continues to have major importance both as an initial therapy and as an adjunct to mechanical recanalization techniques.

Regional intra-arterial thrombolysis involves injecting the thrombolytic agent into the afferent vessel (internal carotid artery [ICA], vertebral artery). Bridging therapy refers to initial intravenous drug injection prior to intraarterial diagnosis and treatment.

Since most patients are in an agitated state, general endotracheal anesthesia is generally recommended to create safe conditions for intracerebral microcatheter manipulation. This applies even more to the use of technically sophisticated mechanical recanalization systems. Often, vascular segments occluded by the thrombus must be catheterized under fluoroscopic guidance alone without benefit of "road map" control. Superselective images and road maps are of key importance in the periphery (e.g., distal to the MCA bifurcation) to avoid vascular perforation. Only general anesthesia can provide these very precise and meticulous working conditions. Especially if complications arise, safe endovascular catheterization cannot be achieved without general anesthesia. In some cases the start of treatment can be expedited by first placing the microcatheter in the thrombus under local anesthesia before general anesthesia is induced. Subsequent endovascular manipulations are then performed under general anesthesia. Even at logistically advanced treatment centers, the interval from hospital admission to start of angiography averages 109 min (Nedeltchev et al. 2003).

Technique

> **Note**
>
> Local intra-arterial thrombolysis has a more complex logistic setup than intravenous thrombolysis, resulting in a longer time to treatment.

Femoral artery catheterization is followed by diagnostic angiography to define the vascular occlusion and collateral circulation. Next, a microcatheter is advanced through an introducer sheath in the afferent cervical artery and navigated to the intracranial occlusion site. The thrombus must be carefully traversed with a thin guidewire to define the length of the occlusion and the peripheral circulation. The microcatheter is positioned in the proximal thrombus, and the thrombolytic agent is locally (superselectively) injected (**Fig. 6.3**). Local intraarterial thrombolysis delivers a higher concentration of the agent to the thrombus than is achieved with intravenous thrombolysis.

> **Practical Tip**
>
> Generally a catheter can be advanced into a fresh atherothrombotic occlusion of the ICA. If the distal ICA is merely collapsed, a causal proximal stenosis can be reopened with a stent (see **Fig. 6.3**). If multiple intraluminal thrombi are detected in the ICA, it is better to consider exclusive local intra-arterial thrombolysis via the ICA or circle of Willis without proximal stenting (**Fig. 6.4**).

Pharmacology

The pharmacologic properties of thrombolytic agents are summarized in **Table 6.1**.

Thrombolytic Agents

Pharmacologically, thrombolytic agents act by dissolving the occluding thrombus, which is held together by a network of fibrin fibers. From a pharmacodynamic standpoint, then, it would be more correct to speak of "fibrinolytic agents," but the term "thrombolysis" is widely used in the literature to describe the pharmacologic dissolution of clots, and so "thrombolysis" and "fibrinolysis" may be considered synonyms. Both terms refer to the dissolution of the fibrin framework by the proteolytic enzyme plasmin, which is generated during endogenous (intrinsic) fibrinolysis but is not sufficiently abundant in proximity to the clot. Thrombolytic agents are plasminogen activators that convert the endogenous proenzyme plasminogen to active plasmin. Besides the fibrin bound in the clot, plasmin also lyses fibrinogen and fibrin monomers into fibrin cleavage products.

> **Caution**
>
> The fibrin cleavage products lead to thrombin inhibition with a prolongation of the partial thromboplastin time, thus increasing the risk of bleeding even after the specific half-life of the plasminogen activator. For this reason, coagulation status should be checked before the femoral sheath is removed.

II

Treatment of Acute Ischemic Stroke

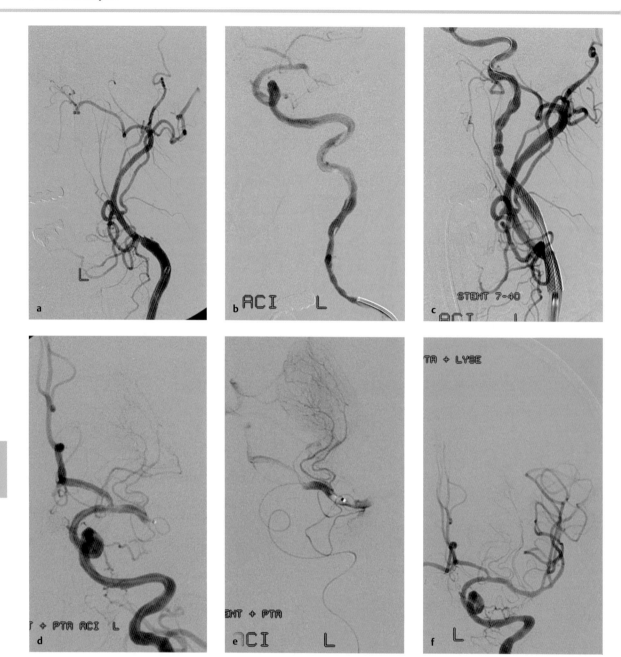

Fig. 6.3a–f   Proximal occlusion of the left ICA with periocclusional embolism of the MCA. Bridging with intravenous tirofiban.

a Complete proximal occlusion of the left ICA.

b After passing the occlusion with a guidewire and 5F diagnostic catheter, angiogram shows the collapsed lumen of the ICA and proximal occlusion of the MCA.

c Stenting of the causal ICA stenosis with reactive vasospasm in the high cervical segment of the ICA.

d Injection via the ICA demonstrates proximal occlusion of the MCA. Microcatheter is in the thrombus.

e Superselective angiogram with optimum catheter placement in the thrombus, followed by local intra-arterial thrombolysis with 20 mg rtPA.

f Complete recanalization of the MCA.

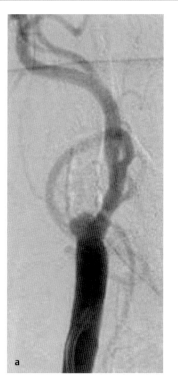
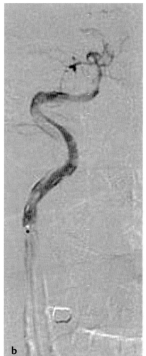
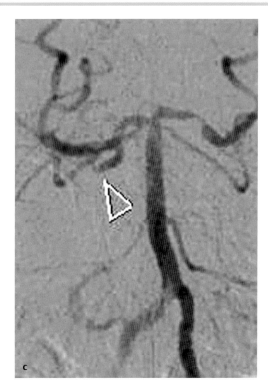

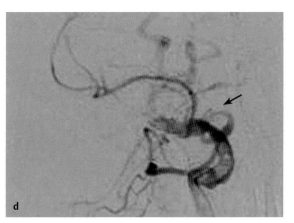
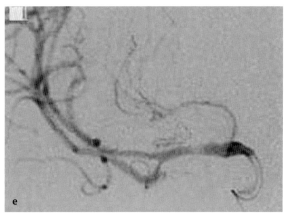

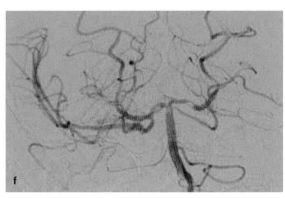

Fig. 6.4a–f Proximal occlusion of the left ICA with perioc-clusional carotid-T embolism (with kind permission of Springer Science + Business Media, Heidelberg; Jakubowska MM, Michels P, Müller-Jensen A, Leppien A, Eckert B. Endovascular treatment in proximal and intracranial carotid occlusion 9 hours after symptom onset. Neuroradiology 2008;50(7):599–604).

a Complete proximal occlusion of the right ICA.

b After passing the occlusion with a microcatheter, superselective angiography demonstrates multiple intraluminal thrombi in the ICA.

c Injection via the left vertebral artery demonstrates a large right posterior communicating artery (*arrow*) prior to local intra-arterial thrombolysis.

d Angiogram after local intra-arterial thrombolysis in the carotid-T segment (20 mg of rtPA) shows partial recanalization with flow re-established to the posterior communicating artery (*arrow*).

e Superselective angiogram shows complete recanalization of the right MCA after an additional 20 mg of rtPA.

f Reperfusion of the right MCA via the right posterior communi-cating artery. The right ICA remained occluded after withdrawal of the microcatheter.

Table 6.1 Pharmacology of agents used for intra-arterial and intravenous thrombolysis

Agent	Trade name	Mechanism of action	Excretion	Half-life	Administration	Randomized stroke studies
Thrombolytic agents						
Streptokinase	Streptase	Protein from β-hemolytic bacteria, plasminogen activator	Metabolized in the liver, metabolites excreted via the kidney	18–23 min	Intra-arterial; intravenous use is obsolete in stroke treatment	ASK (Donnan et al. 1996) MAST-E (Jaillard et al. 1999) MAST-I (Multicenter Acute Stroke Trial–Italy (MAST-I) Group 1995)
Urokinase	Urokinase HS medac, reotromb	Serine protease from human urine, plasminogen activation	Liver	10 min	Intra-arterial	
Prourokinase	Not currently available	Genetically engineered, precursor of urokinase, converted to urokinase in fibrin clots	Liver	20 min	Intra-arterial	PROACT I–II (del Zoppo et al. 1998; Furlan et al. 1999)
rtPA	Actilyse, Activase	Serine protease, genetically engineered recombinant, tissue-specific plasminogen activation	Kidney	3–5 min	Intra-arterial; intravenous	ECASS I–III (Hacke et al. 1995, 1998, 2008) NINDS (National Institute of Neurological Disorders and Stroke rtPA Stroke Study Group 1995)
Reteplase	Rapilysin	Genetically engineered mutant plasminogen activator, less fibrin binding, better clot penetration	Kidney	15–18 min	Intravenous bolus, intra-arterial	
Tenecteplase	Metalyse	Genetically engineered, high fibrin specificity, resistant to inactivation by PAI-1	Kidney	17 min	Intravenous bolus, intra-arterial	

(continued)

Table 6.1 Pharmacology of agents used for intra-arterial and intravenous thrombolysis *(continued)*

Agent	Trade name	Mechanism of action	Excretion	Half-life	Administration	Randomized stroke studies
Desmolase	Currently in clinical trials	Enzyme from vampire bat saliva, produced by recombinant genetic engineering, plasminogen activation, active only in fibrin-bound form	Liver	2.5 h	Intravenous bolus	DIAS I–II (Hacke et al. 2005, 2009)
Ancrod	Viprinex	Produced from venom of Malayan pit viper, proteolysis leads to fibrin cleavage (defibrino-genation), induces anticoagulation	Kidney	3–5 h	Intravenous	STAT (Sherman et al. 2000)
Glycoprotein IIb/IIIa inhibitors						
Abciximab	ReoPro	Genetically engineered; Fab fragment of a monoclonal antibody, binds with strong affinity to GP IIb/IIIa receptor	Binds rapidly (in minutes) and irreversibly to platelets, inhibits platelet function	Plasma half-life: 10–30 min, long duration of action (24–48 h)	Intravenous bolus followed by infusion	AbESTT (Adams et al. 2008)
Tirofiban	Aggrastat	Nonpeptide	Kidney	2 h	Intravenous bolus followed by infusion	SATIS (Siebler et al. 2011)
Eptifibatide	Integrilin	Cyclic peptide	Kidney	2.5 h	Intravenous bolus followed by infusion	

Plasmin itself is not currently available as a thrombolytic agent outside of studies and would break down very quickly after intravenous injection. When injected locally into a thrombus, plasmin binds immediately to fibrin to exert its effect. Plasmin inhibitors would instantly neutralize free, unbound plasmin and would thus prevent a systemic bleeding risk. In theory, then, local plasmin therapy could be used even in stroke patients who have had recent surgery. Animal studies have shown that plasmin has greater efficacy than plasminogen activators with less bleeding risk. In the only clinical study to date involving the local injection of human plasmin into the thrombus (Freitag et al. 1996), PA + Lys-plasminogen (plasmin) accelerated recanalization (68 min vs. 104 min with local intra-arterial

thrombolysis) and led to a markedly higher success rate of 83% (vs. 50% for local intra-arterial thrombolysis) with a comparable risk of hemorrhage (**Fig. 6.5**). A clinical study is currently underway to test plasmin produced by recombinant technology for the local treatment of MCA occlusions.

Approved thrombolytic agents differ mainly in their half-life and fibrin specificity. The first studies on stroke treatment were done with streptokinase, an agent available since 1950. Because of negative study results with increased rates of intracerebral hemorrhage and immunization by the protein derived from β-streptococci, streptokinase is now considered obsolete in the treatment of strokes (see the section on Clinical Studies of Thrombolysis in Acute Stroke, p. 54).

Treatment of Acute Ischemic Stroke

II

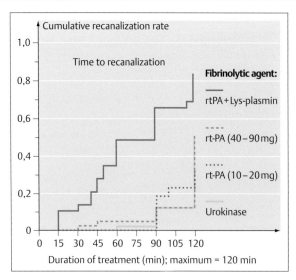

Fig. 6.5 Cumulative probability of recanalization during local intra-arterial thrombolysis (maximum 2 h) of proximal vascular occlusions in the anterior circulation. Total of 137 participants; 44 treated with urokinase and 64 with rtPA (10–20 mg: $n = 22$; 40–90 mg: $n = 42$), with comparable results: late onset of recanalization and maximum recanalization rate of 50%. The addition of Lys-plasmin (plasmin) significantly reduced the time to recanalization and yielded an 83% success rate (with kind permission of S. Karger AG, Basel; Eckert B, Kucinski T, Neumaier-Probst E, Fiehler J, Röther J, Zeumer H. Local intra-arterial fibrinolysis in acute hemispheric stroke: effect of occlusion type and fibrinolytic agent on recanalization success and neurological outcome. Cerebrovasc Dis 2003;15(4):258–263).

Note

Streptokinase and urokinase, the other first-generation thrombolytic agent, carry an increased risk of hypofibrinogenemia due to their low fibrin specificity, leading to an increased risk of hemorrhage.

The second generation of thrombolytic agents are recombinant forms produced by genetic engineering (rtPA, prourokinase) and have significantly higher fibrin specificity. All studies on intravenous thrombolysis to date have employed alteplase (rtPA). Besides the desired high thrombus penetration, however, rtPA was also found to cause neurotoxic effects in experimental animals. rtPA crossing an injured blood–brain barrier and reaching the extracellular space was found to produce neurotoxic effects by acting on the NMDA (N-methyl-D-aspartate) receptor and amplifying the conductance of intracellular calcium channels. Also, activation of the enzyme metalloproteinase by rtPA can further increase the permeability of the blood–brain barrier and promote parenchymal hemorrhage or brain edema (Kaur et al. 2004). Prourokinase was never approved by the FDA despite the successful PROACT II study (local intra-arterial thrombolysis for MCA occlusion; see **Table 6.1**).

The third generation of thrombolytic agents (reteplase, tenecteplase) consists of genetically engineered mutations of tissue-specific plasminogen activators with a longer half-life, higher fibrin specificity, and less neurotoxicity. The newer agents are also more resistant to inactivation by the antagonistic enzyme PAI-1, considered a major reason for the failure of rtPA. Comprehensive study results have not yet been published on these new agents, however.

The desired conversion of plasminogen to plasmin by plasminogen activators also causes an increase of thrombin and consequent platelet activation with increased levels of the antagonistic enzyme PAI-1 and of α-2-antiplasmin. Moreover, residual thrombi left by incomplete recanalization can induce secondary platelet aggregation with thrombus growth. These interactions are considered an important cause of the long recanalization time and relatively high reocclusion rate (~20%) (Qureshi et al. 2004). Reocclusion rates as high as 32% were reported in a Doppler ultrasound study of intravenous thrombolysis.

Glycoprotein IIb/IIIa Receptor Inhibitors

Drawing on clinical cardiologic studies, investigators have combined a half-dose of rtPA with a powerful platelet aggregation inhibitor in an effort to achieve better and faster recanalization.

The first step in platelet aggregation is the formation of cross-bridges at fibrinogen receptors (glycoprotein IIb/IIIa receptors) on the surface of platelets. Glycoprotein IIb/IIIa receptor inhibitors are highly specific antagonists of these fibrinogen receptors and will inhibit almost all platelet aggregation within a few minutes after they are administered. These agents can prevent rethrombosis and growth in thrombus size while also producing a slight thrombolytic effect in platelet-rich thrombi ("white clot"). The ability of glycoprotein IIb/IIIa receptor inhibitors to dissolve fresh, platelet-rich thrombus is a known phenomenon relating to thrombotic complications that may arise in the coil embolization of intracranial aneurysms. Glycoprotein IIb/IIIa receptor inhibitors also reduce the thrombin level, increase the permeability of thrombi, and improve the microcirculation distal to an occlusion. In cases where stenting is also performed, these agents immediately produce the platelet inhibition necessary to prevent stent thrombosis. In the event of incomplete recanalization with residual thrombi on the vessel wall, glycoprotein IIb/IIIa receptor inhibition can effectively prevent secondary reocclusion until complete recanalization has been achieved.

The monoclonal antibody abciximab binds in minutes with high affinity to glycoprotein IIb/IIIa receptors while its free form is quickly eliminated from the plasma. Because it binds almost irreversibly to platelets, the effect of abciximab is tied to the life span of inactivated platelets. As a result, abciximab has a very short plasma half-life but a long biologic half-life. This distinguishes it from other glycoprotein IIb/IIIa receptor inhibitors, which consist of small antibody fragments ("small molecules") that bind reversibly to fibrinogen receptors for a short time. Hence these agents have a much shorter biologic half-life and their pharmacodynamics are easier to control. Patients are operable just 2 h after small-molecule glycoprotein IIb/IIIa receptor inhibitors are discontinued. Platelet concentrates cannot shorten this interval because the large amount of free, unbound small-molecule receptor inhibitors in the plasma would immediately block the fresh platelets as well. By contrast, no free abciximab is available in the plasma after that agent has been administered.

> **Note**
>
> Platelet concentrates given immediately after abciximab use in patients requiring emergency surgery will quickly restore the blood to a coagulable (operable) state.

Previous studies on the intravenous use of glycoprotein IIb/IIIa receptor inhibitors alone in acute stroke have not yielded definitive results. A randomized study of intravenous abciximab vs. placebo during the first 5 h after stroke onset showed no benefit in the patients treated with abciximab (Adams et al. 2008). Patients' inclusion was based on noncontrast cranial CT scans; the vascular occlusion was not visualized. Patients treated with abciximab had a significantly higher rate of symptomatic intracerebral hemorrhage (5.5% vs. 0.5% with placebo), comparable to the studies of intravenous thrombolysis. On the other hand, nonrandomized pilot studies of intravenous tirofiban given to patients with clinically progressive microangiopathic strokes within 24–96 h after symptom onset showed evidence of clinical efficacy without significant bleeding complications (Philipps et al. 2009; Siebler et al. 2011).

Indication

The indication for treatment depends on laboratory, clinical, and neuroimaging factors. In principle, local intra-arterial thrombolysis has the same clinical and radiologic contraindications as intravenous thrombolysis (see p. 52).

The main priority in the anterior circulation is to minimize the neurologic deficit. The risks of intracerebral hemorrhage with clinical deterioration must be rigorously assessed. The therapeutic time window (starting local intra-arterial thrombolysis within 6 h after symptom onset), the extent of known infarct lesions, and the severity of the vascular occlusion are key factors in patient selection and may prompt a decision to withhold local intra-arterial thrombolysis in some cases.

Severe, acute vascular occlusions in the posterior circulation (basilar artery, bilateral vertebral artery occlusion) have an ~90% mortality rate without thrombolytic therapy (Hacke et al. 1988). The collateral supply in the brainstem via the arcades of the perforating pontine arteries is better developed than in the anterior circulation. There are no reliable morphologic imaging criteria in the posterior circulation for evaluating early ischemic changes by CT or MRI. As a result, there should be much less hesitation in recommending local intra-arterial thrombolysis for occlusions in the posterior circulation. Local intra-arterial thrombolysis or other endovascular interventions should be withheld only if the patient has been comatose for several hours or if definite signs of a large, demarcated brainstem infarction are demonstrated by CT or MRI.

Efficacy

Local Intra-Arterial Thrombolysis in the Anterior Circulation

> **Caution**
>
> The goal of treatment is the fastest possible recanalization of the occluded vessel to reperfuse the brain tissue. Successful recanalization does not guarantee a favorable clinical outcome, however.

There may be several reasons for this:
- Recanalization is too late.
- Successful proximal recanalization with a persistent peripheral occlusion (recanalization without reperfusion).
- A large infarction with poor primary collateralization has developed before treatment is started.

There is no question that successful recanalization is essential for clinical success. All recent studies show a direct link between recanalization and clinical outcome. With successful recanalization of proximal vascular occlusions, the mortality rate falls from 50% to 30% while the rate of patients with a good neurologic outcome rises from 9% to 45% (Nogueira et al. 2009).

II

> **Note**
>
> The clinical prognosis depends critically on the location of the occlusion and the thrombus burden.

Occlusion of the intracranial carotid bifurcation (carotid T) has a mortality rate of ~50%. Less than 25% of patients can be successfully recanalized by local intra-arterial or intravenous thrombolysis (Jansen et al. 1995). The recanalization rates for a proximal MCA occlusion are significantly higher and are in the range of 50–70%; the mortality rate is ~30%. More peripheral MCA occlusions have a much lower mortality rate (< 10%) with equal recanalization rates (Eckert et al. 2003). In a study of the mechanical MERCI thrombectomy system for M1/M2 MCA occlusions, 42% of the patients were additionally treated by local intra-arterial thrombolysis. The recanalization rate was 50% with MERCI retrieval alone but rose to 64% when local intra-arterial thrombolysis was added.

The recanalization rates reported in studies on local intra-arterial thrombolysis refer to the immediate angiographic result documented within the 1–2-h duration of treatment. The recanalization data for intravenous thrombolysis are rarely confirmed angiographically; usually they are based on transcranial Doppler ultrasound scans, MRI, or CT performed within 6–24 h after the start of treatment. The angiographic recanalization rate 1 h after intravenous thrombolysis is 9% for carotid-T occlusions and 35% for proximal MCA occlusions. The rates at 24 h based on CTA are 46% for carotid-T occlusions and 53% for proximal MCA occlusions (Tomsick et al. 2010)—although these late recanalization rates would have very little bearing on clinical outcome.

The PROACT II study (prourokinase for acute ischemic stroke) analyzed the efficacy of local intra-arterial thrombolysis in patients with MCA occlusions (Furlan et al. 1999). Patients were randomized to local intra-arterial thrombolysis with prourokinase + systemic heparin vs. diagnostic angiography without local intra-arterial thrombolysis and systemic heparin only (**Table 6.2**). In contrast to the studies on intravenous thrombolysis (ECASS I–III, NINDS; see p. 55–57), the site of the intracranial occlusion was defined angiographically in all patients. Angiography confirmed the clinically presumed MCA occlusion in only 40% of the patients. Nearly 60% of the patients were excluded on the basis of angiographic findings. The reasons for this were either a microangiopathic (lacunar) infarction with no detectable vascular occlusion or an ICA occlusion with a corresponding poor prognosis. The PROACT II study showed a significant clinical benefit in patients with proximal MCA occlusions treated within 6 h of symptom onset (treatment concluded up to 8 h after symptom onset) compared with heparin-only treatment.

To date, there has been no randomized clinical study comparing intravenous thrombolysis with local intra-arterial thrombolysis. One study analyzed clinical data from two stroke units in Switzerland to compare intravenous thrombolysis (started within 3 h after symptom onset) with local intra-arterial thrombolysis (started within 6 h) in patients with a hyperdense MCA sign and comparable clinical severity (intravenous thrombolysis: NIHSS = 18; local intra-arterial thrombolysis: NIHSS = 17). Intra-arterial thrombolysis was found to be significantly more beneficial than intravenous thrombolysis (local intra-arterial thrombolysis: favorable outcome in 53% of patients with 7% mortality; intravenous thrombolysis: favorable outcome in 23% with 23% mortality), even though intra-arterial thrombolysis was started an average of ~90 min later than intravenous thrombolysis (Mattle et al. 2008).

Table 6.2 Various studies on the efficacy of intravenous and intra-arterial thrombolysis in the anterior circulation

Study	Participants (n)	Treatment/ Drug	Median NIHSS on admission Placebo/drug	Time window (h)	Imaging	Good neurologic outcome at 90 days Placebo/ drug (%)	Symptomatic hemorrhage Placebo/drug (%)
NINDS (National Institute of Neurologic Disorders and Stroke rtPA Stroke Study Group 1995)	624	Intravenous thrombolysis/ rtPA	15/14	< 3	Cranial CT	26/39	0.6/6.4
ECASS III (Hacke et al. 2008)	821	Intravenous thrombolysis/ rtPA	9/10	3–4.5	Cranial CT	45.2/52.4	0.2/2.4
PROACT (Furlan et al. 1999)	180	Local intra-arterial thrombolysis/ prourokinase	17/17	< 6	Cranial CT/ angiography	25/40	2/10

Local Intra-arterial Thrombolysis in the Posterior Circulation

Without successful recanalization, the probability of a good neurologic outcome in acute vertebrobasilar occlusions is close to zero and the mortality rate is > 80% (Lindsberg and Mattle 2006). Given this very poor clinical prognosis, it would be unethical to conduct randomized studies with a placebo treatment arm. The therapeutic results of clinically controlled but nonrandomized studies show a definite advantage of local intra-arterial thrombolysis over conservative anticoagulant therapy, but even with successful recanalization, the mortality rate is still 40–60%. No more than one-third of patients survive with a mild neurologic deficit (**Table 6.3**).

As in the anterior circulation, the early initiation of treatment is of key importance for posterior occlusions. If treatment is started within the first 6 h after symptom onset, a good neurologic outcome can be achieved in approximately one-third of patients. After 6 h, this rate declines to <10% while mortality rises from ~50% to > 70%. The risk of fatal hemorrhages also increases markedly during the late treatment phase (Eckert et al. 2002). There are cases, however, in which collateral channels, especially with atherothrombotic occlusions and nonocclusive thrombi, can maintain borderline perfusion for a certain period, thereby extending the time window after symptom onset in which treatment can be initiated. There are even exceptional cases in which a slowly progressive atherothrombotic occlusion with good collateralization may remain asymptomatic (Brandt et al. 1995).

A pilot study on intravenous thrombolysis in patients with MRA-confirmed vertebrobasilar occlusions also showed good treatment results (Lindsberg et al. 2004). One weakness in the study methodology lies in the MRA detection of vascular occlusion, which may be false-positive in patients with high-grade stenosis or a very narrow basilar artery. The study demonstrated that early intravenous thrombolysis is an appropriate therapy and may be preferred over intra-arterial thrombolysis, especially if intra-arterial therapy would involve long delays (e.g., due to patient transport).

There are no comparative studies of intravenous thrombolysis and local intra-arterial thrombolysis in the posterior circulation. Analysis of a prospective, multicenter study registry showed a significant advantage of intravenous thrombolysis and local intra-arterial thrombolysis over antithrombotic aspirin therapy alone (mortality 93%) but did not show a significant difference between intravenous and local intra-arterial thrombolysis. It should be noted, however, that local intra-arterial thrombolysis was performed under less favorable conditions. It was initiated later, and the patients had greater clinical stroke severity than patients treated by intravenous thrombolysis (Schonewille et al. 2009).

II

Table 6.3 Various studies on the efficacy of intravenous and intra-arterial thrombolysis in the posterior circulation

Study	Participants (n)	Treatment	Recanalization (%)	Mortality (%)	Good neurologic outcome (%)	Parenchymal hematoma/ symptomatic intracerebral hemorrhage (%)
Hacke et al. 1988	43	Local intra-arterial thrombolysis	44	67	23	9
Brandt et al. 1996	51	Local intra-arterial thrombolysis	51	68	20	6
Eckert et al. 2002	83	Local intra-arterial thrombolysis	66	60	23	8
Arnold et al. 2004	40	Local intra-arterial thrombolysis	80	42	35	5
Lindsberg et al. 2004	50	Intravenous thrombolysis after MRA	52	40	24	14
Eckert et al. 2005 (multicenter study)	47	Glycoprotein IIb/IIIa receptor inhibitor i.v., local intra-arterial thrombolysis, percutaneous transluminal angioplasty/stent	72	38	34	13
Schulte-Altedorneburg et al. 2006 (multicenter study)	180	Local intra-arterial thrombolysis	74	43	(not stated)	14

Note

Unlike the anterior circulation, in which embolic occlusions predominate, ~30–40% of occlusions in the posterior circulation are caused by the local atherothrombotic occlusion of a preexisting stenosis. Successful and permanent recanalization in these cases generally requires an endovascular intervention (stent implantation).

Practical Tip

Today there is a consensus that patients with acute vertebrobasilar occlusions should be managed by primary endovascular treatment whenever possible. If this requires transport to a neurovascular center, intravenous bridging therapy should be initiated before patient transport and continued until angiography is performed.

Bridging Therapy

Once a stroke patient has been imaged and selected, intravenous thrombolysis is started right away so that causal recanalization therapy can be instituted as quickly as possible. This can bridge the interval to local intra-arterial thrombolysis within the hospital or while the patient is transferred to a stroke center.

A protocol for primary intravenous thrombolysis before transport with subsequent mechanical thrombus extraction has been referred to as "drip, ship and retrieve."

Intravenous + Local Intra-arterial Thrombolysis (rtPA Bridging)

This concept consists of initial intravenous thrombolysis with subsequent angiography. If the occlusion persists, the rest of the rtPA dose is administered locally. Intravenous thrombolysis generally starts with a reduced dose (maximum of 50–60 mg), leaving 20–30 mg available for local intra-arterial thrombolysis. Two pilot studies in patients with MCA occlusions showed a combined recanalization rate of 83%, a low rate of intracranial hemorrhage, and a favorable clinical outcome in 56% of the patients (Tomsick et al. 2010). The IMS III trial (Interventional Management of Stroke III: intravenous thrombolysis vs. intravenous + local intra-arterial thrombolysis [bridging]; patients recruited since June 2006) is expected to provide definitive data on this combined approach.

One study showed that even when a full dose of rtPA was administered for intravenous thrombolysis (60–90 mg of rtPA), subsequent local intra-arterial thrombolysis could

improve recanalization without increasing the hemorrhage rate. On average, the patients were treated by local intra-arterial thrombolysis 140 min after intravenous thrombolysis (average dose for local intra-arterial thrombolysis: 2.8 IU reteplase or 8.6 mg rtPA, or 700 000 IU urokinase). The rate of symptomatic intracranial hemorrhage was 5.8%, the recanalization rate was 73%, and 55% of patients had a favorable neurologic outcome (Shaltoni et al. 2007).

A comparative study in transported patients with basilar artery thrombosis showed significantly better outcomes with this combined treatment approach (intravenous thrombolysis + subsequent mechanical endovascular therapy) than with endovascular therapy alone, not preceded by intravenous thrombolysis. The angiographically confirmed recanalization rate after intravenous thrombolysis was 38% (Pfefferkorn et al. 2010). These patients required no additional endovascular therapy.

Intravenous Glycoprotein IIb/IIIa Receptor Inhibitor + Local Intra-arterial Thrombolysis (Bridging)

Another treatment approach consists of initial intravenous administration of a glycoprotein IIb/IIIa receptor inhibitor (see **Table 6.1**) and subsequent local intra-arterial thrombolysis with a reduced dose of rtPA (maximum of 40 mg).

Caution

This combination therapy is an absolute contraindication to heparin use because the decrease in thrombin and prolonged partial thromboplastin time would greatly increase the risk of hemorrhage.

The glycoprotein IIb/IIIa receptor inhibitor prevents enlargement of the thrombus and can maintain leptomeningeal collateral circulation for a certain period of time. Intravenous administration of a glycoprotein IIb/IIIa receptor inhibitor may even reopen the occluded vessel (**Fig. 6.6**), although the direct recanalization effect is presumably less than that of intravenous thrombolysis. In any case, intravenous recanalization is likely to occur only with smaller thrombi (volume ~0.1 mL). Intravenous thrombolysis is extremely unlikely to recanalize large thrombi in the carotid-T segment or basilar artery. One study of local intra-arterial thrombolysis in basilar artery thrombosis found significantly poorer recanalization when the thrombus volume exceeded 0.3 mL (Schulte-Altedorneburg et al. 2006).

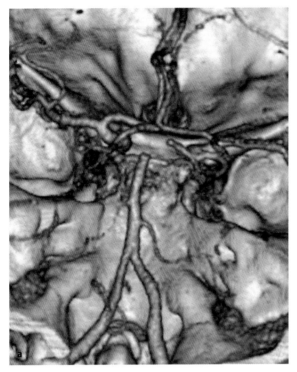
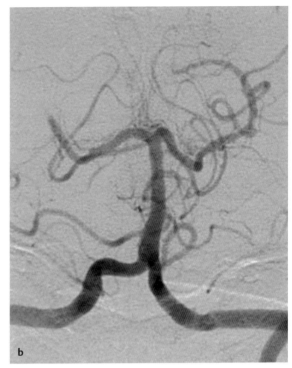

Fig. 6.6a, b Bridging therapy with intravenous tirofiban for distal basilar artery embolism.

a Three-dimensional CTA shows an embolism at the tip of the basilar artery with no filling of the posterior cerebral artery. Intravenous tirofiban was administered at once.

b Angiography after intubation 60 minutes later shows recanalization of the distal basilar artery and left posterior cerebral artery, with persistent peripheral occlusion of the right posterior cerebral artery.

> **Note**
>
> Stent implantation is an essential adjunct for the successful recanalization of an atherothrombotic vertebrobasilar occlusion or a proximal stenosis (carotid artery, vertebral artery) as origin of intracranial arterioarterial embolism.

Intravenous glycoprotein IIb/IIIa receptor inhibition is desirable in this setting because it immediately provides the platelet aggregation inhibition that stenting requires. Moreover, the glycoprotein IIb/IIIa receptor inhibitor is likely to have a greater recanalization effect on fresh, platelet-rich thrombi (white clots). Two studies on intravenous bridging therapy with glycoprotein IIb/IIIa receptor inhibitor and local intra-arterial thrombolysis for vertebrobasilar occlusions showed a marked improvement in neurologic outcomes compared with local intra-arterial thrombolysis alone (good neurologic outcome 34% vs. 17%; mortality 38% vs. 68%). The effect was particularly striking for atherothrombotic occlusions (Eckert et al. 2005).

At present we cannot say which bridging therapy has the greatest benefit, and this decision must be made on a case-by-case basis. Bridging with intravenous thrombolysis during the first 3 h after symptom onset conforms to guidelines and is especially preferred for embolic occlusions. If the full dose of rtPA has already been administered, the added use of a glycoprotein IIb/IIIa receptor inhibitor will increase the risk of intracerebral hemorrhage.

The initial intravenous administration of a glycoprotein IIb/IIIa receptor inhibitor is recommended for atherothrombotic occlusions and arterioarterial embolisms with platelet-rich thrombi. The advantage of bridging with an intravenous glycoprotein IIb/IIIa receptor inhibitor is that it will allow for all subsequent endovascular options including local intra-arterial thrombolysis (maximum of 40 mg). There is a consensus on the fundamental need for rapid initiation of intravenous therapy to utilize the time to endovascular treatment.

> **Practical Tip**
>
> Bridging scenarios in patients with proximal vascular occlusions (basilar artery, CT, M1 segment of MCA):
> - rtPA bridging with intravenous thrombolysis and local intra-arterial thrombolysis:
>   – Start intravenous thrombolysis (IVT) with rtPA (transport to stroke center)
>   – After external transport: control by cranial CT and CTA: recanalization/early infarct signs

- In-hospital, start IVT, immediate transport to angiography; intubation
- Persistent occlusion: transport to angiography; intubation
- Local intra-arterial thrombolysis with remaining rtPA (if full intravenous dose already administered, give maximum of 10–15 mg rtPA)
- Mechanical recanalization
- Optional in cases with stent implantation or poor reperfusion: final intravenous dose of glycoprotein IIb/IIIa receptor inhibitor (caution: increased bleeding risk)
- Bridging with an intravenous glycoprotein IIb/IIIa receptor inhibitor and local intra-arterial thrombolysis:
  - Intravenous bolus of glycoprotein IIb/IIIa receptor inhibitor followed by continuous infusion (transport to stroke center)
  - After external transport: assess by cranial CT and CTA: recanalization/early infarct signs
  - In-hospital: immediate transport to angiography; intubation
  - Start local intra-arterial thrombolysis (maximum total dose 40 mg rtPA)
  - Mechanical recanalization, accompanied if necessary by regional thrombolysis via introducer sheath
  - If mechanical recanalization is unsuccessful: local intra-arterial thrombolysis with the remaining dose
  - Continue intravenous infusion of glycoprotein IIb/IIIa receptor inhibitor, depending on success of recanalization and on stent implantation

Complications

> **Caution**
>
> Most complications result from arterial catheterization problems, intracranial hemorrhage, and secondary peripheral embolism.

Pronounced vascular elongation may hamper access for the introducer sheath and microcatheter placement, and may significantly delay treatment. Failure to reach the occlusion site with a microcatheter occurs in no more than 5% of cases, however.

A subarachnoid or intracerebral hemorrhage may be caused by the guidewire or microcatheter perforating or dissecting the vessel wall, or it may result from ischemic tissue damage after successful reperfusion, much as in intravenous thrombolysis. It has also been suggested that superselective contrast injection may cause harm to the blood–brain barrier. The incidence of intracranial hemorrhages with clinical deterioration (symptomatic intracerebral hemorrhage) is ~10–12% for local intra-arterial thrombolysis—higher than the 6% hemorrhage rate reported for intravenous thrombolysis (Tomsick et al. 2010). In both procedures, symptomatic intracerebral hemorrhage has a fatal outcome in more than 50% of cases. Surgical decompression is not an option, due to the coagulation-inhibiting effect produced by the thrombolysis. Pharmacologic therapies such as the administration of a thrombolysis antagonist (tranexamic acid), coagulation factors, or platelet concentrates usually come too late to produce clinical improvement or restore operability. In the rare complication of persistent subarachnoid hemorrhage from a perforated vessel, endovascular occlusion of the vessel with coils or tissue adhesive may be the only option available for achieving hemostasis. Manipulation with a mechanical thrombectomy system is more technically demanding and presumably carries a somewhat higher procedural risk than microcatheter placement alone in the setting of local intra-arterial thrombolysis. No reliable data have yet been published on this issue. In contrast to cardiac interventions, extracerebral hemorrhage and local complications at the femoral puncture site are of minor importance.

Secondary embolism due to endovascular manipulation is possible in theory, but when it occurs in local intra-arterial thrombolysis it most likely describes a situation where proximal thrombi migrate to peripheral sites. In these cases the proximal circulation is cleared, but terminal branches supplying the parenchyma are not adequately reperfused. In the case of a carotid-T occlusion, intra-arterial manipulations may redistribute portions of the embolus to an anterior cerebral artery previously perfused from the opposite site, causing a secondary embolism. It may also be possible to recanalize the secondary embolisms during the endovascular procedure, however.

Demand for Local Intra-arterial Thrombolysis

A study on local intra-arterial thrombolysis in the United States, based on an incidence of 645 000 ischemic strokes per year, predicted that no more than 20 000 cases per year will be amenable to intra-arterial thrombolysis. An estimated 20% of patients (~126 000) have severe ischemic strokes with NIHSS 10. In 2004, 2% of the stroke population in the United States (~12 000 patients) received intravenous thrombolysis and 1100 patients were treated by local intra-arterial thrombolysis. With optimum logistics, the rate of intravenous thrombolysis could be increased to 9% of acute stroke patients (58 000) during the first 3 h after stroke onset. Even with a broad logistic network staffed by qualified neurointerventionalists, it is estimated that a maximum of 20000 patients per year will qualify for local intra-arterial thrombolysis based on clinical severity and a time window of up to 6 h after symptom onset (Cloft et al. 2009).

Summary

Besides clinical criteria, the indications for endovascular stroke therapy depend on the severity of the vascular occlusion and the extent of infarction detectable by morphologic imaging. Local intra-arterial thrombolysis delays the start of treatment and is not fast or efficient enough to achieve rapid recanalization when used alone. The most promising approach to the recanalization of proximal intracranial vascular occlusions appears to be a combination of primary intravenous therapy and subsequent endovascular treatment. This bridging approach, which combines the rapid initiation of treatment with local thrombolysis, will continue to be an important pillar of stroke therapy. During mechanical recanalization, local intra-arterial thrombolysis can even be combined with simultaneous regional thrombolysis in the afferent vessel with an agent administered through the introducer sheath.

Factors crucial for a favorable clinical outcome in patients with proximal intracranial vascular occlusions are prompt baseline imaging, intravenous bridging therapy, and rapid transfer to a neurovascular center. An effective telemedicine network and the establishment of standard medical treatment protocols will be instrumental in shaping the future of stroke therapy.

References

Intravenous Thrombolysis

Adams HP, del Zoppo G, Alberts MJ, et al. Guidelines for the early management of adults with ischemic stroke: a guideline from the American Heart Association/American Stroke Association Stroke Council, Clinical Cardiology Council, Cardiovascular Radiology and Intervention Council, and the Atherosclerosis Peripheral Vascular Disease and Quality of Care Outcome in Research Interdisciplinary Working Group: The American Academy of Neurology affirms the value of this guideline as an educational tool for neurologists. Circulation 2007;115(20):e478–e534

Ad Hoc Committee representing the National Stroke Foundation and the Stroke Society of Australasia. The implementation of intravenous tissue plasminogen activator in acute ischaemic stroke—a scientific position statement from the National Stroke Foundation and the Stroke Society of Australasia. Intern Med J 2009;39(5):317–324

Alexandrov AV, Molina CA, Grotta JC, et al; CLOTBUST Investigators. Ultrasound-enhanced systemic thrombolysis for acute ischemic stroke. N Engl J Med 2004;351(21):2170–2178

Amaro S, Soy D, Obach V, Cervera A, Planas AM, Chamorro A. A pilot study of dual treatment with recombinant tissue plasminogen activator and uric acid in acute ischemic stroke. Stroke 2007;38(7):2173–2175

Anderson BE, Rafferty AP, Lyon-Callo S, Fussman C, Reeves MJ. Knowledge of tissue plasminogen activator for acute stroke among Michigan adults. Stroke 2009;40(7):2564–2567

Arenillas JF, Sandoval P, Pérez de la Ossa N, et al. The metabolic syndrome is associated with a higher resistance to intravenous thrombolysis for acute ischemic stroke in women than in men. Stroke 2009;40(2):344–349

Ariës MJ, Uyttenboogaart M, Vroomen PC, De Keyser J, Luijckx GJ. tPA treatment for acute ischaemic stroke in patients with leukoaraiosis. Eur J Neurol 2010;17(6):866–870

Berrouschot J, Röther J, Glahn J, Kucinski T, Fiehler J, Thomalla G. Outcome and severe hemorrhagic complications of intravenous thrombolysis with tissue plasminogen activator in very old (> or =80 years) stroke patients. Stroke 2005;36(11):2421–2425

Bluhmki E, Chamorro A, Dávalos A, et al. Stroke treatment with alteplase given 3.0-4.5 h after onset of acute ischaemic stroke (ECASS III): additional outcomes and subgroup analysis of a randomised controlled trial. Lancet Neurol 2009;8(12):1095–1102

Brott TG, Haley EC Jr, Levy DE, et al. Urgent therapy for stroke. Part I. Pilot study of tissue plasminogen activator administered within 90 minutes. Stroke 1992;23(5):632–640

Burggraf D, Martens HK, Jäger G, Hamann GF. Recombinant human tissue plasminogen activator protects the basal lamina in experimental focal cerebral ischemia. Thromb Haemost 2003;89(6):1072–1080

Burggraf D, Vosko MR, Schubert M, Stassen JM, Hamann GF. Different therapy options protecting microvasculature after experimental cerebral ischaemia and reperfusion. Thromb Haemost 2010;103(5):891–900

Clark WM, Madden KP, Lyden PD, Zivin JA. Cerebral hemorrhagic risk of aspirin or heparin therapy with thrombolytic treatment in rabbits. Stroke 1991;22(7):872–876

Clark WM, Wissman S, Albers GW, Jhamandas JH, Madden KP, Hamilton S. Recombinant tissue-type plasminogen activator (Alteplase) for ischemic stroke 3 to 5 hours after symptom onset. The ATLANTIS Study: a randomized controlled trial. Alteplase Thrombolysis for Acute Noninterventional Therapy in Ischemic Stroke. JAMA 1999;282(21):2019–2026

Cronin CA, Weisman CJ, Llinas RH. Stroke treatment: beyond the three-hour window and in the pregnant patient. Ann N Y Acad Sci 2008;1142:159–178

Daffertshofer M, Gass A, Ringleb P, et al. Transcranial low-frequency ultrasound-mediated thrombolysis in brain ischemia: increased risk of hemorrhage with combined ultrasound and tissue plasminogen activator: results of a phase II clinical trial. Stroke 2005;36(7):1441–1446 del Zoppo GJ, Copeland BR, Waltz TA, Zyroff J, Plow EF, Harker LA. The beneficial effect of intracarotid urokinase on acute stroke in a baboon model. Stroke 1986;17(4):638–643

del Zoppo GJ, Poeck K, Pessin MS, et al. Recombinant tissue plasminogen activator in acute thrombotic and embolic stroke. Ann Neurol 1992;32(1):78–86

del Zoppo GJ, Saver JL, Jauch EC, Adams HP Jr. Expansion of the time window for treatment of acute ischemic stroke with intravenous tissue plasminogen activator. a science advisory from the American Heart Association/American Stroke Association. Stroke 2009;40(8):2945–2948

Demchuk AM, Tanne D, Hill MD et al. Predictors of good outcome after intravenous tPA for acute ischemic stroke. Neurology 2001;57(3):474–480

Demchuk AM, Khan F, Hill MD, et al; NINDS rt-PA Stroke Study Group. Importance of leukoaraiosis on CT for tissue plasminogen activator decision making: evaluation of the NINDS rt-PA Stroke Study. Cerebrovasc Dis 2008;26(2):120–125

De Silva DA, Brekenfeld C, Ebinger M, et al; Echoplanar Imaging Thrombolytic Evaluation Trial (EPITHET) Investigators. The benefits of intravenous thrombolysis relate to the site of baseline arterial occlusion in the Echoplanar Imaging Thrombolytic Evaluation Trial (EPITHET). Stroke 2010;41(2): 295–299

Diedler J, Ahmed N, Sykora M, et al. Safety of intravenous thrombolysis for acute ischemic stroke in patients receiving antiplatelet therapy at stroke onset. Stroke 2010;41(2):288–294

Donnan GA, Davis SM, Chambers BR, et al. Streptokinase for acute ischemic stroke with relationship to time of administration: Australian Streptokinase (ASK) Trial Study Group. JAMA 1996;276(12):961–966

Engelter ST, Fluri F, Buitrago-Téllez C, et al. Life-threatening orolingual angioedema during thrombolysis in acute ischemic stroke. J Neurol 2005;252(10):1167–1170

Engelter ST, Rutgers MP, Hatz F, et al. Intravenous thrombolysis in stroke attributable to cervical artery dissection. Stroke 2009;40(12):3772–3776

Fletcher AP, Alkjaersig N, Lewis M, et al. A pilot study of urokinase therapy in cerebral infarction. Stroke 1976;7(2):135–142

Fluri F, Hatz F, Rutgers MP, et al. Intravenous thrombolysis in patients with stroke attributable to small artery occlusion. Eur J Neurol 2010;17(8):1054–1060

Furlan AJ, Eyding D, Albers GW, et al; DEDAS Investigators. Dose Escalation of Desmoteplase for Acute Ischemic Stroke (DEDAS): evidence of safety and efficacy 3 to 9 hours after stroke onset. Stroke 2006;37(5):1227–1231

Gladstone DJ, Rodan LH, Sahlas DJ, et al. A citywide prehospital protocol increases access to stroke thrombolysis in Toronto. Stroke 2009;40(12):3841–3844

Hachinski V, Donnan GA, Gorelick PB, et al; Stroke Synergium. Stroke: working toward a prioritized world agenda. Cerebrovasc Dis 2010;30(2):127–147

Hacke W, Kaste M, Fieschi C, et al; The European Cooperative Acute Stroke Study (ECASS). Intravenous thrombolysis with recombinant tissue plasminogen activator for acute hemispheric stroke. JAMA 1995;274(13):1017–1025

Hacke W, Kaste M, Fieschi C, et al; Second European-Australasian Acute Stroke Study Investigators. Randomised double-blind placebo-controlled trial of thrombolytic therapy with intravenous alteplase in acute ischaemic stroke (ECASS II). Lancet 1998;352(9136):1245–1251

Hacke W, Albers G, Al-Rawi Y, et al; DIAS Study Group. The Desmoteplase in Acute Ischemic Stroke Trial (DIAS): a phase II MRI-based 9-hour window acute stroke thrombolysis trial with intravenous desmoteplase. Stroke 2005;36(1):66–73

Hacke W, Aichner F, Bode C, et al. Akuttherapie des ischämischen Schlaganfalls. In: Kommission Leitlinien der Deutschen Gesellschaft für Neurologie, ed. Leitlinien für Diagnostik und Therapie in der Neurologie. Stuttgart: Thieme; 2008a: 243–257

Hacke W, Kaste M, Bluhmki E, et al; ECASS Investigators. Thrombolysis with alteplase 3 to 4.5 hours after acute ischemic stroke. N Engl J Med 2008b;359(13):1317–1329

Hacke W, Furlan AJ, Al-Rawi Y, et al. Intravenous desmoteplase in patients with acute ischaemic stroke selected by MRI perfusion-diffusion weighted imaging or perfusion CT (DIAS-2): a prospective, randomised, double-blind, placebo-controlled study. Lancet Neurol 2009;8(2):141–150

Haley EC Jr, Levy DE, Brott TG, et al. Urgent therapy for stroke. Part II. Pilot study of tissue plasminogen activator administered 91-180 minutes from onset. Stroke 1992;23(5): 641–645

Haley EC Jr, Brott TG, Sheppard GL, et al; The TPA Bridging Study Group. Pilot randomized trial of tissue plasminogen activator in acute ischemic stroke. Stroke 1993;24(7): 1000–1004

Haley EC Jr, Thompson JL, Grotta JC, et al; Tenecteplase in Stroke Investigators. Phase IIB/III trial of tenecteplase in acute ischemic stroke: results of a prematurely terminated randomized clinical trial. Stroke 2010;41(4):707–711

Hamann GF. Thrombophilien. In: Hermann D, Steiner T, Diener HCH, eds. Vaskuläre Neurologie. Stuttgart: Thieme; 2010: 77–82

Hill MD, Buchan AM; Canadian Alteplase for Stroke Effectiveness Study (CASES) Investigators. Thrombolysis for acute ischemic stroke: results of the Canadian Alteplase for Stroke Effectiveness Study. CMAJ 2005;172(10):1307–1312

Kimura K, Iguchi Y, Shibazaki K, Iwanaga T, Yamashita S, Aoki J. IV t-PA therapy in acute stroke patients with atrial fibrillation. J Neurol Sci 2009a;276(1-2):6–8

Kimura K, Iguchi Y, Shibazaki K, Terasawa Y, Aoki J, Matsumoto N. The presence of a right-to-left shunt is associated with dramatic improvement after thrombolytic therapy in patients with acute ischemic stroke. Stroke 2009b;40(1):303–305

Köhrmann M, Nowe T, Huttner HB, et al. Safety and outcome after thrombolysis in stroke patients with mild symptoms. Cerebrovasc Dis 2009;27(2):160–166

Kwiatkowski TG, Libman RB, Frankel M, et al; National Institute of Neurological Disorders and Stroke Recombinant Tissue Plasminogen Activator Stroke Study Group. Effects of tissue plasminogen activator for acute ischemic stroke at one year. N Engl J Med 1999;340(23):1781–1787

Lees KR, Bluhmki E, von Kummer R, et al; ECASS, ATLANTIS, NINDS and EPITHET rt-PA Study Group. Time to treatment with intravenous alteplase and outcome in stroke: an updated pooled analysis of ECASS, ATLANTIS, NINDS, and EPITHET trials. Lancet 2010;375(9727):1695–1703

Lyden PD, Zivin JA, Clark WA, et al. Tissue plasminogen activator-mediated thrombolysis of cerebral emboli and its effect on hemorrhagic infarction in rabbits. Neurology 1989;39(5):703–708

Lyden PD, Madden KP, Clark WM, Sasse KC, Zivin JA. Incidence of cerebral hemorrhage after treatment with tissue plasminogen activator or streptokinase following embolic stroke in rabbits [corrected]. Stroke 1990;21(11):1589–1593

Martí-Fàbregas J, Bravo Y, Cocho D, et al. Frequency and predictors of symptomatic intracerebral hemorrhage in patients with ischemic stroke treated with recombinant tissue plasminogen activator outside clinical trials. Cerebrovasc Dis 2007;23(2-3):85–90

Martin-Schild S, Hallevi H, Shaltoni H, et al. Combined neuroprotective modalities coupled with thrombolysis in acute ischemic stroke: a pilot study of caffeinol and mild hypothermia. J Stroke Cerebrovasc Dis 2009;18(2):86–96

Meretoja A, Putaala J, Tatlisumak T, et al. Off-label thrombolysis is not associated with poor outcome in patients with stroke. Stroke 2010;41(7):1450–1458

Meseguer E, Mazighi M, Labreuche J, et al. Outcomes of intravenous recombinant tissue plasminogen activator therapy according to gender: a clinical registry study and systematic review. Stroke 2009;40(6):2104–2110

Meyer JS, Gilroy J, Barnahrt ME, et al. Therapeutic thrombolysis in cerebral thromboembolism. In: Siekert RG, Wishnant JGS, eds. Cerebral Vascular Diseases. Philadelphia: Grune & Stratton; 1961: 160–175

Meyer JS, Gilroy J, Barnhart MI, Johnson JF. Therapeutic thrombolysis in cerebral thromboembolism: double-blind evaluation of intravenous plasmin therapy in carotid and middle cerebral arterial occlusion. Neurology 1963;13:927–937

Meyer JS, Gilroy J, Barnahrt ME, et al. Therapeutic thrombolysis in cerebral thromboembolism: Randomized evaluation of intravenous streptokinase. In: Millikan CH, Siekert RG, Wishnant JGS, eds. Cerebral Vascular Diseases. Fourth Princeton Conference. New York: Grune & Stratton; 1965: 200–213

Mishra NK, Albers GW, Davis SM, et al. Mismatch-based delayed thrombolysis: a meta-analysis. Stroke 2010;41(1):e25–e33

Molina CA, Barreto AD, Tsivgoulis G, et al. Transcranial ultrasound in clinical sonothrombolysis (TUCSON) trial. Ann Neurol 2009;66(1):28–38

Mori E, Yoneda Y, Tabuchi M, et al. Intravenous recombinant tissue plasminogen activator in acute carotid artery territory stroke. Neurology 1992;42(5):976–982

Mori E, Minematsu K, Nakagawara J, Yamaguchi T, Sasaki M, Hirano T; Japan Alteplase Clinical Trial II Group. Effects of 0.6 mg/kg intravenous alteplase on vascular and clinical outcomes in middle cerebral artery occlusion: Japan Alteplase Clinical Trial II (J-ACT II). Stroke 2010;41(3):461–465

Multicentre Acute Stroke Trial—Italy (MAST-I) Group. Randomised controlled trial of streptokinase, aspirin, and combination of both in treatment of acute ischaemic stroke. Lancet 1995;346(8989):1509–1514

Multicenter Acute Stroke Trial—Europe Study Group. Thrombolytic therapy with streptokinase in acute ischemic stroke. N Engl J Med 1996;335(3):145–150

National Institute of Neurological Disorders and Stroke rt-PA Stroke Study Group. Tissue plasminogen activator for acute ischemic stroke. N Engl J Med 1995;333(24):1581–1587

Naess H, Idicula T, Lagallo N, Brogger J, Waje-Andreassen U, Thomassen L. Inverse relationship of baseline body temperature and outcome between ischemic stroke patients treated and not treated with thrombolysis: the Bergen stroke study. Acta Neurol Scand 2010;122(6):414–417

Paciaroni M, Agnelli G, Caso V, et al. Acute hyperglycemia and early hemorrhagic transformation in ischemic stroke. Cerebrovasc Dis 2009;28(2):119–123

Palumbo V, Boulanger JM, Hill MD, Inzitari D, Buchan AM; CASES Investigators. Leukoaraiosis and intracerebral hemorrhage after thrombolysis in acute stroke. Neurology 2007; 68(13):1020–1024

Pérez de la Ossa N, Millán M, Arenillas JF, et al. Influence of direct admission to Comprehensive Stroke Centers on the outcome of acute stroke patients treated with intravenous thrombolysis. J Neurol 2009;256(8):1270–1276

Poppe AY, Buchan AM, Hill MD. Intravenous thrombolysis for acute ischaemic stroke in young adult patients. Can J Neurol Sci 2009a;36(2):161–167

Poppe AY, Majumdar SR, Jeerakathil T, Ghali W, Buchan AM, Hill MD; Canadian Alteplase for Stroke Effectiveness Study Investigators. Admission hyperglycemia predicts a worse outcome in stroke patients treated with intravenous thrombolysis. Diabetes Care 2009b;32(4):617–622

Preissner KT. Biochemistry and physiology of blood coagulation and fibrinolysis. [Article in German] Hamostaseologie 2004;24(2):84–93

Putaala J, Metso TM, Metso AJ, et al. Thrombolysis in young adults with ischemic stroke. Stroke 2009;40(6):2085–2091

Reeves M, Bhatt A, Jajou P, Brown M, Lisabeth L. Sex differences in the use of intravenous rt-PA thrombolysis treatment for acute ischemic stroke: a meta-analysis. Stroke 2009; 40(5):1743–1749

Sanák D, Herzig R, Král M, et al. Is atrial fibrillation associated with poor outcome after thrombolysis? J Neurol 2010; 257(6):999–1003

Schonewille WJ, Wijman CA, Michel P, et al; BASICS study group. Treatment and outcomes of acute basilar artery occlusion in the Basilar Artery International Cooperation Study (BASICS): a prospective registry study. Lancet Neurol 2009; 8(8):724–730

Slivka A, Pulsinelli W. Hemorrhagic complications of thrombolytic therapy in experimental stroke. Stroke 1987;18(6):1148–1156

Smith EE, Abdullah AR, Petkovska I, Rosenthal E, Koroshetz WJ, Schwamm LH. Poor outcomes in patients who do not receive

6 Thrombolysis

Treatment of Acute Ischemic Stroke

II

intravenous tissue plasminogen activator because of mild or improving ischemic stroke. Stroke 2005;36(11):2497–2499

Thijs VN, Peeters A, Vosko M, et al. Randomized, placebo-controlled, dose-ranging clinical trial of intravenous microplasmin in patients with acute ischemic stroke. Stroke 2009;40(12):3789–3795

Thomalla G, Schwark C, Sobesky J, et al; MRI in Acute Stroke Study Group of the German Competence Network Stroke. Outcome and symptomatic bleeding complications of intravenous thrombolysis within 6 hours in MRI-selected stroke patients: comparison of a German multicenter study with the pooled data of ATLANTIS, ECASS, and NINDS tPA trials. Stroke 2006;37(3):852–858

National Institute of Neurological Disorders and Stroke rt-PA Stroke Study Group. Tissue plasminogen activator for acute ischemic stroke. N Engl J Med 1995;333(24):1581–1587

Toni D, Lorenzano S, Agnelli G, et al. Intravenous thrombolysis with rt-PA in acute ischemic stroke patients aged older than 80 years in Italy. Cerebrovasc Dis 2008;25(1-2):129–135

Tsivgoulis G, Frey JL, Flaster M, et al. Pre-tissue plasminogen activator blood pressure levels and risk of symptomatic intracerebral hemorrhage. Stroke 2009;40(11):3631–3634

Tsivgoulis G, Eggers J, Ribo M, et al. Safety and efficacy of ultrasound-enhanced thrombolysis: a comprehensive review and meta-analysis of randomized and nonrandomized studies. Stroke 2010;41(2):280–287

Uyttenboogaart M, Koch MW, Koopman K, Vroomen PC, De Keyser J, Luijckx GJ. Safety of antiplatelet therapy prior to intravenous thrombolysis in acute ischemic stroke. Arch Neurol 2008;65(5):607–611

Wahlgren N, Ahmed N, Dávalos A, et al; SITS-MOST investigators. Thrombolysis with alteplase for acute ischaemic stroke in the Safe Implementation of Thrombolysis in Stroke-Monitoring Study (SITS-MOST): an observational study. Lancet 2007;369(9558):275–282

Wahlgren N, Ahmed N, Dávalos A, et al; SITS investigators. Thrombolysis with alteplase 3-4.5 h after acute ischaemic stroke (SITS-ISTR): an observational study. Lancet 2008;372(9646):1303–1309

Wardlaw JM, Zoppo G, Yamaguchi T, et al. Thrombolysis for acute ischaemic stroke. Cochrane Database Syst Rev 2003;3:CD 000213

Wardlaw JM, Murray V, Berge E, et al. Thrombolysis for acute ischaemic stroke. Cochrane Database Syst Rev 2009;4:CD 000213

Winkler DT, Fluri F, Fuhr P, et al. Thrombolysis in stroke mimics: frequency, clinical characteristics, and outcome. Stroke 2009;40(4):1522–1525

Yamaguchi T, Mori E, Minematsu K, et al; Japan Alteplase Clinical Trial (J-ACT) Group. Alteplase at 0.6 mg/kg for acute ischemic stroke within 3 hours of onset: Japan Alteplase Clinical Trial (J-ACT). Stroke 2006;37(7):1810–1815

Zhang L, Zhang ZG, Buller B, et al. Combination treatment with VELCADE and low-dose tissue plasminogen activator provides potent neuroprotection in aged rats after embolic focal ischemia. Stroke 2010;41(5):1001–1007

Zivin JA, Fisher M, DeGirolami U, Hemenway CC, Stashak JA. Tissue plasminogen activator reduces neurological damage after cerebral embolism. Science 1985;230(4731):1289–1292

Intra-arterial Thrombolysis

Adams HP Jr, Effron MB, Torner J, et al; AbESTT-II Investigators. Emergency administration of abciximab for treatment of patients with acute ischemic stroke: results of an international phase III trial: Abciximab in Emergency Treatment of Stroke Trial (AbESTT-II). Stroke 2008;39(1):87–99

Arnold M, Nedeltchev K, Schroth G, et al. Clinical and radiological predictors of recanalisation and outcome of 40 patients with acute basilar artery occlusion treated with intra-arterial thrombolysis. J Neurol Neurosurg Psychiatry 2004;75(6):857–862

Brandt T, Pessin M, Kwan A, et al. Survival with basilar artery occlusion. Cerebrovasc Dis 1995;5:182–187

Brandt T, von Kummer R, Müller-Küppers M, Hacke W. Thrombolytic therapy of acute basilar artery occlusion. Variables affecting recanalization and outcome. Stroke 1996;27(5):875–881

Cloft HJ, Rabinstein A, Lanzino G, Kallmes DF. Intra-arterial stroke therapy: an assessment of demand and available work force. AJNR Am J Neuroradiol 2009;30(3):453–458

del Zoppo GJ, Higashida RT, Furlan AJ, Pessin MS, Rowley HA, Gent M. PROACT: a phase II randomized trial of recombinant pro-urokinase by direct arterial delivery in acute middle cerebral artery stroke. PROACT Investigators. Prolyse in Acute Cerebral Thromboembolism. Stroke 1998;29(1):4–11

Donnan GA, Davis SM, Chambers BR, et al. Streptokinase for acute ischemic stroke with relationship to time of administration: Australian Streptokinase (ASK) Trial Study Group. JAMA 1996;276(12):961–966

Eckert B, Kucinski T, Pfeiffer G, Groden C, Zeumer H. Endovascular therapy of acute vertebrobasilar occlusion: early treatment onset as the most important factor. Cerebrovasc Dis 2002;14(1):42–50

Eckert B, Kucinski T, Neumaier-Probst E, Fiehler J, Röther J, Zeumer H. Local intra-arterial fibrinolysis in acute hemispheric stroke: effect of occlusion type and fibrinolytic agent on recanalization success and neurological outcome. Cerebrovasc Dis 2003;15(4):258–263

Eckert B, Koch C, Thomalla G, et al. Aggressive therapy with intravenous abciximab and intra-arterial rtPA and additional PTA/stenting improves clinical outcome in acute vertebrobasilar occlusion: combined local fibrinolysis and intravenous abciximab in acute vertebrobasilar stroke treatment (FAST): results of a multicenter study. Stroke 2005;36(6):1160–1165

Freitag HJ, Becker VU, Thie A, et al. Lys-plasminogen as an adjunct to local intra-arterial fibrinolysis for carotid territory stroke: laboratory and clinical findings. Neuroradiology 1996;38(2):181–185

Furlan A, Higashida R, Wechsler L, et al. Intra-arterial prourokinase for acute ischemic stroke. The PROACT II study: a randomized controlled trial. Prolyse in Acute Cerebral Thromboembolism. JAMA 1999;282(21):2003–2011

Hacke W, Zeumer H, Ferbert A, Brückmann H, del Zoppo GJ. Intra-arterial thrombolytic therapy improves outcome in patients with acute vertebrobasilar occlusive disease. Stroke 1988;19(10):1216–1222

Hacke W, Kaste M, Fieschi C, et al; The European Cooperative Acute Stroke Study (ECASS). Intravenous thrombolysis with recombinant tissue plasminogen activator for acute hemispheric stroke. JAMA 1995;274(13):1017–1025

Hacke W, Kaste M, Fieschi C, et al; Second European-Australasian Acute Stroke Study Investigators. Randomised double-blind placebo-controlled trial of thrombolytic therapy with intravenous alteplase in acute ischaemic stroke (ECASS II). Lancet 1998;352(9136):1245–1251

Hacke W, Albers G, Al-Rawi Y, et al; DIAS Study Group. The Desmoteplase in Acute Ischemic Stroke Trial (DIAS): a phase II MRI-based 9-hour window acute stroke thrombolysis trial with intravenous desmoteplase. Stroke 2005;36(1):66–73

Hacke W, Kaste M, Bluhmki E, et al; ECASS Investigators. Thrombolysis with alteplase 3 to 4.5 hours after acute ischemic stroke. N Engl J Med 2008;359(13):1317–1329

Hacke W, Furlan AJ, Al-Rawi Y, et al. Intravenous desmoteplase in patients with acute ischaemic stroke selected by MRI perfusion-diffusion weighted imaging or perfusion CT (DIAS-2): a prospective, randomised, double-blind, placebo-controlled study. Lancet Neurol 2009;8(2):141–150

Jaillard A, Cornu C, Durieux A, et al; MAST-E Group. Hemorrhagic transformation in acute ischemic stroke. The MAST-E study. Stroke 1999;30(7):1326–1332

Jakubowska MM, Michels P, Müller-Jensen A, Leppien A, Eckert B. Endovascular treatment in proximal and intracranial carotid occlusion 9 hours after symptom onset. Neuroradiology 2008;50(7):599–604

Jansen O, von Kummer R, Forsting M, Hacke W, Sartor K. Thrombolytic therapy in acute occlusion of the intracranial internal carotid artery bifurcation. AJNR Am J Neuroradiol 1995;16(10):1977–1986

Kaur J, Zhao Z, Klein GM, Lo EH, Buchan AM. The neurotoxicity of tissue plasminogen activator? J Cereb Blood Flow Metab 2004;24(9):945–963

Lindsberg PJ, Soinne L, Tatlisumak T, et al. Long-term outcome after intravenous thrombolysis of basilar artery occlusion. JAMA 2004;292(15):1862–1866

Lindsberg PJ, Mattle HP. Therapy of basilar artery occlusion: a systematic analysis comparing intra-arterial and intravenous thrombolysis. Stroke 2006;37(3):922–928

Mattle HP, Arnold M, Georgiadis D, et al. Comparison of intra-arterial and intravenous thrombolysis for ischemic stroke with hyperdense middle cerebral artery sign. Stroke 2008;39(2):379–383

Multicentre Acute Stroke Trial—Italy (MAST-I) Group. Randomised controlled trial of streptokinase, aspirin, and combination of both in treatment of acute ischaemic stroke. Lancet 1995;346(8989):1509–1514

National Institute of Neurological Disorders and Stroke rtPA Stroke Study Group. Tissue plasminogen activator for acute ischemic stroke. N Engl J Med 1995;333(24):1581–1587

Nedeltchev K, Arnold M, Brekenfeld C, et al. Pre- and in-hospital delays from stroke onset to intra-arterial thrombolysis. Stroke 2003;34(5):1230–1234

Nogueira RG, Yoo AJ, Buonanno FS, Hirsch JA. Endovascular approaches to acute stroke, part 2: a comprehensive review of studies and trials. AJNR Am J Neuroradiol 2009;30(5):859–875

Pfefferkorn T, Holtmannspötter M, Schmidt C, et al. Drip, ship, and retrieve: cooperative recanalization therapy in acute basilar artery occlusion. Stroke 2010;41(4):722–726

Philipps J, Thomalla G, Glahn J, Schwarze M, Rother J. Treatment of progressive stroke with tirofiban—experience in 35 patients. Cerebrovasc Dis 2009;28(5):435–438

Qureshi AI, Siddiqui AM, Kim SH, et al. Reocclusion of recanalized arteries during intra-arterial thrombolysis for acute ischemic stroke. AJNR Am J Neuroradiol 2004;25(2):322–328

Schonewille WJ, Wijman CA, Michel P, et al; BASICS study group. Treatment and outcomes of acute basilar artery occlusion in the Basilar Artery International Cooperation Study (BASICS): a prospective registry study. Lancet Neurol 2009;8(8):724–730

Schulte-Altedorneburg G, Hamann GF, Mull M, et al. Outcome of acute vertebrobasilar occlusions treated with intra-arterial fibrinolysis in 180 patients. AJNR Am J Neuroradiol 2006;27(10):2042–2047

Shaltoni HM, Albright KC, Gonzales NR, et al. Is intra-arterial thrombolysis safe after full-dose intravenous recombinant tissue plasminogen activator for acute ischemic stroke? Stroke 2007;38(1):80–84

Sherman DG, Atkinson RP, Chippendale T, et al. Intravenous ancrod for treatment of acute ischemic stroke: the STAT study: a randomized controlled trial. Stroke Treatment with Ancrod Trial. JAMA 2000;283(18):2395–2403

Siebler M, Hennerici MG, Schneider D, et al. Safety of tirofiban in acute ischemic stroke: The SaTIS trial. Stroke 2011;42(9):2388–2392

Tomsick TA, Khatri P, Jovin T, et al; IMS III Executive Committee. Equipoise among recanalization strategies. Neurology 2010;74(13):1069–1076

Zeumer H, Hacke W, Kolmann HL, Poeck K. Local fibrinolysis in basilar artery thrombosis (author's transl). [Article in German] Dtsch Med Wochenschr 1982;107(19):728–731

II

7 Mechanical Recanalization Materials

Aspiration Thrombectomy

A. Kreusch and M. Knauth

Introduction

The standard treatment for acute ischemic stroke is systemic (intravenous) pharmacologic thrombolysis. This therapy is widely practiced and is rapidly available following the exclusion of intracranial hemorrhage. Large, randomized, placebo-controlled double-blind studies on intravenous thrombolysis (ECASS, NINDS, ATLANTIS; **Table 7.1**) have shown, however, that no more than 1 in 8 patients (13%) will benefit from this therapy compared with placebo and will be able to live a (largely) independent life with no disability in daily activities (mRS $\leq$ 2) (National Institute of Neurological Disorders and Stroke tPA Stroke Study Group 1995). Only patients treated within the first 3 h of stroke onset were enrolled in the NINDS study.

The ECASS III study showed that stroke patients can benefit from intravenous thrombolysis even beyond a time window of 4.5 h after symptom onset (Hacke et al. 2008). Longer periods of time to (intravenous) treatment are associated with higher mortality and decreased benefit from intravenous thrombolysis (Lees et al. 2010).

In a meta-analysis of 53 studies on the importance of vascular recanalization in acute ischemic stroke, Rha and Saver (2007) found that recanalization had a high correlation with good functional outcomes and reduced mortality. Intra-arterial recanalization techniques were associated with significantly higher success rates than intravenous thrombolysis.

The length of a vascular occlusion is a limiting factor in the efficacy of systemic intravenous thrombolysis. While intravenous thrombolysis can produce recanalization in 63% of cases where thrombus length was < 4 mm, the recanalization rate fell to 1% when thrombus length was > 8 mm (Riedel and Jansen 2009).

> **Note**
>
> In these cases, and/or cases treated outside the time window, mechanical recanalization is a potentially important option that can be used alone or in conjunction with systemic thrombolysis to achieve complete recanalization. Mechanical recanalization may employ any of three main principles: thrombus aspiration, thrombus extraction, or thrombus fragmentation.

Mechanical recanalization systems currently on the market can be subdivided into three groups based on their relationship to the intravascular thrombus:
- *Proximal systems:* These devices engage and remove the clot from the proximal side (e.g., Penumbra System, Snare, Alligator, AngioJet, EPAR).
- *Distal systems:* These devices are deployed past the thrombus—that is, they must first be advanced through the thrombus and positioned behind it (e.g., MERCI, Catch, Phenox pCR/CRC, Lazarus, Neuronet, Snare).
- *On-the-spot systems:* These devices are deployed within the thrombus (e.g., EKOS, stents, stent-like retrievers such as Solitaire, Bonnet, Trevo, Mindframe, ReVive, and the Penumbra System).

The first aspiration thrombectomies were successfully performed with simple catheters which were particularly useful in the vertebrobasilar system.

The AngioJet device (Minneapolis, MN) was developed for cardiologic and peripheral vascular recanalizations. To date, most published reports on the device have dealt with cerebrovascular applications for venous sinus thrombosis. A directional fluid jet in the catheter creates a suction effect that draws pieces of the thrombus into side holes where they are fragmented and evacuated through the catheter.

Penumbra System

The Penumbra System is widely used for mechanical recanalization in acute ischemic stroke. Classified as a proximal or on-the-spot system, it employs a combined principle of thrombus aspiration and extraction. However, based on the practice at our hospital and surveys of neurointerventionalist colleagues, we find that, at least in Germany, the system is used almost exclusively in the aspiration mode and is very rarely used for clot extraction.

The Penumbra System was developed by Penumbra, Inc. (Alameda, CA, USA) and received FDA approval in late 2007. Besides the MERCI Retriever from Concentric Medical, Inc. (Mountain View, CA, USA), the Penumbra System is currently the only device approved by the United States Food and Drug Administration (FDA) for the mechanical recanalization of patients with acute ischemic stroke in cases where intravenous thrombolysis is contraindicated or unsuccessful.

Table 7.1 Overview of key studies dealing with the treatment of acute ischemic stroke

Therapy	Studies	Number of patients and initial NIHSS	Mean time to treatment (min)	Recanalization rate (%)	Good clinical outcome (mRS ≤ 2 at 90 days; %)	Mortality (at 90 days; %)	Symptomatic intracerebral hemorrhage (%)
Intravenous thrombolysis	NINDS (NINDS rtPA Stroke Study Group 1997)	n = 312 Ø NIHSS = 14	115 ± 36.7	n.s.	50.3	17	6.4
Intravenous thrombolysis	ATLANTIS (Clark et al. 1999)	n = 272 Ø NIHSS = 11	276	n.s.	42.3 (mRS = 0–1)	11	10
	ECASS (Hacke et al. 1995)	n = 313 Ø NIHSS = 14	264	n.s.	35.7 (mRS = 0–1)	22.4	(?)
	ECASS II (Hacke et al. 1998)	n = 409 Ø NIHSS = 11	n.s.	n.s.	40.3 (mRS = 0–1)	10.5	8.8
	ECASS III (Hacke et al. 2008)	n = 418 Ø NIHSS = 9	236	n.s.	52.4 (mRS = 0–1)	7.7	2.4
Intra-arterial thrombolysis	PROACT I (del Zoppo et al. 1998)	n = 26 Ø NIHSS = 17	324	57.7	30.8 (mRS = 0–1)	26.9	15.4
	PROACT II (Furlan et al. 1999)	n = 121 Ø NIHSS = 17	282	66	40	25	10
	MELT (Ogawa et al. 2007)	n = 114 Ø NIHSS = 14	199 ± 61	73.7	49.1	5.3	9
Intravenous + intra-arterial thrombolysis	IMS I (IMS Study Investigators 2004)	n = 80 Ø NIHSS = 18	IVT: 136 ± 30 IAT: 217 ± 46	56	43	16	6.3
	IMS II (IMS II Trial Investigators 2007)	n = 81 Ø NIHSS = 19	140 ± 31	58	46	16	9.9
Intravenous thrombolysis + mechanical	RECANALISE (Mazighi et al. 2009)	n = 46 Ø NIHSS = 14	132	87	57	17	9
Intravenous vs. intra-arterial thrombolysis	Mattle et al. (2008)	IVT: n = 57; Ø NIHSS = 18 IAT: n = 55; Ø NIHSS = 17	IVT: 156 ± 21 IAT: 244 ± 63	IVT: n.s. IAT: 71	IVT: 23 IAT: 53	IVT: 23 IAT: 7	IVT: 2 IVT: 7

(continued)

Treatment of Acute Ischemic Stroke

Table 7.1 Overview of key studies dealing with the treatment of acute ischemic stroke *(continued)*

Therapy	Studies	Number of patients and initial NIHSS	Mean time to treatment (min)	Recanalization rate (%)	Good clinical outcome (mRS ≤ 2 at 90 days; %)	Mortality (at 90 days; %)	Symptomatic intracerebral hemorrhage (%)
Penumbra System	Bose et al. (2008)	N = 23 Ø NIHSS = 21	n.s.	100	45 (at 30 days)	45 (at 30 days)	10
	Huded et al. (2009)	n = 5 Ø NIHSS = 26.8	348	100	40	40	0
	Penumbra Pivotal Stroke Trial (Penumbra Pivotal Stroke Trial Investigators 2009)	n = 125 Ø NIHSS = 17.6	258 ± 90	81.6	25	32.8	11.2
	Struffert et al. (2009)	n = 15 Ø NIHSS = 15	151	80	42	25	0
	Grunwald et al. (2009)	n = 29 Ø NIHSS = 20	312 ± 107	86.2	37.9	13.9 (at 30 days)	7
	Kulcsár et al. (2010a)	n = 27 Ø NIHSS = 14	266	93	48	11	0
	Menon et al. (2011)	n = 27 Ø NIHSS = 18	192	67	48.1	18.5	7.4
	Our results (2010)	n = 86 Ø NIHSS = 18	321	77.9	33	23.2	4.6
MERCI	MERCI (Smith et al. 2005)	n = 141 Ø NIHSS = 20	258 ± 102	60.3	27.7	44	7.8
	Multi-MERCI (Smith et al. 2008)	n = 164 Ø NIHSS = 19	258	68	36	34	9.8
	Kim et al. (2006)	n = 24 Ø NIHSS = 21	303	63	25	29	8
	Devlin et al. (2007)	n = 25 Ø NIHSS = 18	258	56	24	36	4

Ø, average; IVT, intravenous thrombolysis; mRS, modified Rankin Scale; n.s., not stated; IAT, intra-arterial thrombolysis; NIHSS, National Institute of Health Stroke Scale.

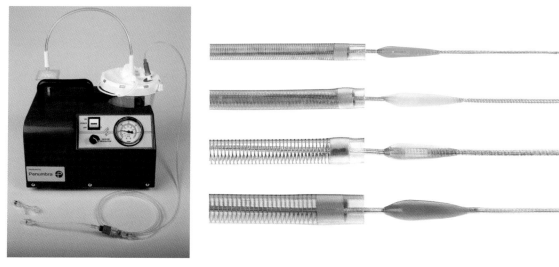

Fig. 7.1 Components of the Penumbra System (with kind permission of Penumbra Europe GmbH, Berlin, Germany).

The Penumbra System consists of five main components (**Fig. 7.1**):

- Reperfusion catheter
- Separator
- Aspiration pump
- Aspiration tubing
- Canister

Since the Penumbra System was introduced, seven studies and single-center study results have been published on this new treatment option; a randomized control study has not yet been conducted (see **Table 7.1**).

Indications and Contraindications

Practical Tip
Before mechanical recanalization starts, it must be confirmed that the patient has suffered a (symptomatic) ischemic stroke in the intracranial vascular system. Intracranial hemorrhage must be excluded. Patient selection requires an imaging study that can demonstrate the vascular occlusion and assess the size of the definitive infarction.

The Penumbra System is designed for the revascularization of large intracranial vessels—the internal carotid artery (ICA), the M1 and M2 segments of the middle cerebral artery (MCA), the basilar artery, and the vertebral arteries. The manufacturer states that the device should be used within the first 8 h from stroke onset, although there are no hard data to support this recommendation. There are patients who will no longer benefit from recanalization within a considerably shorter time frame because the entire territory supplied by the occluded vessel is already infarcted. Conversely, imaging criteria may identify patients who will still benefit from (mechanical) recanalization even after a longer interval from symptom onset. This particularly applies to vertebrobasilar strokes.

Technique

Percutaneous arterial access is established at a peripheral site, usually the right common femoral artery, using aseptic technique, and a sheath is introduced. Next, a guide catheter or long sheath, flushed continuously with heparinized saline solution, is introduced over a guidewire. This is followed by selective catheterization and angiographic visualization of the intracranial vessels to determine the location and extent of the thrombotic occlusion and assess collateral circulation.

When perfusion status has been assessed and the decision to proceed with mechanical recanalization has been made, the reperfusion catheter is advanced to the primary occlusion site with the help of a micro-guidewire. The selected size of the reperfusion catheter depends on the site of the occlusion, the vessel diameter at that site, and the tortuosity of the approach. Penumbra reperfusion catheters and separators are available in four different sizes for vessels ranging from < 2 to > 4 mm in diameter (**Table 7.2**).

Table 7.2 Available catheter sizes of the Penumbra System

Reperfusion catheter	Outer diameter (F)	Inner diameter (mm)	Length (cm)
026	2.8	0.66	154
032	3.4	0.81	154
041	4.1	1.04	141
054	5.0	1.37	136

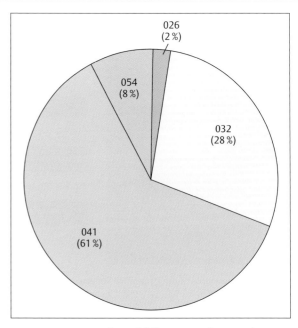

Fig. 7.3   Frequency of use of different reperfusion catheter sizes in the Penumbra System. The 041 reperfusion catheter, with an outer diameter of 4.1F and a luminal diameter of 1.04 mm, is most commonly used.

The reperfusion catheter is navigated to the site of the vascular occlusion, and the separator is advanced through the reperfusion catheter. Its function is to facilitate aspiration of the thrombus and prevent clogging of the aspiration catheter.

The aspiration pump, which is connected to the reperfusion catheter by tubing, generates a continuous suction of −20 inches of mercury (= −677.2 mbar). Mechanical recanalization is achieved by repeatedly advancing and retracting the separator through the reperfusion catheter and thrombus while the fragments are aspirated through the catheter (**Fig. 7.2**).

The 041 reperfusion catheter is the size most often used at our hospital in Göttingen, Germany. To date we have used it in 61% of interventions. The 041 catheter can reach occlusions as far as the M1 segment of the MCA and in the vertebrobasilar system, depending on individual circumstances. The 032 and 026 catheter sizes are better for accessing more distal thrombi or secondary emboli (**Fig. 7.3**).

An average of 1.47 Penumbra Systems are used per intervention at our center. Exchanges may be necessitated by a distal taper of the vessel diameter or the fragility of the separator tip, which should be replaced after several reperfusion maneuvers.

Various grading scales can be used to document vascular status before and after mechanical recanalization. The TICI score (Thrombolysis in Cerebral Infarction; **Table 7.3**) is widely employed (Higashida et al. 2003). Other scoring systems are the TIMI (Thrombolysis in Myocardial Infarction; see the section on Concepts, and **Table 8.1**, p. 111) and the Qureshi Grading System.

Complications

> **Note**
>
> On the whole, it has been our experience that few complications arise during mechanical recanalization.

The most frequent complication in our patients was intracerebral vasospasm, which occurred in 8.1% of interventions but was easily managed with drug therapy. Symptomatic intracranial hemorrhage occurred in 4.6% of our patients. Incidences of 0–11.2% have been reported in previous publications on the Penumbra System (see **Table 7.1**). Thus, the rates of symptomatic intracranial hemorrhage at our center are no higher than the rates reported in large studies of intravenous thrombolysis (e.g., ECASS III). We experienced a 4.6% rate of periprocedural iatrogenic dissections of the ICA. In all of these cases, significant disruption of blood flow was prevented by careful stenting of the dissection. We have had two cases of separator breakage (2.3%) at our center. Because the break occurred at a proximal site, retrieval was easily accomplished in both cases. In another published case (Kulcsár et al. 2010) the distal tip of the separator broke off and was lost in the thrombus of the M2 segment. Menon et al. (2011) observed distal emboli in 48.1% of their patients treated with the Penumbra System. Other publications did not make significant mention of this phenomenon.

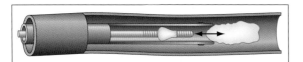

Fig. 7.2   Functional principle of the Penumbra System (with kind permission of Penumbra Europe GmbH, Berlin, Germany).

Table 7.3 TICI perfusion categories (after Higashida et al. 2003)

TICI grade	Perfusion	Description
0	No perfusion	No antegrade flow beyond the point of occlusion
1	Penetration with minimal perfusion	The contrast material passes beyond the area of obstruction but fails to opacify the entire cerebral bed distal to the obstruction for the duration of the angiographic run
2	Partial perfusion	The contrast material passes beyond the obstruction and opacifies the arterial bed distal to the obstruction. However, the rate of entry of contrast into the vessel distal to the obstruction and/or its rate of clearance from the distal bed are perceptibly slower than its entry into and/or clearance from comparable areas not perfused by the previously occluded vessel, e.g., the opposite cerebral artery or the arterial bed proximal to the obstruction
2a		Only partial filling ($<\frac{2}{3}$) of the entire vascular territory is visualized
2b		Complete filling of all of the expected vascular territory is visualized, but the filling is slower than normal
3	Complete perfusion	Antegrade flow into the bed distal to the obstruction occurs as promptly as into the obstruction and clearance of contrast material from the involved bed is as rapid as from an uninvolved bed of the same vessel or the opposite cerebral artery

Other complications have been reported in a few sporadic cases:
- Inguinal hematoma
- Reocclusion of the target vessel
- Vascular perforation
- Vascular dissection
- Infarction in a new vascular territory

Recanalization Rate and Neurologic Outcome

Among the patients treated at our center, 79% of the vascular occlusions were located in the anterior circulation and 21% were in the vertebrobasilar system. Partial or complete recanalization, corresponding to a TICI score of 2 or 3, was achieved in 77.9% of the interventions with the Penumbra System. The following treatment modalities were used:
- Mechanical only: 18.2%
- Intravenous thrombolysis + mechanical: 11.4%
- Intra-arterial thrombolysis + mechanical: 34.1%
- Intravenous thrombolysis + intra-arterial thrombolysis + mechanical: 36.4%

In the studies published thus far, the Penumbra System, usually combined with chemical thrombolysis, has achieved high recanalization rates with a weighted average of 82.25% (67–100%; see **Table 7.1**). To date, these high recanalization rates have been matched only by stent-like recanalization systems such as Solitaire or Trevo used in small experimental series. In an initial trial of the MERCI Retriever, also approved for mechanical thrombectomy, recanalization was achieved in 48% of patients in whom the device was deployed (Smith et al. 2005). The subsequent Multi MERCI trial (Smith et al. 2008) achieved a recanalization rate of 69.5%. In both trials, thrombolytic agents were used as an adjunct to recanalization with the MERCI device.

Thus, the rates for recanalizing cerebral vessels with aspiration systems are considerably higher than the rates reported in a meta-analysis by Rha and Saver (2007) for spontaneous (24.1%), intravenous (46.2%), and intra-arterial fibrinolysis (63.2% of patients treated).

At our center, we documented a good clinical outcome after rehabilitation (mRS $\leq$ 2) in 33% of the patients treated with the Penumbra System. While 39% of the successfully recanalized patients achieved an mRS $\leq$ 2, only 19% of patients did so in the cohort without successful recanalization. Previously published clinical data on the Penumbra System also indicate a weighted average of 33.55% (25–48.1%) for a good clinical outcome 90 days after the stroke event. An average of 31.1% (24–36%) of patients treated with the MERCI Retriever had a good clinical outcome at 90 days.

A more striking difference was found in the weighted mortality rates at 90 days: 27.49% (11–40%) for the Penumbra System vs. 37.78% (29–44%) for the MERCI Retriever.

In a direct comparison of intravenous and intra-arterial thrombolysis in comparable patients with a HMCAS on cranial CT, Mattle et al. (2008) documented a significantly better outcome in patients treated with intra-arterial thrombolysis. When we compare these findings with the results in our own patients with carotid-T and MCA occlusions that would be expected to have a HMCAS on cranial CT, we find a similarly good clinical outcome in patients who were successfully recanalized (TICI score of 2–3; **Fig. 7.4**).

II

Treatment of Acute Ischemic Stroke

II

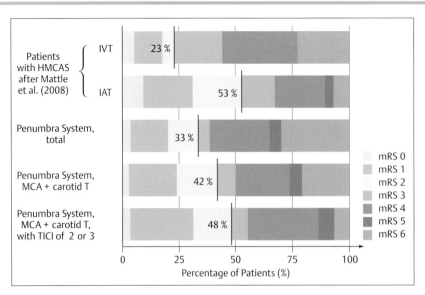

Fig. 7.4 Comparison of clinical outcomes of treatment with intravenous and intra-arterial fibrinolysis (after Mattle et al. 2008) or after mechanical recanalization with the Penumbra System in patients with a HMCAS. An mRS of 2 or less at 90 days after the stroke event is interpreted as a good outcome. HMCAS, hyperdense middle cerebral artery sign; IAT, intra-arterial thrombolysis; IVT, intravenous thrombolysis; TICI, thrombolysis in Cerebral Infarction Score (after Higashida et al. 2003).

Combination Therapies

In principle, it should be possible to combine aspiration therapy with other recanalization techniques. **Table 7.4** shows the possible combinations that may be used in clinical practice.

A combination of pharmacologic and mechanical thrombolysis in the patients at our center yielded a higher recanalization rate (average of 75.0%; $n = 58$) than with use of the aspiration system alone (average of 72.2%; $n = 18$).

Practical Tip

We achieved particularly good recanalization results by combining copious intravenous bridging thrombolysis (> 20 mg rtPA) with subsequent use of the Penumbra System. One possible explanation is that preliminary rtPA therapy "softened" the thrombus and made it easier to aspirate.

The addition of intra-arterial thrombolysis should further reduce the thrombus burden at the primary occlusion site, further improve perfusion beyond the revascularized occlusion, and dissolve any distal emboli that may be present.

Table 7.4 Possible combinations of the Penumbra System with other treatment modalities

	Possible combinations			
	1	2	3	4
Penumbra System	x	x	x	x
Intravenous thrombolysis		x	x	
Intra-arterial thrombolysis			x	x

Case Report

A 25-year-old woman was transferred from another hospital with a suspected left hemispheric stroke marked by a progressive decline in vigilance, decreased movement on the right side of the body, and positive pyramidal tract signs on the right side (NIHSS = 14, mRS = 5). Multimodal MRI revealed an occlusion of the left MCA (**Fig. 7.5a**) with a significant perfusion delay in the affected territory; the diffusion abnormality was still relatively small (**Fig. 7.5b, c**). After the exclusion of intracranial hemorrhage, the patient was selected for mechanical thrombolysis. Angiography commenced at 4.5 h after symptom onset using a 6F Envoy catheter to define the intracranial vessels. Angiograms confirmed a complete occlusion of the M1 segment of the MCA with a TICI score of 0 (**Fig. 7.5d**). The Penumbra 041 reperfusion catheter was positioned proximal to the thrombus, and the clot aspirated swiftly and without difficulty over a period of 24 min. Control angiograms showed complete recanalization of the MCA trunk (**Fig. 7.5e**). Then 20 mg of rtPA was slowly infused into the MCA through the indwelling guide catheter. Cranial CT on the day after mechanical thrombectomy showed a circumscribed infarction of the left basal ganglia with minimal associated hemorrhage (**Fig. 7.5f**). The infarcted area did not extend beyond the diffusion abnormality detected before the intervention.

Eighteen days later, after a period of early inpatient rehabilitation, the patient was discharged from acute hospital care to a rehabilitation facility with her clinical neurologic status significantly improved (NIHSS = 5, mRS = 2). Mild coordination problems and word-finding difficulties were still present at discharge but were successfully addressed in the 22-day rehabilitation program. The patient returned home without significant disability and is able to live an independent life (NIHSS = 0, mRS = 1).

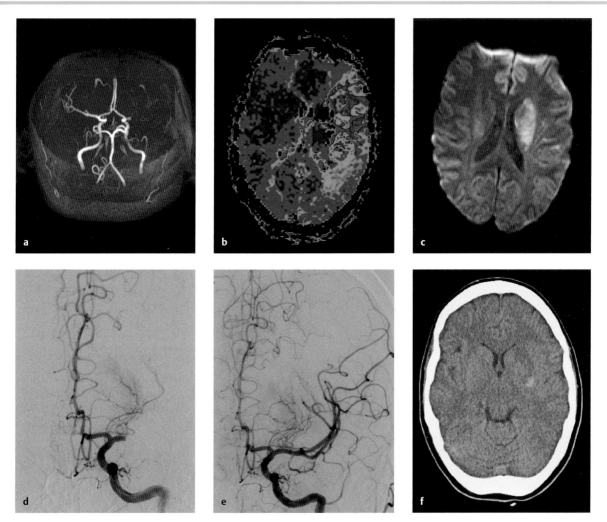

Fig. 7.5a–f   Case report of an aspiration thrombectomy with the Penumbra System.

a Initial MRA shows a complete occlusion of the left MCA.

b TTP map shows a large perfusion delay in the MCA territory.

c DWI (b = 1000) displays the hyperintense core of the infarction. The core appears small relative to the MCA territory and the area of the perfusion deficit.

d DSA confirms a complete occlusion of the M1 segment of the MCA.

e Status following successful recanalization of the M1 segment.

f Next-day cranial CT shows a left basal ganglia infarction with small associated hemorrhage. The infarcted area does not extend beyond the diffusion abnormality seen on preinterventional images.

Summary

Mechanical recanalization is already widely practiced at larger hospitals with expertise in interventional neuroradiology. The application of mechanical recanalization techniques requires a trained and experienced team of neuroradiologists who can administer the treatment safely and effectively. Nevertheless, there is still a lack of large, randomized, placebo-controlled studies on mechanical recanalization that would enable a direct comparison of functional outcomes with intravenous thrombolysis.

The Penumbra System has shown an effective recanalization success rate in clinical practice in patients with long-segment intracranial vascular occlusions, even when used beyond 4.5 h from symptom onset. Very distal occlusions are difficult to reach with the Penumbra System and therefore limit the applications of the device. Vascular kinking is another potential difficulty.

Aspiration thrombectomy is a safe procedure associated with few complications. The maximum incidence of symptomatic intracranial hemorrhage is ~10%. On the other hand, Rha and Saver (2007) found that there was no significant difference in the incidence of symptomatic hemorrhages between successfully recanalized patients and nonrecanalized patients.

Since intra-arterial therapies are performed under angiographic control, the times to treatment are longer than with intravenous thrombolysis. But this delay can be effectively offset by bridging therapy, which may consist of a single bolus injection of the fibrinolytic agent (1/10 the standard dose) or the infusion of a complete dose prior to the intervention. Early intravenous thrombolysis after the exclusion of contraindications appears to be an effective strategy based on available data and can reduce the impact of the time delay for intra-arterial therapy. Initial bridging therapy followed by mechanical thrombectomy combines the two advantages of each modality: rapid availability and high recanalization rates. In a study of stroke patients with HMCAS, Mattle et al. (2008) found that the group of patients treated by intra-arterial fibrinolysis had a significantly better outcome at 90 days than the group treated intravenously, despite the average time to treatment being 88 min longer.

Study data indicate that not all patients undergoing successful mechanical recanalization benefit from the procedure (Hussein et al. 2010). It is important, however, to distinguish between successful recanalization at the site of the arterial occlusion and successful reperfusion of the brain tissue supplied by the occluded vessel (Rha and Saver 2007). Reperfusion is probably the critical factor in terms of patient benefit. Furthermore, improved patient selection is probably one of the most important issues to achieve a higher proportion of patients with a favorable clinical outcome.

> **Note**
>
> This underscores the importance of the prompt identification and selection of patients who may potentially benefit from endovascular recanalization.

imposes strict limits for initiating an established form of recanalization therapy (see the section on Bridging Therapy, p. 76). The severity of the stroke and the site of the vascular occlusion will determine the indication for intensive multimodal intra-arterial recanalization measures, which should be instituted promptly and with the necessary technical expertise in patients with an NIHSS score $\geq$ 12 and a confirmed M1, carotid-T, or basilar artery occlusion. Self-expanding stents for the acute treatment of ischemic stroke are a promising tool in this scenario owing to the improved outcomes that result from acute recanalization (Khatri et al. 2009). Stenting has assumed greater importance since the development of retrievable self-expanding stents (Sauvageau and Levy 2006; Levy et al. 2006) and can at least provide a temporary endovascular bypass (Levy et al. 2009). The Solitaire FR system in particular goes beyond this endovascular bypass function and removes the clot distally, prompting (Seifert et al. 2011) coinage of the term "removable stent-assistant revascularization" (RSAR).

> **Note**
>
> RSAR combines the advantages of temporary stenting for immediate restoration of patency (regardless of clot composition) with those of a subsequent definitive mechanical thrombectomy. It also appears that temporary stenting can increase the efficacy of pharmacologic thrombolysis by making more surface area of the thrombus accessible to the agent and to coagulation-inhibiting blood constituents, and by enabling a faster and more effective lysis of fragmented clot residues at peripheral sites.

Temporary Stenting in Stroke Patients

J. Klisch

Introduction

Mechanical thrombectomy using the (detachable) Solitaire AB (off-label) or Solitaire FR device system (Covidien/ev3 Inc, Irvine, CA, USA), like all other endovascular recanalization techniques, should be one component of a multimodal treatment concept for acute ischemic stroke that is marked by the establishment of well-structured regional and interregional treatment pathways (Ickenstein et al. 2008). Thus, the 3-h (or 4.5-h) time window for intravenous thrombolysis with rtPA or even a 6- or 8-h time window (off-label)

At present it is unclear how the relatively high radial force exerted by the Solitaire FR device may influence the efficacy of recanalization. The Solitaire FR device exerts a radial force of 0.0106 N/mm of device length, which is ~30% greater than that exerted by the Enterprise stent, for example (Cordis Neurovascular, Miami Lakes, FL, USA).

An animal study conducted by a group of authors in Bern, Switzerland, showed that deployment of the Solitaire FR device produced immediate flow restoration across a thromboembolic occlusion in 80% of all cases. Early reocclusion occurred in one-third of the cases. Complete recanalization after retrieval of the Solitaire FR device was achieved in 86.7% of cases (Mordasini et al. 2011).

In a recent prospective single-center study of 20 patients with vascular occlusions in the anterior circulation treated within 8 h from stroke onset, Castaño et al. (2010) with the Solitaire AB device achieved a 90% recanalization rate to TIMI 2b or 3 immediately after device deployment, thus confirming the animal data cited above. Although the initial NIHSS score was 19 in this patient study, 45% of the patients still exhibited a good outcome at 3 months (mRS ≤ 2). Similar results were recently reported in small case series published by Nayak et al. (2010) with Solitaire AB and Venker et al. (2010) with Solitaire FR.

Although results from larger case series or controlled therapeutic trials are still lacking, the outlook is promising based on the results of small case series published to date and on positive experience with stent-based recanalization. Available published results also suggest that the rates of technical complications and symptomatic intracranial hemorrhage are no higher than in comparable thrombectomy studies. It should be added that several studies have already been initiated or are in preparation:

- *SWIFT study* (SOLITAIRE FR With the Intention For Thrombectomy): FDA, randomized, prospective. For more information see http://clinicaltrials.gov/ct2/show/NCT01054560.
- *STAR study* (SOLITAIRE FR Thrombectomy for Acute Recanalization: single-arm, prospective, multicenter trial, 15–20 centers, ~200 patients, time window up to 8 h from onset, follow-up at 3 months. For more information see http://clinicaltrials.gov/ct2/show/NCT01327989.

Based on personal experience and the results published to date, there is reason to believe that the RSAR principle, with its capacity for very rapid recanalization, may become a first-line modality in multimodal escalating recanalization, especially when combined with intra-arterial fibrinolysis (Castaño et al. 2009; Venker et al. 2010), and that it can be readily combined with other devices such as the Penumbra System, Phenox Clot Retriever, or MERCI Retriever and also with percutaneous transluminal angioplasty.

Patient Preparation

Although patients can undergo neurologic evaluation while awake, many patients with high NIHSS scores who are referred for mechanical thrombectomy are uncooperative, agitated, and at risk for poor outcomes due mainly to aspiration. There is also a risk that head movements may induce intracranial vascular injury during or after device deployment. For these reasons, clot removal with the Solitaire FR system should be performed under general anesthesia. Based on the results of the PROACT II study (see **Table 6.1** and **Table 7.1**), no more than 2000 IU of heparin is administered by bolus injection.

> **Caution**
>
> It is important to avoid blood pressure spikes during and after the recanalization procedure to help minimize the risk of periprocedural hemorrhage. The blood sugar level should also be closely monitored, during the intervention if possible, and should be adjusted as needed (Natarajan et al. 2011). The procedure is performed under general anesthesia.

Access

When a multiple coaxial catheter system is used (Kulcsár et al. 2010b), the recanalization measures can be safely escalated at any time without delay. In the anterior circulation, an 8F or 7F guide catheter (alternative: Cello balloon catheter for flow occlusion, Covidien/ev3 Inc, Irvine, CA, USA) is introduced into the ICA via a large-bore 8F sheath, aided by a 4F or 5F diagnostic catheter of suitable length (**Fig. 7.6a**). After the coaxial catheter has been placed in the ICA, initial aspiration is applied with two 50-mL syringes to remove relatively fresh thrombus material. An antegrade arterial flush is not used in these guide catheter systems, and the arterial saline flush serves only to prevent reflux into the guide catheter. A second catheter with the largest possible lumen is advanced coaxially through the guide catheter to provide close-up access to the intracranial occlusion site. We routinely use the 054 reperfusion catheter of the Penumbra System for this purpose (Penumbra Inc, San Leandro, CA, USA), which has a luminal diameter of 0.054 inches (1.37 mm). Other large-bore microcatheters may also be used (**Fig. 7.6b**). This later catheter is advanced over a Rebar 18 microcatheter (Covidien/ev3 Inc, Irvine, CA, USA) with a luminal diameter of 0.021 inches (0.53 mm) using a standard 0.014-inch (0.35 mm) microwire (**Fig. 7.6b, c**). A large-bore 6F guide catheter system (e.g., Envoy, Cordis Corporation, Miami Lakes, FL, USA) is used in the posterior circulation, and the other components of the coaxial system are sized accordingly (**Fig. 7.7**). Distal access catheters (DACs) are increasingly used in place of the Penumbra System.

Crossing and Extracting the Thrombus

The Rebar 18 microcatheter is very carefully advanced through the thrombus, and the Solitaire FR device is deployed. This maneuver is not technically difficult since there is no need to use an exchange wire. Continuous aspiration is applied to the 054 reperfusion catheter during this time. Just before deploying the stent, we recommend road mapping through the Rebar 18 microcatheter to help position the stent accurately with respect to thrombus length. In a study of 20 patients treated with the Solitaire device, Castaño et al. (2010) found that thrombus length appeared to be an important factor influencing the ability to achieve immediate flow restoration after stent deployment. If the thrombus is longer than the Solitaire FR device, temporary stenting should be preceded by mechanical thrombectomy in multiple passes to ensure complete recanalization.

II

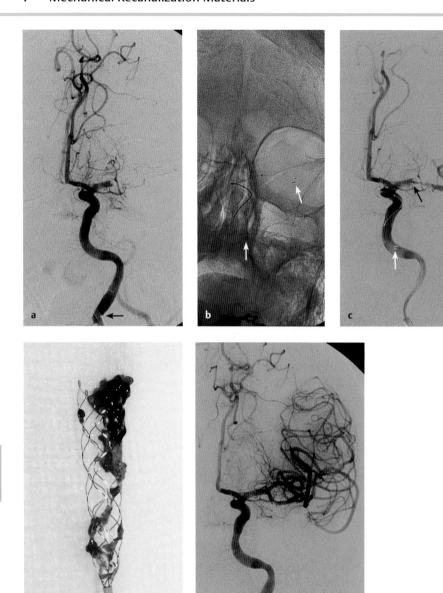

Fig. 7.6a–e   Occlusion of the left MCA trunk with NIHSS = 20 within the 3-h thrombolytic window in a 76-year-old woman.

Initial bridging was done with 20 mg of intravenous rtPA. Patient was immediately placed on the angiography table, and general anesthesia was induced.

a Initial angiogram shows the 7F guide catheter placed as far distally as possible in the left ICA.

b The thrombus has been crossed with the Rebar 18 microcatheter, and the stent has been deployed. The three distal markers (*arrow*) are just proximal to the MCA bifurcation. Up to this point, continuous aspiration has been applied through the Penumbra 054 reperfusion catheter (*arrowhead*). Note: according to Castaño et al. (2010), deployment of the Solitaire stent often provides immediate flow restoration to the lenticulostriate branches of the MCA in patients with an M1 occlusion.

c The Rebar 18 microcatheter with the collapsed stent is advanced to the thrombus (*arrow*). Aspiration through the Penumbra System is turned off, and 10 mg of rtPA is infused through

the Rebar 18 microcatheter over a 5-min period. Then the Penumbra System with expanded stent (*arrowhead*) is advanced into the proximal MCA trunk; the expanded stent makes this maneuver easy to perform even in elongated vessels. While maximum manual aspiration is applied to the Penumbra catheter system with a 50-mL syringe, the stent is carefully retracted into the Penumbra catheter. Caution: do not retrieve the stent through the Rebar 18 microcatheter, but secure the detachment site with the Rebar before withdrawing.

d Following extraction, thrombus material will consistently be found on the stent and clot fragments will be present within the Penumbra catheter system. Therefore the entire system should be removed and freed of possible clots.

e The total duration of this TICI-3 recanalization procedure was 10 min. The patient was extubated without difficulty and showed a very rapid and almost complete resolution of stroke symptoms.

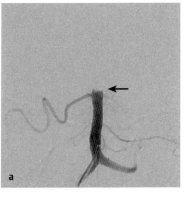
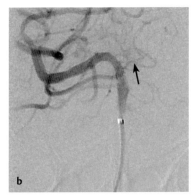
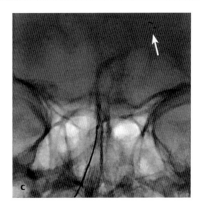
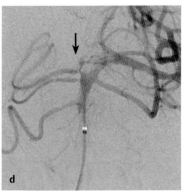
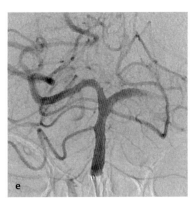

Fig. 7.7a–e Conscious 70-year-old woman had exhibited signs of left-sided Horner syndrome for 8 h.
She presented with right facial paralysis, bilateral saccadic pursuit, bilateral gaze-evoked nystagmus, dysarthria, right arm weakness, and dissociated sensory loss on the right side. Cranial CT/CTA showed no evidence of hemorrhage or infarction. A thrombus at the tip of the basilar artery was suspected.

a Baseline angiogram shows a thromboembolic occlusion of the distal basilar artery (*arrow*).

b Survey angiogram shows the posterior cerebral artery supplied on both sides by a posterior communicating branch from the associated carotid territory. The left vertebral artery has a large caliber and shows marked proximal elongation. A 6F Envoy guide catheter (Envoy, Cordis Cooperation, Miami Lakes, FL, USA) is introduced on the right side, and a Rebar 27 microcatheter is advanced into the thrombus. A total of 70 mg of rtPA is administered by local intra-arterial injection. The thrombus is disrupted with a microwire and multiple aspirations with the Rebar 27 catheter (ev3 Inc, Irvine, CA) and the Penumbra System. Next came a total of three mechanical thrombectomies each in the left and right posterior cerebral arteries using the Phenox CRC clot retriever, leaving a persistent occlusion of the P1 segment of the left posterior cerebral artery (*arrow*).

c A stent has been deployed in the left posterior cerebral artery. The three distal markers (*arrow*) can be seen.

d Repeated stent passes and thrombectomies in the posterior cerebral artery have reopened the tip of the basilar artery. The left posterior cerebral artery still contains thrombus residues. The right posterior cerebral artery is occluded (*arrow*).

e Repositioning the stent again has restored full patency to the distal basilar artery. Residual thrombus material is still visible in the left posterior cerebral artery. The total duration of the recanalization procedure was 50 min. The patient recovered except for a mild residual deficit consisting of slight right-sided weakness.

Caution
Before the device is deployed, friction should be removed from the guide catheter system to prevent uncontrolled advancement of the opening stent at the moment it is deployed. This could potentially cause vascular injury at the level of the MCA bifurcation, for example (see **Fig. 7.6b**). Care should also be taken that the three distal markers of the deploying stent do not accidentally occlude, say, a perforating branch of the MCA.

Once these microcatheter manipulations have been completed and the device is deployed in position, the Penumbra aspiration system is first flushed with saline solution to prevent clogging and is then turned off. Additional rtPA may be administered through the Rebar 18 microcatheter at this time, depending on the specific multimodal treatment setting in which stent-based recanalization is used. Local intra-arterial fibrinolysis may be applied as needed before, during, and after device deployment. From personal experience, we have consistently found that the recanalization times are significantly shorter than with conventional intra-arterial fibrinolysis or with bridging therapy alone.

> **Practical Tip**
>
> The Rebar 18 microcatheter should always be advanced very close to the proximal end of the stent to achieve maximum pharmacologic effect (**Fig. 7.6c**). The work of Schroth et al. suggests that it is advantageous to leave the Solitaire FR device within the thrombus for 5 min without altering its position (Mordasini et al. 2011).

Actual thrombus extraction takes place in two consecutive steps: While maximum aspiration is applied to the 054 reperfusion catheter with a 50-mL perfusor syringe, the catheter is slowly advanced to the proximal marker of the device, and the expanded stent is withdrawn not into the Rebar 18 microcatheter but into the 054 reperfusion catheter, always proceeding very slowly and carefully. With maximum aspiration still applied, the device is removed along with the retrieved thrombus (**Fig. 7.6d**). If the device cannot be withdrawn into the 054 reperfusion microcatheter in the expanded state, an attempt can be made to retrieve the device with the Rebar 18 microcatheter using standard technique. If this is also unsuccessful, it may be prudent to leave the stent in place since further manipulations could pose a risk of vascular dissection, hemorrhage, or both.

> **Practical Tip**
>
> Even if access to the intracranial target vessel is lost at this point in the procedure, the device should still be retrieved and the entire 054 reperfusion catheter removed under suction, since experience has shown that the bulk of the thrombus mass will usually be removed with the catheter. After the system has been cleaned, recanalization may be reattempted or a suitable escalation tried later in the intervention. It should be noted, however, that Castaño et al. (2010) required an average of 1.4 pass attempts with the stent to obtain adequate recanalization in the anterior circulation (see **Fig. 7.7b, d**).

Retrievers and Other Thrombectomy Systems

T. Struffert and A. Doerfler

Introduction

The treatment options for acute ischemic stroke have improved significantly in recent years. One reason for this is that many centers have round-the-clock availability of multimodal stroke imaging by CT, CTA, CTP, MRI, MRA, DWI, and PWI. Application of the mismatch principle can often expand the therapeutic time window. Moreover, the occlusion of a vessel can be positively identified and it can be determined whether patients are likely to benefit from an adjunctive mechanical procedure. The goal of recanalizing an occlusion is to restore perfusion so that structurally intact but critically hypoperfused tissue can be salvaged.

An important milestone in endovascular stroke therapy was the development of intra-arterial thrombolysis (PROACT study; Furlan et al. 1999; see p. 111), although mechanical manipulations of the thrombus itself were not approved in that study.

The first mechanical technique was to perforate the thrombus with ordinary microwires and balloons. This can mechanically disrupt the structure of the clot while increasing the surface area available for attack by thrombolytic drugs. This also allows for direct injection of the thrombolytic agent into the thrombus (Qureshi et al. 2002). Repeated passes of a microwire through the thrombus can create a channel that restores initial blood flow to the dependent territory, even before the affected vascular segment has been completely recanalized. This effect can be enhanced by an inflatable balloon. This can provide a degree of recanalization that will at least reduce the adverse effects of ischemia. It is also believed that flow restoration can prevent further growth of the thrombus while disrupting its structure and enlarging its surface area, making it more accessible to thrombolysis. However, mechanical recanalization techniques are suitable for cases in which thrombolysis is contraindicated, or intravenous or intra-arterial thrombolysis has been used without success.

> **Note**
>
> Treatment with microwires and balloons cannot remove the thrombus, however. So while these devices are classified as mechanical techniques, they do not qualify as thrombectomy procedures, which employ various mechanisms to remove the thrombus itself.

Besides the aspiration systems and stent-based techniques described earlier in this chapter (see pp. 84 and 92), other devices are available that may be used for mechanical recanalization of acute vascular occlusions. While some of these devices were developed initially for retrieving foreign bodies rather than treating vascular occlusions, they have yielded good recanalization rates in individual case reports of stroke patients.

Technique

Owing in part to favorable reimbursement policies, several manufacturers have introduced a variety of new endovascular devices for thrombus removal. Their modes of action are highly diverse and range from thrombus extraction to thrombus fragmentation.

Thrombus Extraction

Extraction devices act by firmly grasping a thrombus and then removing it from the vessel, preferably in one piece. Most systems employ a balloon guide catheter so that the thrombus can be extracted under conditions of flow arrest. This is intended to prevent the embolization of clot fragments (Mayer et al. 2002). Various systems with retrieval baskets, wire loops, or grasping jaws are available on the market.

Thrombus Fragmentation

The goal of this process is mechanical fragmentation of the clot to increase its surface area, similar to the microwire and balloon methods. This makes the thrombus more accessible to attack by thrombolytic agents, increasing their effectiveness. Consequently, these therapies are often used in conjunction with intra-arterial thrombolysis.

Caution
The fragmentation of a thrombus increases the risk of clot fragments embolizing to more distal vessels, resulting in peripheral thromboembolism.

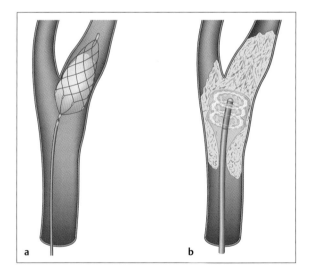

Fig. 7.8a, b Distal and proximal thrombectomy systems.
a Distal thrombectomy system: A small basket (example: Catch, Balt) is deployed "behind" the thrombus and then pulled back toward the operator.
b Proximal thrombectomy system: This type of system (example: EKOS System) acts proximal to or within the thrombus; it is unnecessary to cross the thrombus.

Classification of Systems

Because the devices have such varied modes of action, it is common practice to classify them into proximal and distal systems, regardless of their functional principle:
- With *distal systems* (**Fig. 7.8a**), it is first necessary to cross the thrombus so that the device can be deployed and used "behind" the occlusion.
- With *proximal systems*, it is unnecessary to cross the thrombus because the device can produce mechanical recanalization from the proximal aspect of the thrombus (**Fig. 7.8b**).

Below we look at various techniques for the endovascular treatment of acute stroke, describing their functional principles and finally assessing the efficacy of the different systems. We confine our attention to systems addressed in publications cited by PubMed (as of January 2012).

Proximal Systems

Microsnare Device

This device (Microsnare, Microvena, White Bear Lake, MN, USA) is shaped like a small wire loop and was originally designed for retrieving foreign bodies from the vascular system (e.g., displaced coils or broken catheters). The snare is advanced through a previously placed microcatheter, opens at it emerges from the tip, and is looped over the thrombus. The microcatheter is then advanced further so that the snare can be tightened to secure and extract the clot. Reports from small case series indicate recanalization rates up to 80% (Kerber et al. 2002; Wikholm 2003).

Alligator Device

The Alligator Retrieval Device (Chestnut Medical Technologies, Menlo Park, CA, USA) was also originally designed for retrieving foreign bodies such as displaced coils. When the device is advanced past the tip of a microcatheter, its jaws open and can be used to grasp the thrombus (**Fig. 7.9**). Again, published case reports show recanalization rates > 70% (Kerber et al. 2007; Hussain et al. 2009). This device appears to be most effective and easy to use in straight vascular segments.

Ultrasonic Thrombectomy

With the EKOS system (EKOS MicroLysUS Infusion Catheter, EKOS Corporation, Bothwell, WA, USA), a low-energy ultrasound source (2.01–2.2 MHz) mounted at the tip

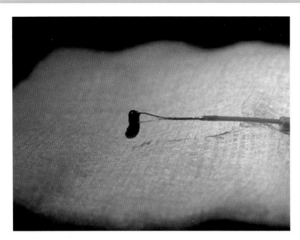

Fig. 7.9 The Alligator Retrieval Device has small jaws for removing foreign bodies from vessels. In principle, however, the device can also be used for thrombectomies.

of a microcatheter is advanced into the thrombus (see **Fig. 7.8b**). The device also has a working channel that permits the simultaneous intra-arterial injection of a thrombolytic agent. The pulsating energy of the ultrasound source is designed to fragment the thrombus while providing optimal dispersion and delivery of the thrombolytic agent. Thus, the ultrasound pulses support the penetration of the agent into the thrombus material. A pilot study in 14 patients showed a recanalization rate of 57% over an average period of 46 min (Mahon et al. 2003). A pooled data analysis of the IMS I and IMS II studies (IMS Study Investigators 2004; Tomsick et al. 2008) confirmed a trend toward an increased recanalization rate using the EKOS system (Tomsick et al. 2008). A recanalization rate of 69% was achieved within 120 min in the anterior circulation (carotid T, MCA). This study also showed a definite trend for successfully treated patients to have better clinical outcomes.

Laser Thrombectomy

In this technique the energy from a laser light source is delivered fiberoptically to the tip of a microcatheter (EPAR = endovascular photoacoustic recanalization, Endovasix Inc, Belmont, CA, USA). This technique does not involve direct laser ablation; rather, the energy of the laser light is converted into acoustic energy. Liquefaction of the thrombus material at the catheter tip produces a continuous suction effect that draws in new thrombus material. The thrombus is disintegrated into minute particles 1–10 μm in size, which are on a subcapillary scale. A feasibility and safety study in 34 patients found that this system achieved a recanalization rate of 41%. The stated average treatment time during laser operation was just 10 min. The mortality rate was 38.2% (Berlis et al. 2004). The development of this device is not being pursued at present.

Distal Systems

Catch Device

The Catch device (Balt, Montmorency, France) comes in two different designs for different vessel diameters (**Fig. 7.10a**). The device is deployed distal to the occlusion to capture and retrieve the thrombus. Results in animal studies indicate a high recanalization rate (Brekenfeld et al. 2008). Though this is described in the literature as a

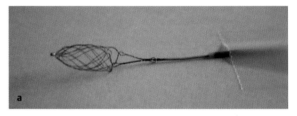
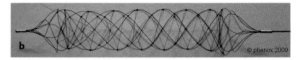
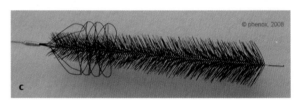
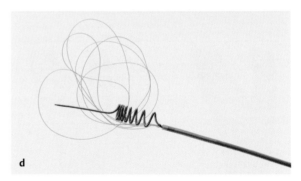

Fig. 7.10a–d Various distal thrombectomy systems.
a The small retrieval basket (Catch, Balt) is deployed distal to the thrombus and pulled back to capture and retrieve the clot (with kind permission of Balt Extrusion, Montmorency, France).
b The Phenox System (Bonnet) functions by a similar principle (with kind permission of Phenox GmbH, Bochum, Germany; http://www.phenox.info).
c Phenox System: CRC Phenox Clot Retriever. The small basket formed by microfilaments at the distal end of the device helps stabilize the thrombus for retrieval (with kind permission of Phenox GmbH, Bochum, Germany; http://www.phenox.info).
d The MERCI Retriever (V series) resembles a corkscrew, which is used to engage and extract the thrombus from the vessel. Monofilaments are added to increase the adhesion rate of the thrombus to the device (with kind permission of Concentric Medical Inc, Mountain View, CA, USA).

stroke device, application studies in large case numbers have not yet been published (Benmira et al. 2011).

Phenox System

Phenox GmbH (Bochum, Germany) offers two different systems in the pCR Clot Retriever, the CRC Clot Retriever Cage (**Fig. 7.10c**) and the Bonnet device (**Fig. 7.10b**). The Clot Retriever system (pCR and CRC) consists of a wire brush, which has been expanded in the Clot Retriever Cage device to include a small basket. The Bonnet device is a small microwire basket that is deployed distal to the thrombus and, like the pCR and Cage devices, is pulled proximally to capture and remove the clot (see **Fig. 7.10b**). Initial applications are very promising (Henkes et al. 2006; see illustrative case in **Fig. 7.11**). Application has been safe and effective, at least in experimental animals (Mordasini et al. 2010). As with other devices, there is a lack of clinical data and no application study has been done in large numbers of patients.

MERCI Retriever

The MERCI Retriever (V Series; Concentric, Mountain View, CA) is a coiled retrieval basket, resembling a corkscrew (**Fig. 7.10d**), that engages the thrombus from the distal side for capture and extraction. The technical success rate is high.

Two large application studies have been published on this device. In the MERCI trial, the system could be deployed in 141 of 151 patients (Smith et al. 2005). Recanalization was achieved in 48% of the 141 patients treated with the first-generation MERCI system within 8h of stroke onset. The need for adjuvant therapy (thrombolytics, etc.) after deployment was high, while the rate of procedural complications, at 7.1%, was relatively low. Subsequent to this trial, the MERCI Retriever was granted FDA approval. A subsequent study evaluated a technically advanced version of the device, which was improved by adding monofilaments to the coiled basket. The Multi MERCI trial was conducted in 164 patients treated within 8h of symptom onset (Smith et al. 2008). Only patients who had persistent occlusion after intravenous thrombolysis were enrolled. Recanalization was achieved in 57.3% of the patients by using the MERCI Retriever alone. The recanalization rate increased to 69.5% when the MERCI device was combined with thrombolytic agents or other mechanical techniques. The rate of procedural complications, at 5.5%, was lower than in the first MERCI trial. A good outcome, defined as mRS ≥ 2 at 90 days, was achieved in 36% of the patients (Smith et al. 2008). Today the system is widely utilized, especially in the United States.

Summary

In summary, there are many different endovascular options for the treatment of acute cerebrovascular occlusions. Almost all of these systems are effective in restoring

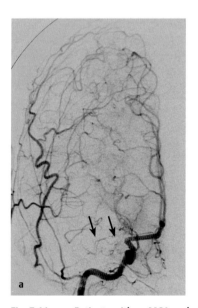 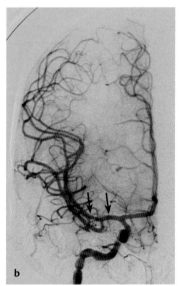 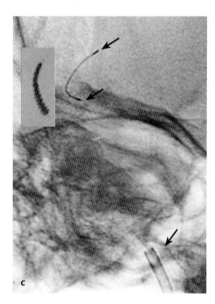

Fig. 7.11a–c   Patients with an MCA occlusion.

a The *arrows* indicate the site of the complete occlusion.

b The pCR Phenox Clot Retriever (brush without filaments) was used in this patient. Combined intravenous and intra-arterial thrombolysis had been unsuccessful. After two passes, the vessel is completely recanalized (*arrows*).

c Fluoroscopic image clearly shows the location of the device by its proximal and distal markers (*arrows*). *Inset* shows the "bottle brush" structure of the pCR Phenox Clot Retriever.

patency, with recanalization rates ranging from 50 to 80%. Several of the devices in this chapter have been evaluated in feasibility studies designed to demonstrate the technical safety and efficacy of the systems (see above). Ultimately, however, all of these endovascular techniques must be measured by their clinical benefit for stroke patients, meaning an improvement in neurologic outcome. There are insufficient data on this score, owing in part to the very heterogeneous use of these techniques. Our goal, then, must be to clarify questions relating to patient selection and especially to outcomes within well-defined study protocols and probably within the framework of a randomized trial.

References

Aspiration Systems

Bose A, Henkes H, Alfke K, et al; Penumbra Phase 1 Stroke Trial Investigators. The Penumbra System: a mechanical device for the treatment of acute stroke due to thromboembolism. AJNR Am J Neuroradiol 2008;29(7):1409–1413

Clark WM, Wissman S, Albers GW, Jhamandas JH, Madden KP, Hamilton S. Recombinant tissue-type plasminogen activator (Alteplase) for ischemic stroke 3 to 5 hours after symptom onset. The ATLANTIS Study: a randomized controlled trial. Alteplase Thrombolysis for Acute Noninterventional Therapy in Ischemic Stroke. JAMA 1999;282(21):2019–2026

del Zoppo GJ, Higashida RT, Furlan AJ, Pessin MS, Rowley HA, Gent M. PROACT: a phase II randomized trial of recombinant pro-urokinase by direct arterial delivery in acute middle cerebral artery stroke. PROACT Investigators. Prolyse in Acute Cerebral Thromboembolism. Stroke 1998;29(1):4–11

Devlin TG, Baxter BW, Feintuch TA, Desbiens NA. The Merci Retrieval System for acute stroke: the Southeast Regional Stroke Center experience. Neurocrit Care 2007;6(1):11–21

Furlan A, Higashida R, Wechsler L, et al. Intra-arterial prourokinase for acute ischemic stroke. The PROACT II study: a randomized controlled trial. Prolyse in Acute Cerebral Thromboembolism. JAMA 1999;282(21):2003–2011

Grunwald IQ, Walter S, Papanagiotou P, et al. Revascularization in acute ischaemic stroke using the penumbra system: the first single center experience. Eur J Neurol 2009;16(11):1210–1216

Hacke W, Kaste M, Fieschi C, et al; The European Cooperative Acute Stroke Study (ECASS). Intravenous thrombolysis with recombinant tissue plasminogen activator for acute hemispheric stroke. JAMA 1995;274(13):1017–1025

Hacke W, Kaste M, Fieschi C, et al; Second European-Australasian Acute Stroke Study Investigators. Randomised double-blind placebo-controlled trial of thrombolytic therapy with intravenous alteplase in acute ischaemic stroke (ECASS II). Lancet 1998;352(9136):1245–1251

Hacke W, Kaste M, Bluhmki E, et al; ECASS Investigators. Thrombolysis with alteplase 3 to 4.5 hours after acute ischemic stroke. N Engl J Med 2008;359(13):1317–1329

Higashida RT, Furlan AJ, Roberts H, et al; Technology Assessment Committee of the American Society of Interventional and Therapeutic Neuroradiology; Technology Assessment Committee of the Society of Interventional Radiology. Trial design and reporting standards for intra-arterial cerebral thrombolysis for acute ischemic stroke. Stroke 2003;34(8):e109–e137

Huded V, Saraf R, Limaye U. Mechanical device the Penumbra system in the management of acute stroke: report of five cases. Neurol India 2009;57(3):310–312

Hussein HM, Georgiadis AL, Vazquez G, et al. Occurrence and predictors of futile recanalization following endovascular treatment among patients with acute ischemic stroke: a multicenter study. AJNR Am J Neuroradiol 2010;31(3):454–458

IMS Study Investigators. Combined intravenous and intra-arterial recanalization for acute ischemic stroke: the Interventional Management of Stroke Study. Stroke 2004;35(4):904–911

IMS II Trial Investigators. The Interventional Management of Stroke (IMS) II Study. Stroke 2007;38(7):2127–2135

Kim D, Jahan R, Starkman S, et al. Endovascular mechanical clot retrieval in a broad ischemic stroke cohort. AJNR Am J Neuroradiol 2006;27(10):2048–2052

Kulcsár Z, Bonvin C, Pereira VM, et al. Penumbra system: a novel mechanical thrombectomy device for large-vessel occlusions in acute stroke. AJNR Am J Neuroradiol 2010;31(4):628–633

Lees KR, Bluhmki E, von Kummer R, et al; ECASS, ATLANTIS, NINDS and EPITHET rt-PA Study Group. Time to treatment with intravenous alteplase and outcome in stroke: an updated pooled analysis of ECASS, ATLANTIS, NINDS, and EPITHET trials. Lancet 2010;375(9727):1695–1703

Mazighi M, Serfaty JM, Labreuche J, et al; RECANALISE investigators. Comparison of intravenous alteplase with a combined intravenous-endovascular approach in patients with stroke and confirmed arterial occlusion (RECANALISE study): a prospective cohort study. Lancet Neurol 2009;8(9):802–809. Correction: Lancet Neurol 2009;8(11):981

Mattle HP, Arnold M, Georgiadis D, et al. Comparison of intraarterial and intravenous thrombolysis for ischemic stroke with hyperdense middle cerebral artery sign. Stroke 2008;39(2):379–383

Menon BK, Hill MD, Eesa M, et al. Initial experience with the Penumbra Stroke System for recanalization of large vessel occlusions in acute ischemic stroke. Neuroradiology 2011;53(4):261–266

NINDS tPA Stroke Study Group. Intracerebral hemorrhage after intravenous t-PA therapy for ischemic stroke. Stroke 1997;28(11):2109–2118

Ogawa A, Mori E, Minematsu K, et al; MELT Japan Study Group. Randomized trial of intraarterial infusion of urokinase within 6 hours of middle cerebral artery stroke: the middle cerebral artery embolism local fibrinolytic intervention trial (MELT) Japan. Stroke 2007;38(10):2633–2639

Rha JH, Saver JL. The impact of recanalization on ischemic stroke outcome: a meta-analysis. Stroke 2007;38(3):967–973

Riedel CH, Jansen O. Thrombuslängenmessung im CCT beim akuten Schlaganfall zur Vorhersage der Rekanalisierungsrate durch systemische Lysetherapie. DGNR-Jahrestagung; 2009

Smith WS, Sung G, Starkman S, et al; MERCI Trial Investigators. Safety and efficacy of mechanical embolectomy in acute ischemic stroke: results of the MERCI trial. Stroke 2005;36(7):1432–1438

Smith WS, Sung G, Saver J, et al; Multi MERCI Investigators. Mechanical thrombectomy for acute ischemic stroke: final results of the Multi MERCI trial. Stroke 2008;39(4):1205–1212

Struffert T, Köhrmann M, Engelhorn T, et al. Penumbra Stroke System as an "add-on" for the treatment of large vessel occlusive disease following thrombolysis: first results. Eur Radiol 2009;19(9):2286–2293

National Institute of Neurological Disorders and Stroke rt-PA Stroke Study Group. Tissue plasminogen activator for acute ischemic stroke. N Engl J Med 1995;333(24):1581–1587

Penumbra Pivotal Stroke Trial Investigators. The penumbra pivotal stroke trial: safety and effectiveness of a new generation of mechanical devices for clot removal in intracranial large vessel occlusive disease. Stroke 2009;40(8):2761–2768

Tempory Stenting in Stroke Patients

Castaño C, Serena J, Dávalos A. Use of the New Solitaire (TM) AB device for mechanical thrombectomy when Merci Clot Retriever has failed to remove the clot. A case report. Interv Neuroradiol 2009;15(2):209–214

Castaño C, Dorado L, Guerrero C, et al. Mechanical thrombectomy with the Solitaire AB device in large artery occlusions of the anterior circulation: a pilot study. Stroke 2010;41(8):1836–1840

Ickenstein GW, Isenmann S, Fiehler J, et al. Thrombolysis in neuromedicine. Bridging concepts for the management of acute brain infarction with occlusion of intracranial vessels. Clin Neuroradiol 2008;2:23–28

Khatri P, Abruzzo T, Yeatts SD, Nichols C, Broderick JP, Tomsick TA; IMS I and II Investigators. Good clinical outcome after ischemic stroke with successful revascularization is time-dependent. Neurology 2009;73(13):1066–1072

Kulcsár Z, Bonvin C, Lovblad KO, et al. Use of the Enterprise Intracranial Stent for revascularization of large vessel occlusions in acute stroke. Clin Neuroradiol 2010a;20(1)204–214

Kulcsár Z, Yilmaz H, Bonvin C, Lovblad KO, Rüfenacht DA. Multiple coaxial catheter system for reliable access in interventional stroke therapy. Cardiovasc Intervent Radiol 2010b;33(6):1205–1209

Levy EI, Ecker RD, Horowitz MB, et al. Stent-assisted intracranial recanalization for acute stroke: early results. Neurosurgery 2006;58(3):458–463, discussion 458–463

Levy EI, Siddiqui AH, Crumlish A, et al. First Food and Drug Administration-approved prospective trial of primary intracranial stenting for acute stroke: SARIS (stent-assisted recanalization in acute ischemic stroke). Stroke 2009;40(11):3552–3556

Mordasini P, Frabetti N, Gralla J, et al. In vivo evaluation of the first dedicated combined flow-restoration and mechanical thrombectomy device in a swine model of acute vessel occlusion. AJNR Am J Neuroradiol 2011;32(2):294–300

Natarajan SK, Dandona P, Karmon Y, et al. Prediction of adverse outcomes by blood glucose level after endovascular therapy for acute ischemic stroke. J Neurosurg 2011; ;114(6):1785–1799

Nayak S, Ladurner G, Killer M. Treatment of acute middle cerebral artery occlusion with a Solitaire AB stent: preliminary experience. Br J Radiol 2010;83(996):1017–1022

Sauvageau E, Levy EI. Self-expanding stent-assisted middle cerebral artery recanalization: technical note. Neuroradiology 2006;48(6):405–408

Seifert M, Ahlbrecht A, Dohmen C, Spuentrup E, Moeller-Hartmann W. Combined interventional stroke therapy using intracranial stent and local intraarterial thrombolysis (LIT). Neuroradiology 2011;53(4):273–282

Venker C, Stracke P, Berlit P, et al. New options in the therapeutic management of acute ischaemic stroke. Good results with combined i.v. and i.a. lysis and mechanical thrombectomy. [Article in German] Fortschr Neurol Psychiatr 2010;78(11):652–657

Retrievers and Other Thrombectomy Systems

Benmira S, Banda ZK, Bhattacharya V. The start of a new era for stroke treatment: mechanical thrombectomy devices. Curr Neurovasc Res 2011;8(1):75–85

Berlis A, Lutsep H, Barnwell S, et al. Mechanical thrombolysis in acute ischemic stroke with endovascular photoacoustic recanalization. Stroke 2004;35(5):1112–1116

Brekenfeld C, Schroth G, El-Koussy M, et al. Mechanical thromboembolectomy for acute ischemic stroke: comparison of the catch thrombectomy device and the Merci Retriever in vivo. Stroke 2008;39(4):1213–1219

Furlan A, Higashida R, Wechsler L, et al. Intra-arterial prourokinase for acute ischemic stroke. The PROACT II study: a randomized controlled trial. Prolyse in Acute Cerebral Thromboembolism. JAMA 1999;282(21):2003–2011

Henkes H, Reinartz J, Lowens S, et al. A device for fast mechanical clot retrieval from intracranial arteries (Phenox clot retriever). Neurocrit Care 2006;5(2):134–140

Hussain MS, Kelly ME, Moskowitz SI, et al. Mechanical thrombectomy for acute stroke with the alligator retrieval device. Stroke 2009;40(12):3784–3788

IMS Study Investigators. Combined intravenous and intra-arterial recanalization for acute ischemic stroke: the Interventional Management of Stroke Study. Stroke 2004;35(4):904–911

Kerber CW, Barr JD, Berger RM, Chopko BW. Snare retrieval of intracranial thrombus in patients with acute stroke. J Vasc Interv Radiol 2002;13(12):1269–1274

Kerber CW, Wanke I, Bernard J Jr, Woo HH, Liu MW, Nelson PK. Rapid intracranial clot removal with a new device: the alligator retriever. AJNR Am J Neuroradiol 2007;28(5):860–863

Mahon BR, Nesbit GM, Barnwell SL, et al. North American clinical experience with the EKOS MicroLysUS infusion catheter for the treatment of embolic stroke. AJNR Am J Neuroradiol 2003;24(3):534–538

Mayer TE, Hamann GF, Brueckmann HJ. Treatment of basilar artery embolism with a mechanical extraction device: necessity of flow reversal. Stroke 2002;33(9):2232–2235

Mordasini P, Hiller M, Brekenfeld C, et al. In vivo evaluation of the Phenox CRC mechanical thrombectomy device in a swine model of acute vessel occlusion. AJNR Am J Neuroradiol 2010;31(5):972–978

Smith WS, Sung G, Starkman S, et al; MERCI Trial Investigators. Safety and efficacy of mechanical embolectomy in acute ischemic stroke: results of the MERCI trial. Stroke 2005;36(7):1432–1438

Smith WS, Sung G, Saver J, et al; Multi MERCI Investigators. Mechanical thrombectomy for acute ischemic stroke: final results of the Multi MERCI trial. Stroke 2008;39(4):1205–1212

Qureshi AI, Siddiqui AM, Suri MF, et al. Aggressive mechanical clot disruption and low-dose intra-arterial third-generation thrombolytic agent for ischemic stroke: a prospective study. Neurosurgery 2002;51(5):1319–1327, discussion 1327–1329

Tomsick T, Broderick J, Carrozella J, et al; Interventional Management of Stroke II Investigators. Revascularization results in the Interventional Management of Stroke II trial. AJNR Am J Neuroradiol 2008;29(3):582–587

Wikholm G. Transarterial embolectomy in acute stroke. AJNR Am J Neuroradiol 2003;24(5):892–894

8 Treatment Concepts and Results

Carotid-T Occlusion

G. Fesl

Introduction

The intracranial bifurcation of the internal carotid artery (ICA), called the carotid terminus (carotid T), plays a central role in the blood supply to the brain. It is the site where the ICA divides into the middle cerebral artery (MCA) and anterior cerebral artery (ACA), which are the main suppliers of one cerebral hemisphere. As part of the circle of Willis, the carotid T is also critically involved in the collateral blood supply to the hemispheres.

An acute occlusion of the carotid T is most often caused by an embolus of cardiac origin. Less frequent causes are arterioarterial emboli arising from a proximal stenosis or atherosclerotic plaque. Generally these thrombi extend from the supraclinoid portion of the carotid siphon into the proximal portions of the MCA (M1 segment) and ACA (A1 segment), blocking antegrade blood flow to the peripheral branches of those arteries. Lenticulostriate perforators from the M1 segment, central branches of A1 (e.g., the medial striate artery), the anterior choroidal artery, and the posterior communicating branch may be obstructed, depending on the extent of the thrombus. Adequate collateral circulation may be maintained through leptomeningeal branches of the ACA or through choroidal and leptomeningeal branches of the posterior cerebral artery (PCA), but this is uncommon. Most acute occlusions of the carotid T cause an extensive infarction involving the basal ganglia, internal capsule, and large portions of the frontal, temporal, and parietal lobes. This results in a very severe, acute hemispheric neurologic syndrome with permanent disability. Carotid-T occlusions have a high mortality rate (Jansen et al. 1995).

> **Note**
>
> Acute carotid-T occlusions typically cause a major stroke with high morbidity and mortality. The prime therapeutic goal is to restore flow through the occluded vessel as quickly as possible to salvage tissue that is still structurally intact ("time is brain").

Treatment

An acute cerebrovascular occlusion should be treated without delay. The goal of prompt recanalization is to salvage brain tissue that has already sustained a degree of functional damage but is still structurally intact (penumbra). Treatment options during the early postocclusion period are pharmacologic thrombolysis and mechanical recanalization techniques.

Intravenous Thrombolysis

Intravenous thrombolysis was approved by the U.S. Food and Drug Administration (FDA) in 1996 for the treatment of acute stroke. This approval is based on the study results of the National Institute of Neurologic Disorders (NINDS) and the rtPA Stroke Study Group (National Institute of Neurologic Disorders and Stroke rtPA Stroke Study Group 1995). Since then, intravenous thrombolysis has become established as the standard treatment for stroke within the first 3 h after symptom onset. Based on the results of the ECASS III study, it was later suggested that the time window for intravenous thrombolysis be expanded from 3 h to 4.5 h (Hacke et al. 2008b).

A major advantage of intravenous thrombolysis is its technical simplicity, which allows for rapid initiation of treatment in stroke victims. It does not require complex technology or special interventional training like that needed for mechanical recanalization, for example.

Intra-arterial Thrombolysis

In this therapy (see p. 66) the fibrinolytic agent is delivered directly to the site of the thrombus through a microcatheter. This allows a much higher local concentration of the fibrinolytic agent to be delivered to the clot than is possible with intravenous thrombolysis. This selective application also allows the total dose of the fibrinolytic agent to be reduced, thereby lessening the risk of intracranial hemorrhage. In turn, this lower hemorrhage risk allows the therapeutic window to be expanded past the time frame recommended for intravenous thrombolysis (see PROACT I and II trials; del Zoppo et al. 1998; Furlan et al. 1999). The principal agent used for intravenous and intra-arterial thrombolysis is rtPA (alteplase). Urokinase is less commonly used.

Treatment of Acute Ischemic Stroke

II

Mechanical Recanalization Techniques

Mechanical, catheter-based recanalization techniques (see Chapter 7) permit the rapid and safe restoration of blood flow through an acutely occluded vessel. They can even be used in patients who are not eligible for thrombolysis because of contraindications, or have shown poor response to primary thrombolysis. The therapeutic time window for mechanical recanalization alone is considerably longer than that for classic intravenous thrombolysis because the risk of bleeding into a possible infarcted area is lower when thrombolytic agents are not used. For example, patients enrolled in the MERCI and Penumbra trials were treated up to 8 h after onset of clinical symptoms (Smith et al. 2005, 2008; Penumbra Pivotal Stroke Trial Investigators 2009).

Of course, mechanical recanalization is more costly and complex than intravenous thrombolysis. It is an interventional procedure that requires proper training and equipment and carries the risks of a cerebral catheter angiography. Interventional risks include vascular dissection, perforation, and vascular occlusion.

The development of recanalization techniques is proceeding at a rapid pace. Below we review the main functional principles of devices currently available. Some procedures combine several of the techniques described, and readers are referred to specific sections in this book for technical details.

Aspiration Systems

Aspiration systems (see also p. 84) remove the thrombus by suction. The simplest variant is manual aspiration with a large syringe on an aspiration catheter. The ICA can be occluded proximally with a balloon cuff during the aspiration maneuver. More sophisticated systems utilize the Venturi–Bernoulli effect to fragment and aspirate the clot with a saline jet. A widely used system employs a "separator" wire to fragment the clot and simultaneously aspirate the fragments with a pump connected to the guide catheter (**Fig. 8.1b**).

Thrombectomy Systems

Thrombectomy systems are designed to retrieve the thrombus in one piece. The device may use a snare or prongs to grasp the clot from the proximal side and pull it into the guide catheter, or it may capture the clot from the distal side with a brush, corkscrew wire, mesh, or small basket (**Fig. 8.1c**). Intermittent balloon occlusion of the ICA with a cuffed guide catheter, for example, can prevent clot fragments from embolizing to more distal cerebral vessels.

Fragmentation Devices

Fragmentation devices break the clot into small pieces. This treatment is usually supplemented by intra-arterial thrombolysis. Microwires, snares, and soft balloons for peripheral transluminal angioplasty are simple types of fragmentation device. More complex systems employ ultrasound or other mechanisms for clot disruption.

Intracranial Stents

Intracranial stents are designed to provide rapid restoration of antegrade blood flow. Stent placement also increases the surface area of the clot that is accessible to thrombolysis, enabling the clot to be dissolved more quickly by the endogenous plasminogen–plasmin system or by adjuvant thrombolytic therapy.

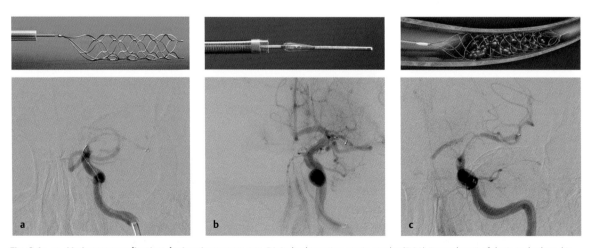

Fig. 8.1a–c   Various recanalization devices in current use. Digital subtraction angiography (DSA) "snapshots" of devices deployed in three patients with an acute carotid-T occlusion.
a Solitaire stent (with kind permission of ev3 GmbH, Bonn, Germany).
b Penumbra System (with kind permission of Penumbra Europe GmbH, Berlin, Germany).
c Bonnet device (with kind permission of Phenox GmbH, Bochum, Germany, http://www.phenox.info).

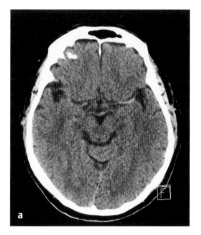 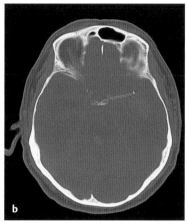 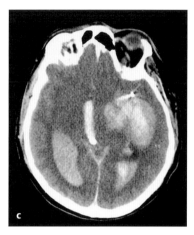

Fig. 8.2a–c   A 70-year-old man who presented with left hemispheric syndrome of 4 h duration.

a Initial CT shows hyperdensity of the left MCA with no evidence of early ischemic changes.

b After several failed thrombectomy attempts using various devices, an intracranial stent was deployed. The stent extends from the distal left ICA into the MCA bifurcation.

c Tirofiban (Aggrastat) was administered. Cranial CT the next day shows a large parenchymal hemorrhage with associated mass effect and ventricular invasion.

> **Caution**
>
> Whenever possible, avoid using stents that are not retrievable from the vessel after deployment. These permanent stents require additional treatment with an antiplatelet drug (e.g., tirofiban), which increases the risk of intracranial hemorrhage (**Fig. 8.2**).

The latest generation of closed-cell stents allow the device to be retrieved after recanalization. Antiplatelet therapy is unnecessary when a temporary stent is used. It has also been found that retractable stents can be successfully used for thrombus extraction. New stentlike systems combine the rapid restoration of antegrade blood flow (temporary bypass function) with the capability for thrombus extraction (**Figs. 8.1a**, **8.3**, and **8.4**).

Combination Therapies

Increasingly, multimodal treatment protocols are being instituted at many centers. Different recanalization methods are combined to increase the speed and efficacy of recanalization. Various combinations are possible: intravenous and intra-arterial thrombolysis, intravenous thrombolysis followed by mechanical recanalization, mechanical recanalization accompanied by intra-arterial thrombolysis, or a combination of all three modalities.

At our institution, patients with an acute carotid-T occlusion receive immediate intravenous thrombolysis after CT scanning, provided they present within the 4.5-h time window and there are no contraindications to lytic therapy. While continuous intravenous thrombolysis is maintained, the patients are intubated and undergo diagnostic angiography. As a rule, intravenous thrombolysis is almost complete by the time the angiograms are available. In the best-case scenario, patency has been restored to the carotid T; however, if the occlusion persists, mechanical recanalization can be performed without further loss of time.

Patients seen initially at a hospital without interventional neuroradiology can be diagnosed and then bridged with intravenous thrombolysis during transport to a stroke center after contraindications have been excluded (see also the section on Bridging Therapy, p. 76). In this way the time to mechanical recanalization is utilized for intravenous thrombolysis, and the clot has already been "softened" or partially dissolved.

Intra-arterial thrombolysis may be done as an adjunct to mechanical recanalization. As noted above, this is an option when retrievable stents are used. The deployed stent restores antegrade blood flow and increases the surface area available for attack by the thrombolytic agent. In turn, the thrombolysis softens the clot and facilitates its extraction.

> **Practical Tip**
>
> Various catheter systems can be used successively during mechanical recanalization. Not all devices are equally suitable for different situations, so it may be advantageous to change materials during recanalization to achieve a better result.

Treatment of Acute Ischemic Stroke

II

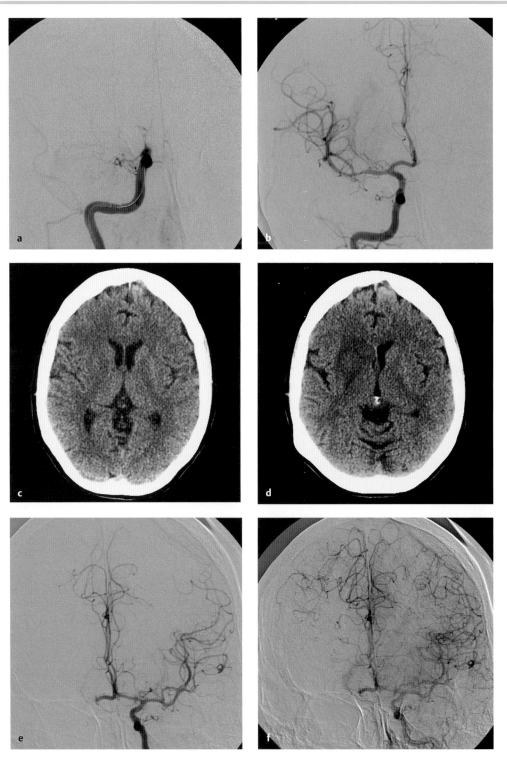

Fig. 8.3a–f   A 66-year-old woman who presented with an acute right hemispheric syndrome of 3 h duration.

a DSA image before mechanical recanalization of the carotid T. The right ICA is still occluded following intravenous thrombolysis.

b DSA image of the right ICA after mechanical recanalization of the carotid T. Complete thrombectomy with a Solitaire stent has restored perfusion to all MCA and ACA branches on the right side.

c Initial cranial CT before recanalization shows no early ischemic changes.

d CT scan 2 days after recanalization shows infarction confined to the right basal ganglia.

e DSA of the left ICA before recanalization shows definite crossflow through the anterior communicating branch to the right side.

f Excellent collateral supply to the right MCA territory has contributed to a good clinical outcome (mRS = 2) in this patient.

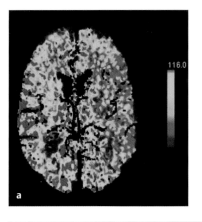
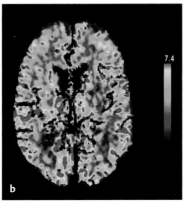
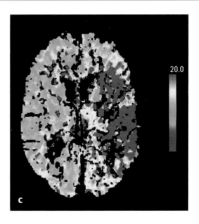

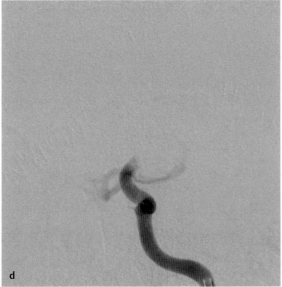
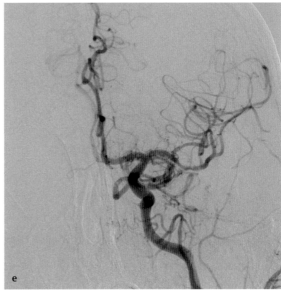

II

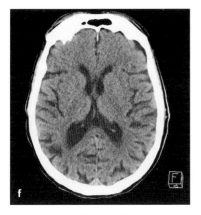
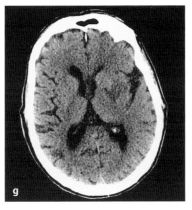

Fig. 8.4a–g   A 78-year-old man who presented 2.5 h after onset of severe aphasia and severe right hemiparesis.

a CT perfusion imaging (CTP) shows markedly decreased blood flow in the left MCA territory.

b CTP shows a mismatch relative to **a** with a small area of decreased blood volume in the left MCA territory.

c CTP shows significant delay of contrast medium transit time throughout the left MCA territory with normal perfusion in the left ACA territory and good collateral flow through the anterior communicating branch (**a–c**).

d DSA of the left ICA before mechanical recanalization of the carotid T. After completion of intravenous thrombolysis, the left ICA is still occluded above the origin of the posterior communicating branch.

e DSA after mechanical recanalization with a Solitaire stent shows normal filling of the MCA and ACA branches on the left side.

f Cranial CT shows no early ischemic changes prior to the intervention.

g CT scan 1 day after recanalization shows small infarction confined to the left basal ganglia.

Study Results

Two main criteria are used to evaluate the efficacy of different treatment methods for acute carotid-T occlusions: recanalization rates and clinical results.

Recanalization Rates

Several studies have confirmed that acute carotid-T occlusions do not respond well to pharmacologic thrombolysis alone. Saqqur et al. (2007) found that intravenous thrombolysis produced complete recanalization of the carotid T by Doppler ultrasound in only 6% of patients treated within the 3-h window. Jansen et al. (1995) reported recanalization rates of only 12.5% after intravenous or intra-arterial thrombolysis. Arnold et al. (2003) found partial recanalization of the ICA in 63% of patients after intra-arterial urokinase, but this treatment restored MCA patency in only 17%. In a comparative study on the efficacy of intra-arterial thrombolysis in different types of occlusion, Eckert et al. (2003) reported a recanalization rate of 23% for carotid-T occlusions, compared with a 70% rate for M1 occlusions of the MCA. Zaidat et al. (2002) described a recanalization rate of 50% for carotid-T occlusions that were treated by intra-arterial thrombolysis or a combination of intravenous plus intra-arterial thrombolysis.

Significantly better recanalization rates for carotid-T occlusions have been reported with mechanical recanalization techniques alone or combined with thrombolysis. For example, the Multi MERCI trial described a recanalization rate of 65% for carotid-T occlusions (Smith et al. 2008). The RECANALISE study noted a definite advantage of combining intravenous thrombolysis with endovascular therapy compared with intravenous thrombolysis alone. In the patient group with an ICA occlusion or combined ICA and MCA occlusion, the combination of intravenous thrombolysis and endovascular therapy yielded a recanalization rate of 69%, vs. only 30% with intravenous thrombolysis alone (Mazighi et al. 2009). Lin et al. (2009) published their results in a series of 75 patients with carotid-T occlusions treated by intra-arterial thrombolysis, the MERCI device, stents, or a combination of these methods. The best recanalization rates (86%) were achieved using a combination of intra-arterial thrombolysis and the MERCI device. This contrasted with a recanalization rate of only 46% after use of the MERCI device alone and 18% after intra-arterial thrombolysis. In our study, consisting of 14 patients with acute carotid-T occlusions, various mechanical recanalization techniques were used alone and in conjunction with pharmacologic thrombolysis. The combined approach restored ICA patency in 93% of cases and recanalized the carotid T and MCA (M1 segment and at least one M2 branch) in 79% of cases (Fesl et al. 2011).

This principle is illustrated by a post-hoc analysis of the MERCI and Multi MERCI trials (Shi et al. 2010), which showed a definite trend toward shorter intervention times in patients that received previous intravenous thrombolysis.

Clinical Results

Several studies have shown that pharmacologic thrombolysis alone does not yield acceptable clinical results. Arnold et al. (2003) found that only 17% of patients achieved a good outcome (mRS ≤ 2) after intra-arterial urokinase therapy alone, with a mortality rate of 42% after 90 days. Eckert et al. (2003) reported a poor clinical outcome in 49% of patients with carotid-T occlusions (Barthel index < 50) and a mortality rate of 43%. Jansen et al. (1995) found a good or moderate outcome (mRS = 1–3) in 16% of patients after intravenous or intra-arterial thrombolysis, with a mortality rate of 53%. Zaidat et al. (2002) described a mortality rate of 70% in patients with acute carotid-T occlusions who had received thrombolytic therapy.

Mechanical recanalization alone and combinations of mechanical thrombectomy with thrombolysis provide very good recanalization rates, but the clinical outcomes often fail to meet expectations. In the Multi MERCI trial, for example, 33% of patients with carotid-T occlusions had a good clinical outcome (mRS ≤ 2) with a mortality rate of 45% (Smith et al. 2008). Lin et al. (2009) described a favorable outcome in 23% of patients with a carotid-T occlusion. The mortality rate in this study was 37%. In the Penumbra study (Penumbra Pivotal Stroke Trial Investigators 2009), 23% of the patients achieved a good or satisfactory outcome (mRS ≤ 3), and the mortality rate at 90 days was 57%. Our results are comparable, with a good clinical outcome in 21% of patients and a mortality rate of 43% (Fesl et al. 2011).

A large meta-analysis of 53 studies in 2066 patients with acute vascular occlusions describes successful recanalization as the most important predictor of a good clinical outcome (Rha and Saver 2007). An analysis of the

MERCI, Multi MERCI, and RECANALISE studies also indicates that patients with successful recanalization achieve significantly better clinical results (Mazighi et al. 2009; Shi et al. 2010).

The time from symptom onset to recanalization also affects clinical outcomes. In the RECANALISE study, for example, patients who had the shortest times to recanalization with a combination of intravenous thrombolysis and endovascular therapy had the best outcomes (Mazighi et al. 2009). A study of pooled data from the MERCI trials found an association between short intervention time and a lower mortality rate at 90 days (Shi et al. 2010).

Conclusion

Most acute carotid-T occlusions are poorly collateralized and cause extensive infarctions with high morbidity and mortality. The key to successful treatment lies in shortening the time from symptom onset to recanalization and restoring flow before a large infarction can develop.

Pharmacologic thrombolysis alone generally does not provide effective recanalization or a satisfactory clinical outcome. As a result, acute carotid-T occlusions should be reopened by mechanical recanalization as quickly as possible. Prior intravenous thrombolysis or concomitant intra-arterial thrombolysis may support successful recanalization and shorten the time to flow restoration.

Practical Tip

If there are no contraindications to thrombolysis, we recommend a combination of intravenous thrombolysis and endovascular therapy. Intravenous thrombolysis can be started immediately after the clinical and CT examination and continued while the intervention is prepared. If mechanical recanalization is not available on site, then the patient, while still on thrombolysis, should be transferred to a neurovascular center where endovascular recanalization can be performed without further loss of time.

The current trend in mechanical recanalization is toward the use of temporary stents, which permit the very rapid and safe recanalization of carotid-T occlusions.

Despite the high recanalization rates, the clinical outcomes of acute carotid-T occlusions are often unsatisfactory. This is due partly to the central location of the occlusion combined with a usually poor collateral supply, creating an enormous time pressure for initiating treatment. Another crucial factor is patient selection. For example, a patient's age and initial clinical status will greatly influence the clinical outcome of recanalization.

Besides the technical advancement of recanalization therapies, future research should focus on identifying clinical and imaging criteria that will enable better patient selection. Controlled, randomized multicenter studies such as the Interventional Management of Stroke Study III (IMS III) now under way will certainly make a valuable contribution to optimizing the acute management of stroke (Khatri et al. 2008).

Occlusion of the Middle Cerebral Artery

T. Liebig

Introduction

Two-thirds of all ischemic strokes occur in the anterior circulation, and these strokes commonly involve the MCA. The occlusion may be confined to the MCA or may coexist with a carotid-T occlusion described in the previous section (p. 103). Unlike the symptoms of decreased blood flow in the posterior circulation, which are variable and often take a gradually progressive course since they often result from a preexisting stenosis, most anterior circulation strokes are caused by a sudden thromboembolic vascular occlusion from a cardiac or arterioarterial source. The embolus plugs the vessel abruptly like a cork in a bottle and may continue to move, depending on its size and malleability. Agglutination clots may additionally form due to the proximal or distal stagnation of flow. The severity of clinical manifestations depends on the thrombus burden, the site of the occlusion, and individual angioarchitecture. The last of these factors will determine the involvement of the noncollateralized perforators, which supply the basal ganglia and internal capsule, as well as the degree of collateral flow from nonoccluded vascular territories. These circumstances critically define the factors that will determine the success or failure of conservative intravenous or interventional treatment techniques.

Note

Thrombus burden, thrombus location, and individual angioarchitecture are key factors determining the clinical severity of a stroke.

Anatomy

Because an accurate description of the occlusion pattern is necessary in daily communications between clinical colleagues and in the interpretation of study results, and because that pattern will dictate clinical presentation and therapeutic strategies, especially with MCA occlusions, it is important to review briefly the anatomy of the middle cerebral artery (see also the section on Segmental Anatomy of the MCA, p. 8).

The MCA is typically divided into four segments:
- M1: sphenoidal
- M2: insular
- M3: opercular
- M4: multiple cortical segments

This classification is based upon classic, systematic neurosurgical analyses of vascular variants. Initial publications on MCA segmental anatomy date back to the late 1930s (Agarwal et al. 2004) and based the nomenclature on the relationship of the vessel to anatomic landmarks, rather than on hemodynamics. Moreover, the great variability of the MCA bifurcation (e.g., it may form a trifurcation or a large temporal branch with a far proximal origin) has long been recognized, but is sometimes ignored in everyday practice and even in studies. Especially in distinguishing the M1 and M2 segments, it is widely assumed that the M1 segment terminates at its bifurcation. In fact, however, this classification defines one prebifurcation segment and two or more postbifurcation M1 segments, which become M2 only after passing the limen insulae and entering the sylvian fissure.

As noted above, involvement of the lenticulostriate perforators, which are end arteries without a collateral supply, has a major bearing on clinical outcome and on the time frame within which recanalization can positively affect the outcome. Like the main trunks of the MCA itself, however, the perforators are also subject to anatomic variations, both in their number and in their origin relative to, say, the M1 bifurcation. Given this variability, a proximal M1 occlusion in one patient may have relatively mild symptoms or at least a favorable clinical outcome even without successful recanalization, owing to adequate retrograde flow from lenticulostriate perforators arising at far lateral sites. Meanwhile, a different patient may suffer an infarction or hemorrhage despite early recanalization because all the perforators arise from the occluded segment. Since studies have shown that perforator infarctions are likely to bleed in response to systemic thrombolysis, radiologically detected involvement of the area supplied by the perforators (the basal ganglia) would provide a strong rationale for mechanical recanalization. In a study by Vora et al. (2007) of 185 multimodal stroke treatments, this rationale is supported by the fact that 51% of patients with M1 occlusions showed hemorrhagic imbibition of the infarcted area and 42% had a parenchymal hemorrhage. The figures in patients with M2 occlusions were only 7% and 4%, respectively. Hemorrhages were particularly common in cases where multimodal therapy included intravenous or combined intravenous plus intra-arterial fibrinolysis.

Caution

Involvement of the lenticulostriate perforators means a greater risk of hemorrhage in response to thrombolysis and recanalization!

For the same reason, an important goal of mechanical recanalization is to reopen the perforator-bearing segment—usually the proximal M1 segment—as quickly as possible. When a thrombus is manipulated by balloon angioplasty or stenting, care should be taken that the clot moves away from the perforators, which usually arise posterosuperiorly, to avoid the prolonged occlusion of these small vessels, which can no longer be catheterized during the rest of the intervention.

Practical Tip

Early reperfusion of the perforators is an important goal in mechanical recanalization. The placement of a stent or balloon should displace the thrombus in a downward and anterior direction, away from the perforator origins.

A systematic study of angiographic occlusion patterns and NIHSS scores in over 200 patients by a group of authors in Bern, Switzerland (Fischer et al. 2005) clearly documented the strong correlation that exists between the location of a vascular occlusion and the severity of the resulting stroke, despite possible anatomic variants. In patients with an NIHSS score > 12, the positive predictive value for detecting a trunk occlusion, considered here to include the M1 segment, was > 90%.

Note

In more than 90% of cases, a severe stroke with NIHSS > 12 results from an occlusion of the MCA trunk with involvement of the M1 segment.

Imaging Tests

For a review of the imaging features of the various occlusion patterns in stroke, we refer the reader to the corresponding sections in Part I of this book. The technical aspects of MRI and CT examinations are covered in recommendations published in 2008 (Wintermark et al. 2008).

Although MRI is unquestionably the more versatile modality, the majority of studies dealing with stroke therapy are still based on CT. The protocol for both modalities, however, should include vascular imaging and the quantitative assessment of perfusion. Without going into too much detail, current evidence suggests that perfusion is important in predicting both the efficacy of recanalization by systemic thrombolysis and the likelihood of hemorrhagic transformation, at least in patients with an MCA occlusion. For example, in a multivariate analysis of numerous factors, Gupta et al. (2006) found that only a decrease in cerebral blood flow to $< 13\,mL\ 100\,g^{-1}\ min^{-1}$ was associated with a significantly increased likelihood of intracranial hemorrhage in patients who received intra-arterial thrombolysis (odds ratio [OR] 1.58, acquisition with xenon CT). Another analysis of these data showed that perfusion maintained at a level $> 20\,mL\ 100\,g^{-1}\ min^{-1}$ was associated with a significantly greater likelihood of successful thrombolysis (Jovin et al. 2007). These discoveries have definite therapeutic implications. As the treatment modalities for stroke continue to advance, these insights could help to identify patients who would likely benefit from pharmacologic therapy and those who would benefit from primary mechanical recanalization.

> **Practical Tip**
>
> Perfusion in the infarcted area correlates not only with survival of the penumbra but also with the risk of hemorrhage and the likelihood of successful thrombolysis. Whenever possible, therefore, the CT or MRI examination should include perfusion imaging.

Concepts: Intravenous or Intra-arterial Thrombolysis or Mechanical Extraction?

Major studies on intravenous fibrinolysis with rtPA have been mentioned throughout this book. For MCA occlusions too, intravenous thrombolysis up to 4.5 h after symptom onset is considered the current treatment standard according to the NINDS (National Institute of Neurological Disorders and Stroke rtPA Stroke Study Group 1995) and ECASS III trials (Hacke et al. 2008b). Details may be found in the sections dealing with thrombolysis (see Chapter 6). The fact that intravenous rtPA has very limited effectiveness for MCA trunk occlusions, presumably depending on the thrombus burden and occlusion pattern in NINDS (which implies the presence of a trunk occlusion only on the basis of stroke severity), is also noted earlier in the book (see the section on Intravenous Thrombolysis, p. 52).

Earlier experience on the intra-arterial use of fibrinolytic agents (Hacke et al. 1988) for basilar artery occlusions already demonstrated the theoretical advantages of this procedure, which can directly visualize the occlusion while also delivering significantly higher concentrations

of the fibrinolytic agent to the targeted site. The possibility of combining local intra-arterial fibrinolysis with mechanical manipulation of the thrombus is explored later. It is self-evident that all intra-arterial therapies are more costly and complex because of their invasiveness, the need for specialized training and equipment, and potential complications relating to puncture site, catheter insertion, catheterization of the cerebral arteries, and the use of general anesthesia at some centers.

PROACT I and II Trials

These two studies, published in 1998 and 1999 (del Zoppo et al. 1998; Furlan et al. 1999; see also **Table 6.2**), dealt with the intra-arterial use of prourokinase in patients with an angiographically detected M1 or M2 occlusion. PROACT I was designed to investigate the safety and efficacy of prourokinase. In that study, two groups of 40 patients each received 6 mg of prourokinase or placebo over a 2-h period from 3 to 6 h after onset of stroke symptoms. The agent had to be administered proximal to the thrombus; manipulation with a wire or catheter was not allowed. The TIMI (Thrombolysis in Myocardial Infarction) score (**Table 8.1**) was used to evaluate recanalization. This classification is derived from studies on thrombolysis in acute myocardial infarction, and an original or slightly modified form of the classification is still used in studies today.

In the PROACT I trial, at least partial reperfusion (TIMI = 2 or 3) was demonstrable in 57.7% of the patients vs. only 14.3% of the controls. Although the rate of symptomatic intracranial hemorrhage was more than twice as high in the treated group (15.5%) than in the control group (7.1%), the patients treated with intra-arterial prourokinase had a better clinical outcome and lower mortality. While these advantages were very promising but not statistically significant due to the small case numbers, PROACT II studied 180 patients using the same

Tab. 8.1 Thrombolysis in Myocardial Infarction (TIMI) score for classifying perfusion after the recanalization of a thromboembolic occlusion (TICI classification see Table 7.3)

TIMI score	Description
0	No perfusion, no antegrade flow distal to the occlusion
1	Penetration of the thrombus with minimal distal flow; filling around the thrombus but no distal branch filling
2	Partial perfusion with incomplete or slow distal branch filling
3	Full perfusion with timely filling of arteries and veins

Source: The TIMI Study Group 1985.

II

design except for a higher administered dose (9 mg). Of the 180 patients enrolled, 121 received prourokinase plus intravenous heparin; 59 patients served as a control group and underwent arterial catheterization but received only a saline infusion through the microcatheter plus intravenous heparin. The physicians conducting the study were blinded to the group assignments. As expected, the partial and complete recanalization rates were significantly higher in the prourokinase group (66%) than in the control group (18%). This benefit was also reflected in the percentage of patients who survived and were functionally independent (40% vs. 25%). The higher incidence of intracranial hemorrhage (10% vs. 2% in the control group) did not affect the mortality rate at 90 days, which was 25% compared with 27% in the control group. Despite this obvious benefit, the FDA withheld approval of prourokinase for use in acute stroke pending the results of further studies.

Since PROACT I and II, many studies have been published on local intra-arterial fibrinolysis, some even reporting better reperfusion results with no increased incidence of intracranial hemorrhage. A comparative study of intravenous and intra-arterial thrombolysis between two stroke units in Switzerland published in 2008 again documented the benefit of local fibrinolysis in ischemic stroke patients with a HMCAS (Mattle et al. 2008). With a population of > 50 patients per unit, the group that received local intra-arterial fibrinolysis had > 30% *more* independently surviving patients than the group that underwent intravenous thrombolysis at the other unit. This is all the more remarkable when we note that baseline stroke severity was higher in the group treated with local intra-arterial fibrinolysis, and that the mean time to treatment was considerably longer in the intra-arterial group (244 min) than in the intravenous group (156 min).

Bridging Therapy

Intravenous thrombolysis can be administered at a reduced dose to bridge the time until the initiation of local fibrinolysis. Bridging therapy is described in an earlier chapter (see p. 76) and does not apply exclusively to MCA occlusions.

Support of Fibrinolysis

A major disadvantage of intravenous as well as intra-arterial fibrinolysis without mechanical manipulation is that, with a complete occlusion, the fibrinolytic agent can interact with the thrombus only to a very limited degree. Thus, it was recognized very early that supportive manipulations could increase the recanalization rate. When the studies on intravenous thrombolysis were published

in the 1990s, initial reports appeared on how simple microwire manipulations during fibrinolysis could support and improve recanalization. Even today, this can still be an effective tool in settings which lack availability or experience with approved mechanical thrombectomy systems. As recently as 2008, a study was published in which 18 of 19 patients were successfully recanalized by urokinase therapy that was aided by microwire manipulation (Kim et al. 2008).

> **Note**
>
> Mechanical manipulations support the effectiveness of fibrinolysis.

Ultrasound

Ultrasound provides a noninvasive mechanical option for supporting fibrinolysis. Similar to its use in cleaning surfaces, ultrasound energy can induce the mixing and movement of fluids without causing grossly visible flow (see also the section on Classification of Symptoms, p. 97). Ultrasound was found to accelerate fibrinolysis in experimental models (Francis and Suchkova 2001). With isolated reports of continuous transcranial Doppler ultrasound improving the efficacy of intravenous thrombolysis, leading to better clinical outcomes, this phenomenon was subsequently investigated in studies. The most important of these studies, CLOTBUST (Alexandrov et al. 2004), is relevant in that it dealt exclusively with occlusions of the MCA. A total of 126 patients were assigned to two equal groups that received either continuous 2-MHz transcranial Doppler ultrasound at the occlusion interface (target group) or a placebo (control group) during continuous intravenous thrombolysis. Both the rate of successful recanalizations and the percentage of patients with little or no disability were higher in the target group than in the control group. Statistical analysis of the results did not indicate a significant trend, however. This concept can be expanded to include the concurrent use of ultrasound contrast agents (microbubbles) to amplify the disruptive effect of the ultrasound. Study results have not yet been published on this refinement.

The intra-arterial counterpart of ultrasound-enhanced thrombolysis involves the use of intravascular ultrasound or the EKOS catheter system (see **Fig. 7.8**), which have been used for example in the IMS II and III trials (IMS II Trial Investigators 2007; Interventional Management of Stroke III: intravenous thrombolysis vs. intravenous plus local intra-arterial thrombolysis [bridging]; patients recruited since June 2006). Again, ultrasound energy supports the interaction of the fibrinolytic agent with the clot but is delivered through the tip of the microcatheter itself.

Mechanical Thrombectomy

Traditional treatment methods have been based wholly or partly on the action of fibrinolytic agents, with or without mechanical support. A large percentage of patients are ineligible for lytic therapy because of possible contraindications or because the time from symptom onset is too long or unknown. Today, devices and systems for primary thrombus extraction have attracted growing interest and are the subject of numerous studies. Because these devices are not specific for thrombus location and are described earlier in some detail, we limit our attention here to a brief review.

MERCI Retriever (Concentric Medical)

The MERCI Retriever is the first thrombectomy system to be approved by the FDA for use in stroke patients (see also the section on Recanalization Rate and Neurologic Outcome, p. 89). The first generation of this device, which is deployed distal to the clot through a microcatheter and has a corkscrew-like shape, was investigated for its safety and efficacy in a total of 151 patients, 57% of whom had an occlusion of the MCA. The rate of successful recanalizations, at 46% (intention to treat), was not very satisfactory, and the incidence of significant complications, at 7.1%, was unacceptably high from a current perspective. The third-generation MERCI Retriever (V Series) is now being marketed with a design that differs significantly from its predecessors. With regard to MCA occlusions, it is noteworthy that the smallest retriever (2 mm) can even reach the M2 segment. No study results have yet been published on the new design. Based on data in the MERCI Registry, the device has an overall revascularization rate of ~80%.

Phenox

This modular system (see **Fig. 7.10**) consists of a brush-like array of nylon microfilaments radiating from a central wire, which may or may not be combined with a nitinol microcage. It is important in the treatment of MCA occlusions because the smallest version can be deployed in vessels 1–1.5 mm in diameter and, at least in theory, can recanalize occlusions at the M3 level. No clinical studies or comprehensive series have yet been published.

Thrombectomy with Retractable Stents

Stent-based thrombectomy devices are a relatively new and promising approach now being investigated in clinical studies and produced by several manufacturers (see Stenting in Stroke Patients, p. 92). The main goal is not to insert a stent to restore flow but to use its mechanical interaction with the thrombus as a means of extracting the clot. Initial reports and single-center studies have shown that this concept can provide high recanalization rates with few complications (Castaño et al. 2010). Efficacy and safety both depend critically on the mechanical properties of the device such as mesh size, radial pressure, friction during placement, and the surface characteristics of the material, which are currently varied and optimized by various manufacturing firms. At present, the only systems that have received CE (European Community) approval are the Solitaire FR (EV3) and Trevo device (Concentric Medical). It should be added, however, that because these systems also have a temporary endovascular bypass function and are used after or during the administration of fibrinolytic drugs, their success is not based entirely on mechanical clot retrieval, as explained below.

Concept of Temporary Endovascular Bypass

This concept seeks to recanalize the occluded artery as quickly as possible to provide immediate flow restoration to dependent areas, allow local or systemic fibrinolytic agents to reach the thrombus, and clear prothrombogenic substances formed by the clot. Kelly et al. (2008) described a patient with an embolic occlusion of the M1 segment of the right MCA and an associated occlusion of the right cervical ICA that precluded thrombectomy with the MERCI device or other approved system. As an alternative, the authors introduced a microcatheter through the contralateral ICA and advanced it across the anterior communicating artery and through the thrombus in the right MCA. The microcatheter was withdrawn to partially deploy a self-expanding, closed-cell nitinol stent (Enterprise, Codman) across the occlusion site. Two-thirds of the stent was unconstrained to circumferentially displace the thrombus and restore blood flow through the right MCA. Abciximab and rtPA were administered intra-arterially through the microcatheter to dissolve the clot. The stent was then reconstrained and removed.

> **Note**
>
> Besides the minimal need for manipulations (thrombectomy was not done in this case), the advantage of a temporary retractable stent over a permanently implanted stent is that it eliminates the need for long-term platelet inhibition. This can be particularly relevant in stroke patients who are already on anticoagulants for an underlying cardiac arrhythmia.

While the stent used in this initial description was only partially deployed before retrieval, systems are currently being used that are designed almost exclusively for this application. Besides the Trevo and Solitaire systems described earlier, which are designed primarily for thrombectomy (**Fig. 8.5**), today there are systems

II

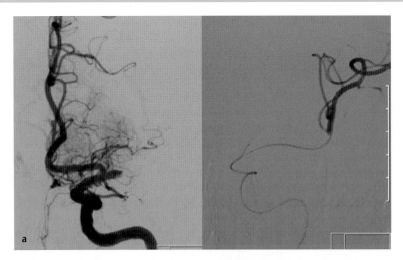

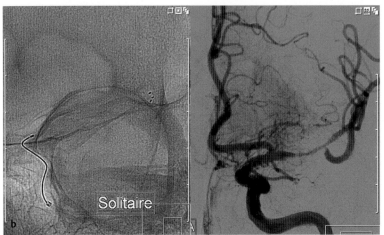

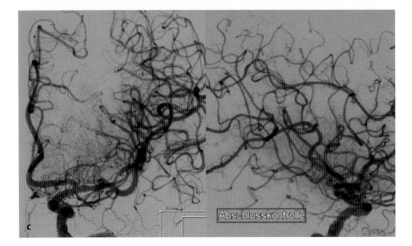

Fig. 8.5a–c   Occlusion of the left MCA.
a The occlusion is crossed with a microcatheter, and contrast medium is injected distal to the thrombus (*right*).
b The microcatheter is carefully withdrawn to deploy the stent in the occluded segment (*left*). Contrast injection through the guide catheter (*right*) shows the efficacy of the temporary endovascular bypass with filling of distal vessels, but with persistent occlusion of lenticulostriate perforators.
c After stent retrieval for mechanical thrombectomy, complete perfusion is restored (TIMI score = 3), including the perforators from the M1 segment.

specifically designed to produce an optimum bypass effect (e.g., MindFrame devices).

Stent or Balloon Thromboplasty

In addition to local intra-arterial fibrinolysis, mechanical support for fibrinolytic agents, mechanical thrombectomy, and stent deployment for temporary bypass, another option is to dilate or "push aside" the occlusive material as in coronary angioplasty. The basic tools available for the purpose are balloons and stents. Initial reports described the use of balloon-expandable coronary stents, particularly in the MCA, but this practice was quickly abandoned due mainly to the stiffness of the stents and the associated risk of vascular rupture. Although the safe use of self-expanding stents for the coiling of aneurysms was already known on the basis of numerous studies and published case series, the first clinical use of a Neuroform 3 stent for recanalizing a postbifurcation M1 occlusion was described in 2006 (Sauvageau and Levy 2006). This concept was investigated somewhat later in a multicenter study of 18 patients, which showed that short segmental occlusions in particular could be recanalized with a self-expanding stent (Wingspan or Neuroform 3) even after previous unsuccessful lytic therapy or thrombectomy. As a result of this study (Levy et al. 2007), an FDA-approved prospective trial of primary intracranial stenting was conducted in 20 stroke patients. Eligibility criteria included contraindications to intravenous fibrinolysis or failure to improve within 1 h after fibrinolysis, a segmental occlusion length no greater than 14 mm, and presentation less than 8 h from symptom onset. Successful revascularization (TIMI 2 or 3) was achieved in all patients. A remarkably high percentage of patients (45%) had little or no disability at 3 months (Levy et al. 2009). These results were reproduced almost contemporaneously by a group of Swiss authors in 12 stroke patients, 5 of whom had an occlusion of the MCA (Brekenfeld et al. 2009).

The concept of permanent intracranial stenting for acute stroke is limited in several respects. One limiting factor is that the occluded segment must be short enough to be encompassed by the stent. Another factor relating to the MCA is that the stent must be positioned between the thrombus and vessel wall in such a way that it separates the thrombus from the perforator origins. Otherwise a good clinical outcome will not be achieved in most patients, even if perfusion has been restored to the distal MCA branches. Another factor to be considered is that permanent stent implantation requires the immediate initiation of antiplatelet medication. Finally, stent implantation in very tortuous or very thin vessels is generally not feasible or leads to potential complications. Another option is to angioplasty the thrombus with a balloon. Gifford et al. (2010) published a successful small series on the use of microballoons (1.5–2.5 mm diameter) in the M2 and M3 branches of the MCA. Tokunaga et al. (2010) described the use of a double-lumen balloon catheter (Gateway) for angioplasty and concurrent fibrinolysis in a total of 59 patients, 33 of whom had MCA occlusions.

Is General Anesthesia Necessary?

Basically there are no specific procedural requirements for MCA occlusions that would differ from other occlusion patterns, aside from the strict time window that applies to anterior circulation strokes (a 6-h window is still observed at most centers). The procedure itself is determined by the particular system that is used for stroke treatment and need not be described here.

We do have access to current study data on endovascular procedures done under conscious sedation or general endotracheal anesthesia. Jumaa et al. (2010) compared general endotracheal anesthesia with the nonintubated state with respect to length of stay on the intensive care unit (ICU), procedural complications, periprocedural mortality, final infarct volume, and clinical outcome at 3 months in 126 consecutive patients with a proximal MCA occlusion. A uni- and multivariate analysis showed that the *nonintubated* patients had significantly better results with respect to mortality, clinical outcome, and final infarct volume. The authors suggest that one reason for this phenomenon may be a brief, transient fall in blood pressure during anesthesia induction, leading to larger infarct volumes in the intubated patients. It is unclear at present whether these findings will be reproducible in further studies or applicable to other occlusion patterns.

Summary

Thromboembolic occlusion of the MCA is the most common form of ischemic stroke. The length and precise location of the segmental occlusion, individual anatomy with regard to collateral circulation, and the involvement of lenticulostriate perforators determine the extent of potential tissue damage. The clinical presentation depends on the hemisphere or brain area affected by the stroke. The ability of recanalization procedures to improve outcomes depends on when and where they are applied, how effective they are, and whether they can actually worsen the patient's condition: for example, as a result of intracranial hemorrhage after fibrinolysis or direct vascular injury from mechanical recanalization.

II

Note

The standard treatment for MCA occlusions in general is still intravenous thrombolysis started within 4.5 h from symptom onset. If the patient is treated at a center where endovascular therapy is available, prompt intra-arterial thrombolysis or mechanical recanalization should be strongly considered separate from intravenous thrombolysis (bridging), at least in patients with M1 involvement or long-segment occlusions, due to the limited efficacy of thrombolytic therapy. Otherwise intravenous thrombolysis should be started and the patient transferred to a neurovascular center ("drip and ship").

Regardless of whether CT or MRI is used, the goal of stroke imaging is no longer limited to excluding hemorrhage but includes visualization of the vessels and the occlusion and the measurement of perfusion. These findings play a major role in planning treatment and identifying possible treatment risks.

Until more study data are available, the selection of systems for mechanical thrombus extraction will be based largely on the individual preferences of interventionalists. It is already becoming apparent, however, that stent-based systems may dominate the field in the future, because of their versatility. Multimodal therapy based on a combination of different strategies also appears to offer advantages. On the basis of current information, patients with an MCA occlusion who undergo endovascular therapy without general anesthesia have at least comparable clinical outcomes, justifying treatment under conscious sedation until further studies become available.

Basilar Artery Thrombosis

G. Schulte-Altedorneburg and

H. Brueckmann

Introduction

The most severe forms of vertebrobasilar occlusion are thrombosis or embolic occlusion of the basilar artery. Untreated basilar artery thrombosis has a mortality rate of 80–90%. As early as 1982, this led Hermann Zeumer to employ selective intra-arterial thrombolysis, which had not previously been used for cerebrovascular occlusions (Zeumer et al. 1982). While this procedure did bring significant improvement in recanalization and mortality rates, the number of patients with a significant neurologic deficit following endovascular therapy was still

high (Hacke et al. 1988; Schulte-Altedorneburg et al. 2006). Delayed recanalization, thrombus migration, and intracerebral hemorrhage were identified as the major shortcomings of intra-arterial thrombolysis alone. This inevitably spurred the development of mechanical recanalization, which had already been tested and partially established for use in peripheral and cardiac vessels. For some years, the different approaches to mechanical or thrombolytic recanalization have been combined with preliminary or overlapping intravenous therapy with a thrombolytic agent or platelet inhibitor (see the section on Bridging Therapy, p. 76).

The sections below explore the factors that should be considered in selecting patients for endovascular therapy as well as the advantages and disadvantages of the various treatment concepts and their results.

Indications for Endovascular Therapy

The indications for endovascular therapy are based on the clinical syndromes described in Chapter 3 and the corresponding vascular occlusions, which are diagnosed by semi-invasive imaging techniques. Although there has been great and undisputed success in the development and testing of mechanical recanalization techniques during the past 5–10 years, neurologists have continued to question the concept because of inconsistencies in clinical outcomes despite complete recanalization (Molina 2010). This applies mainly to the anterior circulation, however. We feel that the disastrous spontaneous prognosis of basilar artery thrombosis obligates every stroke physician to offer maximum endovascular therapy to patients whenever there is any doubt.

Patient Selection

Various groups are working to develop imaging protocols that can improve patient selection for endovascular therapy. Although MR and CT perfusion imaging still do not have sufficient resolution to accurately define circumscribed peripheral deficits in brainstem areas, they can detect a possible perfusion–diffusion mismatch in the thalamus and occipital and temporal lobes, which is crucial in therapeutic decision-making. Additionally, semiautomated algorithms for generating maps of cerebral blood flow, blood volume, mean transit time (MTT), and time to peak (TTP) have become faster and more user-friendly and may provide another useful selection criterion pending systematic studies on the capabilities of perfusion imaging.

Time Window

In contrast to the anterior circulation, studies on the treatment of basilar artery thrombosis, done mostly in retrospective series, have not disclosed a time window for initiating treatment. The two largest retrospective case series on intra-arterial thrombolysis published to date even included patients treated more than 12 h after symptom onset (Eckert et al. 2002b; Schulte-Altedorneburg et al. 2006). Over a wide range of time to treatment, from 3 to 18 h after symptom onset, Eckert et al. (2002b) identified the early initiation of endovascular therapy as the most important factor in achieving a good outcome.

> **Caution**
>
> This led Eckert and his colleagues (Eckert et al. 2002b) to conclude that endovascular therapy is not reasonable in patients with severe neurologic symptoms (tetraplegia, coma) that have been present for more than 6 h. It should be noted, however, that the fluctuation and slow progression of a severe brainstem syndrome often make it difficult to determine the exact time of symptom onset (Ferbert et al. 1990).

Duration of Coma

Coma duration has frequently been cited as an important parameter in therapeutic decision-making. We believe that this is problematic, however, since critical care measures (with protective intubation) often leave no time to determine an accurate neurologic status or elicit a reliable history from the patient or a third party. Unlike strokes in the anterior circulation, then, information on the duration of coma is too imprecise to establish a firm time window for deciding whether to initiate therapeutic actions. It is our practice to document coma duration and correlate it with imaging findings; however, we do not base therapeutic decisions on the duration of coma.

On the other hand, if a neurologic examination by a specialist can be completed prior to intubation, our data indicate that pretreatment neurologic findings are a highly significant parameter in terms of patient outcome (Schulte-Altedorneburg et al. 2006).

Age Limit

As with other cardiovascular diseases and with cancer, we are reluctant to impose a strict age limit when selecting patients for treatment. Given the gains in life expectancy, better health awareness among the public,

and the frequent discrepancy between biological and chronological age in older patients, we feel that all cases should be considered on an individual, interdisciplinary basis taking into account cerebrovascular and parenchymal findings and comorbid conditions.

> **Practical Tip**
>
> In elderly patients with long-segment basilar artery occlusions and comorbid disease, stroke physicians should discuss the possible presence of an advance directive with family members before proceeding with aggressive recanalization therapy.

Diffusion-Weighted MRI

Several stroke centers use diffusion-weighted MRI (DWI) as a prognostic parameter in cases where the time from symptom onset is unknown or exceeds 6 h. Indeed, all patients with suspected basilar artery thrombosis undergo primary MRI at centers where that modality is available on a 24-h basis. There is no question that MRI is the most sensitive modality for detecting brainstem ischemia (Schulte-Altedorneburg and Brückmann 2006). One difficulty, however, is that the detection of intracerebral hemorrhage, especially subarachnoid hemorrhage, requires a suitable MRI protocol that goes beyond the "fast protocol" for stroke patients. At present it is unclear what degree of diffusion abnormality would justify the choice of palliative therapy over a recanalization procedure. The reliability of this parameter is questionable, since the reversibility of DWI lesions after basilar artery recanalization beyond the 6-h limit has been described by case reports (Yoo et al. 2010).

Circumscribed Infarctions

All authors agree that circumscribed infarctions in the cerebellum, the occipital or temporal cortex, or the thalamus that are clearly demarcated on baseline CT do not contraindicate endovascular therapy. Their presence should be considered only in determining the dose of possible thrombolytic agents, to avoid the risk of intracranial hemorrhage.

Treatment Concepts and Results

Figure 8.6 shows the treatment algorithm recommended for patients with clinical suspicion of basilar artery thrombosis.

II

Treatment of Acute Ischemic Stroke

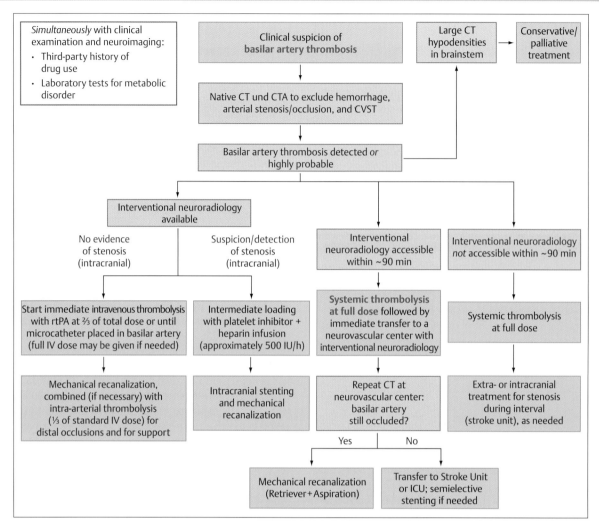

Fig. 8.6 **Algorithm for the management of clinically suspected basilar artery thrombosis.**

Intra-arterial Thrombolysis

The agent used for intra-arterial thrombolysis at most centers is rtPA. The dose depends on whether intra-arterial thrombolysis is used alone or for bridging therapy. Experience has shown that the dose should not exceed the weight-adjusted maximum dose that is standard for intravenous thrombolysis. Whether the dose is given by continuous infusion or in multiple boluses, as well as the rate of administration for continuous infusion (30–45 mg/h), will depend on the progress of recanalization, the frequency of microcatheter position changes, and the experience of the interventionalist.

Some groups use urokinase as an alternative thrombolytic agent to rtPA. Again, the reported maximum doses show a large range of variation (250 000 to 1.5 million IU). There is evidence that intra-arterial rtPA provides a slightly higher recanalization rate than intra-arterial urokinase, but rtPA appears to be linked with a higher rate of intracerebral hemorrhage than urokinase, especially when used at doses

> 80 mg (Brückmann et al. 1986; Zeumer et al. 1993; Eckert et al. 2002b; Schulte-Altedorneburg et al. 2007a).

Practical Tip

It is difficult to convert an rtPA dose to the corresponding urokinase dose, because the chemical properties (molecular weight) of the agent and particularly the direct action of rtPA on the vessel wall presumably contribute to the incidence of intraparenchymal hemorrhage.

A retrospective comparison of results in patient cohorts shows that while recanalization rates improved from 44% to ~75% during the period from 1988 to 2008, the percentage of patients with a good neurologic outcome has remained stagnant at ~25% (**Table 8.2**). Even so, the mortality rate relative to earlier antiplatelet therapy has fallen to ~40%, which represents a major success for intra-arterial thrombolysis alone.

Tab. 8.2 Selected studies from the past 20 years on various approaches to the treatment of basilar artery thrombosis

Study	Treatment modality	Number of patients	Patient age (years)	Mortality (%)	Time to intra-arterial treatment (h)	Recanalization rate (%)	Thrombolytic agent	Good neurologic outcome (mRS = 0–2; %)	Symptomatic parenchymal hemorrhage (%)
Hacke et al. 1988	IAT	43	52	67	n.a.	44	UK. SK	23	9
Eckert et al. 2002b	IAT	83	60	60	8	66	rtPA: n = 41 UK: n=23 rtPA + Lys-plas: n=19	23	8
Arnold et al. 2004	IAT	40	58	42	5.5	80	UK	35	5
Eckert et al. 2005	IAT, PI, PTA/Stent	47	69	38	6	72	rt-PA	34	13
Schulte-Altedorneburg et al. 2006	IAT	180	58	43	n.a.	74	rt-PA: n = 97 UK: n = 75 SK:n = 8	23	12
Nagel et al. 2009	IAT	32	65	75	6	63	rtPA	6	19
Nagel et al. 2009	Bridging: IAT + PI, PTA/Stent	43	65	42	5	84	rtPA	19	14
Pfefferkorn et al. 2010	Bridging: IVT + MT	26	60	31	4.2	85	IV rtPA	38	8

i.a., intra-arterial
IAT, intra-arterial thrombolysis
i.v., intravenous
IVT, intravenous thrombolysis
MT, mechanical thrombectomy
n.a., not applicable
PTA, peripheral transluminal angioplasty
PI, platelet inhibitor (abciximab or tirofiban)
UK, urokinase
SK, streptokinase
Lys-plas, human-derived Lys-plasminogen.

Regardless of improved guide catheters and micro-catheters, which provide better and faster access to the occlusion site, problems of clot migration and intracranial hemorrhage at high thrombolytic doses continue to be intrinsic disadvantages of intra-arterial thrombolysis. Our own analysis of 143 patients showed that the occurrence of any type of intracranial hemorrhage (subarachnoid or intracerebral bleeding, hemorrhagic transformation) was associated with a significantly poorer clinical outcome (Schulte-Altedorneburg et al. 2007a).

Intravenous Thrombolysis

Intravenous thrombolysis is not classified as a endovascular therapy strategy for acute stroke. Several retrospective studies, meta-analyses, and registries on the intravenous treatment of basilar artery thrombosis have been published during the past 5 years. Surprisingly, the publications on recanalization rates and clinical outcomes, authored mainly by neurologists, described results comparable to those of intra-arterial thrombolysis (Lindsberg et al. 2004; Lindsberg and Mattle 2006; Schonewille et al. 2009). On closer analysis of these heterogeneous data, however, we find that the diagnosis of basilar artery thrombosis in patients treated by intravenous thrombolysis was confirmed solely by time-of-flight MR angiography (TOF MRA). It remains unclear, therefore, whether patients actually had basilar artery thrombosis as opposed to only a stenosed artery with a residual flow maintaining the perfusion of the brainstem (with a much better prognosis than occlusion), which was misinterpreted because of the known limitations of TOF MRA in slow and low flow ("skip sign"). In addition, precise data on occlusion length and/or severity of clinical syndrome were not given. Thus, we cannot make a meaningful, systematic comparison with previously published studies on endovascular therapy (Schulte-Altedorneburg et al. 2007b and 2009).

Nevertheless, intravenous thrombolysis alone is still a treatment option for basilar artery thrombosis in less populated areas with poor access to a neurointerventional center. Moreover, intravenous thrombolysis is a key element in protocols that bridge the interval from diagnosis to microcatheter insertion for intra-arterial thrombolysis or mechanical thrombectomy on site (see below). The combined intravenous administration of rtPA and tirofiban has been used successfully in the treatment of MCA occlusions but, to our knowledge, has not been pursued further (Straub et al. 2004).

Mechanical Thrombectomy

During the past decade many different devices have been successfully used for mechanical recanalization, as discussed elsewhere (Mayer et al. 2002 and 2005; Liebig et al. 2008; Chopko et al. 2000; Clarençon et al. 2009; see Chapter 7). It has become clear that none of the thrombectomy devices alone can offer a 100% recanalization rate for all conceivable patterns of vertebrobasilar occlusion. It is equally clear that catheterization laboratories should keep several different recanalization systems in stock. A particular system is selected according to the consistency of the thrombus (soft or hard), the volume and length of the thrombus, vessel wall status (calcification or high-grade stenosis), presumed etiology, the proximal vascular segment (elongation, coiling, extracranial stenosis) and, last but not least, the experience and preferences of the interventionalist.

> **Practical Tip**
>
> Overall, it has been found that aspiration-only systems yield good results in the smooth, straight vessels of young patients (< 40 years), who tend to have cardiogenic emboli. Other devices such as snares, (more rigid) cages, and permanent stents are better for older patients, who tend to have irregular arteries with atherosclerotic and/or hypertensive changes and thrombi with a harder consistency. Temporary stents can provide effective recanalization in any age group.

To date, the migration of thrombotic material is a problem that has not been fully solved even by the current practice of simultaneous aspiration and retrieval (Liebig et al. 2008; **Fig. 8.7**), and there is still the time loss

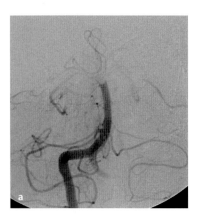
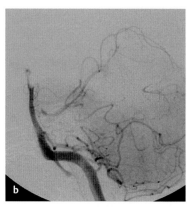

Fig. 8.7a–h Basilar artery thrombosis. A 65-year-old man who presented with fluctuating symptoms of impaired consciousness, dysarthria, and hypoesthesia of the tongue since of ~3 h duration.
CT angiography (CTA) revealed a basilar tip occlusion. The patient was intubated, and right vertebral angiography was performed through a 6F Envoy catheter.
a DSA in the PA projection.
b DSA in the lateral projection. Both views (**a, b**) show nonfilling of the basilar artery and its branches distal to the origin of the superior cerebellar artery.

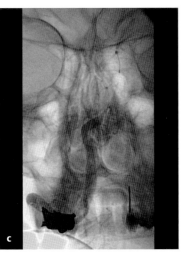

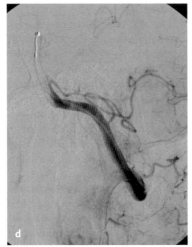

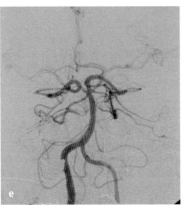

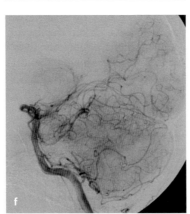

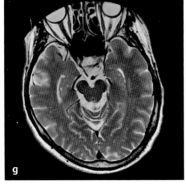

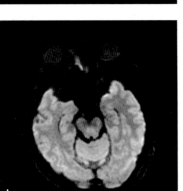

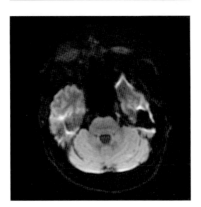

Fig. 8.7c–h (*continued*)

c Recanalization with the Penumbra system (0.041 inches [1.04 mm]). Unsubtracted PA view shows the Penumbra catheter with the separator inside. The tip of the aspiration catheter is within the thrombosed basilar artery segment.

d Corresponding DSA image in the lateral projection.

e Final DSA in the PA projection.

f Final DSA in the lateral projection. Both views (**e, f**) document complete recanalization of the vertebrobasilar system within a few minutes.

g T2w MRI 4 h postintervention.

h DW MRI 4 h postintervention. Both sets of images (**g, h**) show no evidence of restricted diffusion or infarction. The patient was discharged 2 days later with mRS = 0.

II

caused by the need for multiple retriever passes. In reviewing our own cases and the current literature, we note that the use of a mechanical recanalization device is supplemented by low-dose intra-arterial thrombolysis in the great majority of patients treated. This has to be taken in account when evaluating optimistic case reports and (pilot) studies on specific occlusion treatments published during the past 10 years. In general, we find that mechanical recanalization has been able to increase recanalization rates and shorten recanalization times relative to intra-arterial thrombolysis alone in the treatment of basilar artery thrombosis (Pfefferkorn et al. 2010; see also **Table 8.2**).

Bridging Therapy

The rationale for bridging therapy, in which intravenous thrombolysis or platelet inhibition serves as a temporizing prelude to a selective intra-arterial recanalization procedure, is based on the observation that the interval from admission to the start of intra-arterial thrombolysis was too long in many patients. The risk of appositional thrombi and an "occlusion on top of an occlusion" was not prevented by the former practice of administering a heparin bolus. On the basis of positive experience with intravenous thrombolysis with rtPA in the anterior circulation and equally positive cardiologic reports on the effectiveness of platelet aggregation inhibitors (glycoprotein IIb/IIIa receptor inhibitors) in preventing recurrent thrombosis, both of these medications have been incorporated into therapeutic regimens (Eckert et al. 2002a and 2005; Pfefferkorn et al. 2010). Given the risks of intracranial and systemic hemorrhage, this approach calls for even greater care in performing microwire and microcatheter manipulations.

Previous studies on combined intravenous and intra-arterial therapy with a thrombolytic agent pertain exclusively to the anterior circulation (except for occasional retrospective case data), and so we cannot assess the efficacy of this therapy in the vertebrobasilar system (Shaltoni et al. 2007).

Treatment with a glycoprotein IIb/IIIa receptor inhibitor (abciximab) followed by intra-arterial thrombolysis with rtPA at a dose of 20–60 mg and possible stent implantation was investigated in two studies. Both studies found that this combination was superior to intra-arterial thrombolysis alone in terms of recanalization rates and neurologic outcomes (Eckert et al. 2005; Nagel et al. 2009; see also **Table 8.2**). It did not increase the incidence of symptomatic intracranial hemorrhage.

Due in part to many transfers from peripheral hospitals, a group in Munich, Germany, has been working for several years on a bridging protocol consisting of initial intravenous thrombolysis at a standard dose followed later by mechanical recanalization (Pfefferkorn et al. 2010; see also **Table 8.2**). The mechanical recanalization therapy can be escalated from pure aspiration to temporary (**Fig. 8.8**) or permanent stent placement, depending on the volume and consistency of the thrombus. Recanalization is achieved in a full one-third of patients after intravenous thrombolysis alone. The final recanalization rate after mechanical thrombectomy is 80–90%. As for clinical outcomes, this protocol led to reduced mortality and better neurologic status at 3 months compared with patients who had been treated by intra-arterial thrombolysis alone or a combination of intra-arterial thrombolysis and tirofiban (Pfefferkorn et al. 2010).

Unfortunately, the only available American Heart Association (AHA) publication is a scientific statement dating from 2009 regarding "Indications for the performance of intracranial endovascular neurointerventional procedures" (Meyers et al. 2009). Considering the current and ongoing studies on endovascular stroke treatment, we believe that intra-arterial thrombolysis and mechanical revascularization will reach a higher classification of level of evidence in future AHA recommendations.

Fig. 8.8a–j   A 73-year-old woman on anticoagulant therapy had undergone previous cardioablation for atrial fibrillation.
She now presented with markedly decreased vigilance of 2.5 h duration. CTA demonstrated basilar artery thrombosis. It was decided to intubate and proceed with mechanical recanalization.
a DSA in the PA projection.
b DSA in the lateral projection. Both views (**a, b**) show an occlusion of the basilar artery distal to the origin of the AICA.
c Access is established with a reinforced 70-cm 6F sheath, which is advanced into the brachiocephalic trunk.
d A DAC 0.057-inch (1.45-mm) catheter is advanced into the atlas loop.
e The occluded basilar artery is crossed with a Rebar 18 microcatheter, which is advanced into the right P1 segment.

f Corresponding DSA image in the lateral projection.
g Final DSA in the PA projection.   ▷
h Final DSA in the lateral projection. Both views (**g, h**) show complete vertebrobasilar recanalization, which was achieved quickly with a 4-mm × 20-mm Solitaire FR device deployed in the occluded segment. The Solitaire FR was deployed with continuous aspiration on the DAC catheter and was withdrawn on the sheath. Thrombus fragments were present in the aspirate.
i MRI the next day shows a large, bilateral pontine infarction with restricted diffusion.
j Corresponding FLAIR sequence. The patient died a few days later.

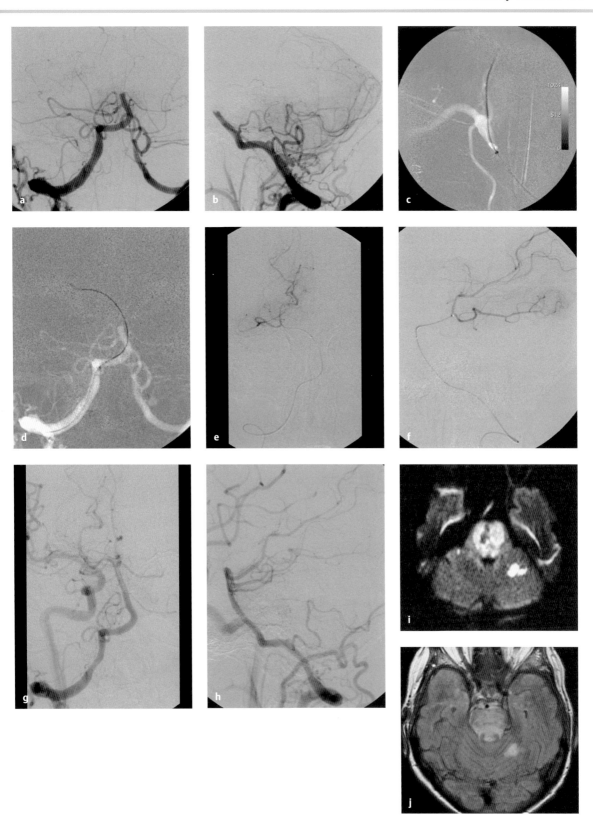

Cervical Artery Dissections

A. Rohr and H. Goerike

Introduction

Dissections of the carotid or vertebral arteries pose a serious health threat to the patient and require immediate therapy. The main treatment options are pharmacologic thromboprophylaxis and interventional radiology. The treatment of choice for a particular patient is an individual decision based on the specific situation. Thus, a traumatic vascular dissection with persistent bleeding, a ruptured intracranial dissecting aneurysm, an impending stroke due to luminal narrowing, a chronic pseudoaneurysm, or a "simple" stenosis are all different manifestations of the same underlying pathology: vascular dissection. While some of these conditions require active measures or even emergency action in the form of a neuroradiologic intervention, other cases are best managed by pharmacologic thromboprophylaxis or simple follow-up. The development of endovascular techniques is progressing swiftly and promises ever newer and better treatment options. But given the nonspecific clinical presentation and diverse neurologic manifestations of cervical artery dissections on the one hand, and the relative rarity of these conditions on the other, we do not have the benefit of well-documented results based on large therapeutic trials.

Note

Because dissections vary, there is no typical dissection patient or standard evidence-based therapy. Patients with dissections must be treated individually, on the basis of the specific situation.

Given the lack of large studies, the results of small case series generally provide the basis for case management in patients with cervical artery dissections (review in Santos-Franco et al. 2008; Goyal and Derdeyn 2009; Kim and Schulman 2009). Treatment planning depends on the individual situation and should include a detailed analysis of vascular status and related pathophysiologic considerations (e.g., collateral circulation, tandem stenosis, bilateral changes, aneurysm configuration, etc.). Treatment decisions are also influenced by the personal experience and skills of the interventionalist—who is preferably part of an interdisciplinary team—and by patient attitudes and preferences regarding anticoagulant medication, for example, which are essential for good compliance.

Study Results and Guidelines

To date, there have been no randomized double-blind studies with a class I level of evidence dealing with the treatment of cervical artery dissections. Nevertheless, several management principles can be identified based on available studies and meta-analyses (Diener and Putzki 2008):

- Acute systemic or local thrombolytic therapy is an option within the usual time window, i.e., a cervical artery dissection does not contraindicate such therapy. Thrombolysis has not been directly proven to be of benefit in dissection patients, however. This is merely suggested by stroke studies in patients without dissections.
- Flow-limiting stenosis caused by a dissection can be treated uneventfully by stent angioplasty, but the benefit of this treatment has not been proven in controlled trials.
- Pharmacologic prophylaxis of stroke following a dissection should employ anticoagulant or antiplatelet drugs. No groups of drugs are superior to any others.
- As a general rule, an intradural dissecting aneurysm should be managed by interventional therapy.

Treatment

Therapeutic Goals

The main therapeutic goals are derived from the pathophysiology and effects of cervical artery dissections:

- With a dissection causing high-grade stenosis: restoration of adequate cerebral blood flow to prevent or limit a hemodynamic infarction.
- With a thromboembolic occlusion distal to the dissection: thrombolysis to prevent or limit a territorial infarction.
- With a frank or impending vascular rupture: angioplasty or occlusion of the vessel or aneurysm.
- Prevention of thrombus formation and thromboembolism due to the intimal injury.

Table 8.3 shows a simplified treatment protocol that reflects the authors' preferred practice.

Pharmacologic Prophylaxis of Thromboembolic Events

It is assumed that most ischemic strokes in the setting of a cervical artery dissection result from an arterioarterial embolism in which a thrombus forms at the site of vascular injury and embolizes to an intracranial site. Such an event appears to be relatively rare in the peracute phase of the dissection, and more than half of patients experience cerebral infarctions or transient ischemic

Table 8.3 Treatment protocols for cervical artery dissections. Main therapeutic goals are thromboprophylaxis (pharmacologic or by angioplasty), hemodynamic restoration (angioplasty of high-grade stenoses with poor collateral flow), the prevention or treatment of vascular or aneurysmal rupture (stenting and/or coiling), and acute stroke therapy with thrombolysis based on the penumbra concept for dissection-induced occlusion with thrombus formation (intravenous or intra-arterial thrombolysis, mechanical recanalization if required)

Type of dissection	Location	Therapy (first choice)	Therapy (second choice)	Remarks
Dissection without significant stenosis or aneurysm	Extradural	Medical[a]		
	Intradural	Low-dose heparin	Stent, endovascular occlusion	Moderate risk of rupture (close-interval follow-ups)
Dissection with stenosis or aneurysm	Extradural	Medical	(Covered) stent, stent and coil	Indicated in patients symptomatic on medical therapy, and in cases with progression or high-grade stenosis
	Intradural	Low-dose heparin or stent (stenosis). Double stent or stent + coil (aneurysm)	Endovascular occlusion	Higher risk of rupture (aneurysm)
Dissection with thrombotic infarction, time window for thrombolysis	Extradural or intradural	Thrombolysis (intravenous, intra-arterial, mechanical)		Stent angioplasty of stenosis or vascular occlusion if required
Dissection with rupture	Extradural	(Covered) stent, stent and coil	Endovascular occlusion	
	Intradural (status post subarachnoid hemorrhage)	Endovascular occlusion	Stent and coil	Very high risk of rerupture

[a] Medical (pharmacologic) thromboprophylaxis, starting with full heparinization adjusted to PTT, then giving oral anticoagulants until vascular remodeling is complete (maximum of 24 months). This is followed by long-term aspirin therapy (100 mg/day).
Note: The treatment regimens outlined above reflect the personal experience of the authors. The protocols are greatly simplified and are for orientation purposes only. For example, the dissections were not subclassified into acute, chronic, symptomatic, or incidental forms.

attacks at a later time (usually during the first week after initial symptoms). This explains why the pharmacologic prophylaxis of thromboembolism plays a major role. Generally speaking, thromboembolism prophylaxis will not cause the intramural hematoma to enlarge and will not cause a pseudoaneurysm to grow or rupture. This is also true of thrombolytic therapy.

The preferred type of thromboprophylaxis—treatment with anticoagulant or antiplatelet drugs—is controversial. Current practice is anticoagulation with unfractionated heparin during the acute phase (adjusted to a two- to threefold increase in PTT) for 7–14 days, followed by oral anticoagulation (INR [Quick value] = 2–3) for a period of 3–6 months. Initial prophylaxis should be discontinued at least by the time the artery has recanalized without hemodynamic sequelae. Finally the patient is placed on long-term aspirin therapy at a dose of 100 mg/day. Alternatively, aspirin may be given at a daily dose of 100–325 mg instead of oral anticoagulants (Sacco et al. 2006).

Caution

Intradural dissections pose a risk of rupture with subarachnoid hemorrhage, and pharmacologic thromboprophylaxis should be used sparingly in these cases. This particularly applies to anticoagulant drugs. Given the increased risk of intracranial hemorrhage, anticoagulants should be withheld even in patients with major strokes (e.g., NIHSS > 14), and antiplatelet drugs should be given instead.

Practical Tip

Uncomplicated extradural dissections generally require only medical treatment. Imaging follow-ups can determine when therapies should be changed.

Interventional Therapy

Indications

No statistically valid studies have yet been done on the benefit of interventional therapies in patients with cervical artery dissections. On the other hand, there is a consensus that interventional techniques are appropriate in many cases and may even be the optimum form of treatment. This particularly applies to a ruptured intracranial dissecting aneurysm, which requires definitive treatment to prevent rebleeding (occurs in ~30% of cases). Interventional therapy is also appropriate for an initially unruptured intradural dissecting aneurysm due to the risk of rupture, and it is an elegant modality for treating an extracranial vascular rupture or fistula. Interventional therapy would also be indicated in the following circumstances:

- Ischemic cerebral events that occur during pharmacologic thromboprophylaxis in patients with an intra- or extracranial dissection (failed conservative therapy).
- Dissection causing a hemodynamically significant stenosis with insufficient collateral flow, especially in symptomatic patients. As an alternative, induced hypertension may be tried over a period of days or weeks under conditions of ICU surveillance.

If prolonged treatment with anticoagulant or antiplatelet drugs is contraindicated or not desired, interventional therapy can provide an alternative for the treatment of dissection-induced stenosis or aneurysm. Interventional vascular therapy may also be considered in cases where an extracranial pseudoaneurysm shows unexpected enlargement or a dissection-induced stenosis narrows further, causing greater risk of thromboembolic or hemodynamic complications. The recurrence of Horner syndrome or lower cranial nerve palsies, or their exacerbation due to redissection or pseudoaneurysm growth, would also justify interventional therapy. Acute interventional thrombus fragmentation or aspiration may be indicated for thromboembolic occlusion of the MCA secondary to a more proximal dissection. Basilar artery thrombosis or carotid-T occlusion are also indications for acute endovascular therapy.

> **Note**
>
> Basically there are three scenarios in which interventional therapy should be considered:
> - Dissections associated with vascular rupture or risk of vascular rupture
> - Failed pharmacologic therapy (or to avoid pharmacologic therapy)
> - Acute treatment of thromboembolic or hemodynamic complications

Methods

Interventional therapy is constantly evolving. There have been no randomized studies comparing the effectiveness of different interventional techniques in the treatment of cervical artery dissections, so we cannot offer clearcut recommendations on preferred techniques. Because interventional therapy is often an acute emergency procedure based on an individual treatment decision, we should choose a technique that is appropriate in principle, is available in the treatment setting, and has proven practical and safe in available studies. Different procedures are available for different conditions.

Intracranial Dissection

Intracranial dissections are rare but carry special risks. Dissecting intracranial aneurysms differ from "ordinary" saccular, nondissecting aneurysms in several respects: They often have an extremely fragile wall (Sasaki et al. 1991; Yasui et al. 1999; Santos-Franco et al. 2008) with up to a 50% risk of rupture. Aneurysms at highest risk are those with associated prestenotic dilatation, lateral dilatations, aneurysms of the posterior inferior cerebellar artery (PICA), and aneurysms proximal to the PICA origin (Takagi et al. 2007). A wait-and-see approach is not justified because of the high risk of rupture (Mizutani et al. 1995; Santos-Franco et al. 2008).

Dissecting aneurysms of the P2 or P3 segment of the PCA are another special case. They may result from trauma that exerts a shearing force on the tentorial margin and are at very high risk for rupture. Therapeutic occlusion of the affected segment while preserving the P1 segment is usually well tolerated without significant posterior infarction owing to the development of a good leptomeningeal collateral circulation from the parieto-occipital branches of the MCA and should therefore be preferred over vessel-conserving treatments.

> **Note**
>
> Ruptured intradural aneurysms should be promptly occluded by endovascular or surgical means.

The very location of vertebrobasilar aneurysms hampers the use of surgical techniques (e.g., clipping or wrapping), increases their complication rate, and may even preclude surgery (Mizutani et al. 1995; Santos-Franco et al. 2008). Interventional techniques are advantageous in several respects: They avoid surgical trauma, prevent ischemic complications, and shorten the procedure time (Santos-Franco et al. 2008). There are, however, some special considerations that apply: Most dissecting aneurysms are fusiform or wide-necked, making them difficult or impossible to treat by coil embolization alone while preserving the parent vessel. An aneurysm often coexists with vascular stenosis. The combined use of endovascular coiling and stenting may therefore be necessary.

Endovascular techniques offer high safety and effectiveness in the treatment of intradural dissections, although there is no consensus on the best procedure for a given situation (Ahn et al. 2006; Shin et al. 2007; Isokangas et al. 2008; Kim et al. 2008; Peluso et al. 2008; Zenteno et al. 2008). *Destructive* techniques that involve occlusion of the parent vessel are distinguished from *reconstructive* techniques in which the aneurysm is occluded while the parent vessel is preserved or even remodeled.

Preservation of the parent vessel would naturally be preferred on principle, but there are arguments and experience that favor occlusion of the parent vessel in some situations. For example, a vertebral artery with an aneurysm can be occluded without hemodynamic problems if an adequate contralateral vertebral artery is present. Interventional occlusion of the vertebral artery or PICA does pose a risk of brainstem or cerebellar infarction, and retrograde reperfusion of the aneurysm may also occur after parent vessel occlusion alone. However, brainstem infarction is a relatively rare complication in practice, apparently because the medulla oblongata has a rich collateral supply. Cerebellar infarctions are more commonly reported after an interventional vascular occlusion, but generally they are well tolerated by the patient. Occlusion of the aneurysm-bearing vertebral artery or PICA is often described as a fast and safe procedure with little risk of periprocedural aneurysm rupture and an excellent outcome (prevention of rerupture and ischemia; Peluso et al. 2008). As a result, several authors regard this procedure as the treatment of first choice, provided that angiography confirms an adequate collateral supply. It may be helpful to test the collateral circulation by temporary balloon occlusion. Another option in patients with an inadequate contralateral vertebral artery is the surgical creation of an extra- or intracranial bypass that will allow for safe occlusion of the vertebral artery bearing the aneurysm.

Caution

Make sure that there are no visible perforators to the brainstem or spinal cord (e.g., the anterior spinal artery) arising from the vascular segment targeted for occlusion. Some authors believe that a reconstructive procedure should generally be favored even in patients with an adequate collateral supply, because it is uncertain whether a new dissection or other problems may eventually occlude the collaterals as well (e.g., the contralateral vertebral artery), with potentially lethal effects on brain perfusion (Ahn et al. 2006; Santos-Franco et al. 2008).

Reconstructive techniques are particularly recommended in cases where the aneurysm has a good neck-to-dome ratio, there has been no active subarachnoid bleeding for several days (relatively stable aneurysm), and the parent artery is relatively large, offering favorable conditions for coil embolization with preservation of the parent vessel. Stent-assisted coiling can obliterate aneurysms that cannot be treated by unprotected coiling. Associated stenosis can be treated in the same sitting. In weighing the procedures, it is important to consider the risks of these technically sophisticated maneuvers in the individual patient.

Reconstructive procedures are strongly recommended in particularly difficult situations such as concomitant involvement of the basilar artery by the aneurysm (Kim et al. 2008). It has been shown that stent placement alone can redirect blood flow in a way that promotes thrombosis and occlusion of the aneurysm, though this is usually a delayed process (sole stenting technique; Ahn et al. 2006; Zenteno et al. 2008). Double overlapping stents (Park et al. 2009) or special flow-diverting stents (Lylyk et al. 2009) can reinforce this effect (**Fig. 8.9**). Another strategy is a two-stage procedure in which a stent is placed initially and, if it is unsuccessful, coil embolization is performed later through the stent interstices. Initially it was hoped that advanced forms of flow-diverting stents would eliminate the need for coil embolization (and its risks) altogether and make "untreatable" aneurysms treatable (e.g., vertebrobasilar dolichoectasia). However, there have been case reports of secondary aneurysm rupture or perforator infarction after the sole stenting of large aneurysms (Pavlisa et al. 2010; van Rooij and Sluzewski 2010). Currently it is recommended that even flow-diverting stents be supplemented by coil embolization. Covered stents carry a special risk of perforator occlusion, and so generally they are not used at the intradural level.

Unruptured intradural dissections and dissecting aneurysms are at less risk for rupture than dissections that have already bled. Unruptured intradural dissections can therefore be managed with low-dose heparin and close radiologic follow-up. On the other hand, acute dissections have a tendency to cause progressive ischemia and develop aneurysmal changes with an associated risk of rupture. Chronic aneurysms may grow, rupture secondarily, or cause a brainstem compression syndrome (Santos-Franco et al. 2008).

Note

As a general principle, aneurysms are managed by endovascular therapy while nonaneurysmal changes are managed conservatively.

Some authors criticize the conservative treatment of nonaneurysmal dissections because the natural history of a dissection is difficult to predict, especially when it causes ischemic symptoms (Santos-Franco et al. 2008). This particularly applies to rare dissections of the basilar artery, which carry a higher risk than dissections of other vessels (Kim et al. 2008; **Fig. 8.10**). If pharmacologic therapy is unsuccessful (e.g., in patients with progressive ischemia), endovascular therapy is indicated.

Treatment of Acute Ischemic Stroke

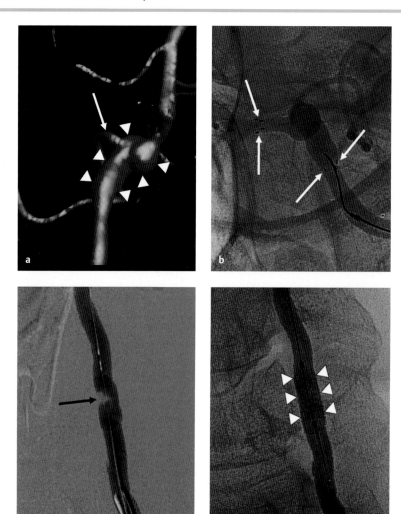

Fig. 8.9a–e   Intradural vertebral artery dissection treated by double stent placement.

a Shaded-surface view of 3D rotational angiography in a 45-year-old woman with an unruptured intradural dissecting aneurysm of the left vertebral artery (*arrowheads*; V4 segment). The PICA (*arrow*) arises from the affected segment. The contralateral vertebral artery is too small to adequately supply the basilar artery (*not shown*).

b Vertebral angiogram, unsubtracted: In the hope of preventing further aneurysm growth by flow diversion while also preserving the vertebral artery and PICA, a self-expanding nitinol stent (Neuroform, Boston Scientific) was placed initially (*arrows:* proximal and distal stent markers). The patient was pretreated with dual antiplatelet medications.

c Vertebral angiogram, unsubtracted: 4 months later, after ingrowth of the first stent, a second nitinol stent of identical design is placed in the same vascular segment for flow modulation (*arrows:* stent markers). The PICA is still perfused (*curved arrow*).

d Vertebral angiogram, subtracted: The aneurysm is not occluded but remains stable during the follow-up period. An ischemic complication with hemiparesis occurred during the intervention, raising suspicion of ischemia in the anterior spinal artery territory. Local thrombolytic therapy with 30 mg of rtPA was unsuccessful. Additionally, the guide catheter caused a dissection in the midcervical portion of the vertebral artery (*arrow*).

e Vertebral angiogram, unsubtracted: A balloon-mounted stainless steel stent is placed across the vertebral artery dissection (Medtronic Driver, *arrowheads*).

If the parent vessel is to be occluded, placing coils or balloons proximal to the dissection site is insufficient for effective occlusion because retrograde filling of the aneurysm may occur (Rabinov et al. 2003). For this reason the aneurysm or dissection, together with the parent vessel, should be occluded locally with coils (Peluso et al. 2008). Small vessels (PICA) can also be occluded with glue (Isokangas et al. 2008). If the parent vessel is to be preserved by treatment with a stent, a flexible self-expanding stent is generally better than a more rigid balloon-expandable stent. Predilatation and/or postdilatation may be necessary. Adjunctive coil embolization through the stent interstices requires an adequate stent pore size. In rare cases, the radial pressure exerted by a

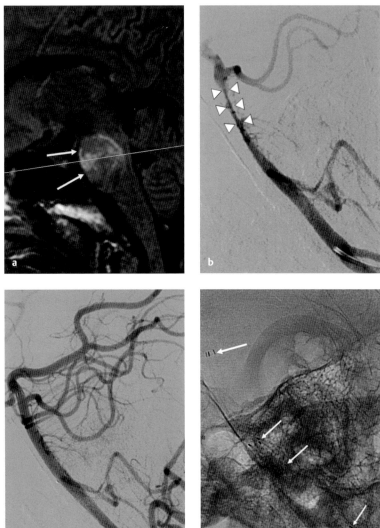

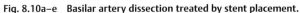

Fig. 8.10a–e Basilar artery dissection treated by stent placement.

a Sagittal FLAIR image in a 34-year-old woman with symptoms of progressive brainstem ischemia due to an acute basilar artery dissection (pontine infarction; *arrows*).

b Lateral vertebrobasilar angiogram, subtracted: Dissection-induced intramural hematoma has caused significant basilar artery stenosis (*arrowheads*), which is successfully treated with a self-expanding nitinol stent (4.5 mm × 28 mm Cordis Enterprise stent).

c Lateral vertebrobasilar angiogram, subtracted: The angioplasty has "milked" the intramural hematoma down the basilar artery, creating a new stenosis at a more proximal level (*arrowheads*).

d Lateral vertebrobasilar angiogram, subtracted: That stenosis is corrected by the overlapping placement of a second nitinol stent (4 mm × 20 mm ev3 Solutions AB Remodeling Device).

e Unsubtracted lateral vertebrobasilar angiogram displays all stent markers (*arrows*).

self-expanding stent may be insufficient to keep the vessel patent.

Extracranial Dissection

The treatment of an extracranial dissection, unlike an intradural dissection, does not require the preservation of perforator vessels, and so an extracranial pseudoaneurysm can be treated most elegantly with a covered stent. This will immediately exclude the aneurysm from the circulation while also relieving the stenosis that often accompanies the aneurysm (**Figs. 8.11** and **8.12**). This procedure can be done quickly at low risk and has a high success rate (Rohr et al. 2007; Yi et al. 2008). Unfortunately, this type of stent is inherently less flexible than a comparable bare stent, so it will not always be possible to maneuver a

Treatment of Acute Ischemic Stroke

II

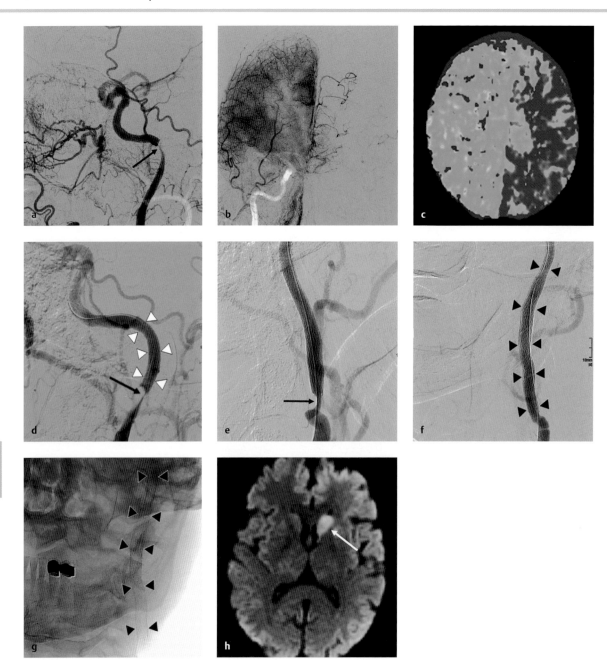

Fig. 8.11a–h   Subpetrous dissection of the ICA treated with four stents.

a   Oblique left carotid angiogram in a 56-year-old man with fluctuating right-sided symptoms present for 6–7 h (with episodes of
complete paralysis and aphasia) caused by an acute, dissection-
induced high-grade stenosis of the subpetrous portion of the
left ICA (*arrow*).

b   PA right carotid angiogram in the capillary phase. The stenosis
shows insufficient collateralization.

c   MTT map from dynamic susceptibility-weighted perfusion MRI
(DSC-PWI) shows that the stenosis has caused hypoperfusion in
the left hemisphere.

d   Left carotid angiography, subtracted: Vascular reconstruction
with a covered balloon-mounted stainless steel stent (arrowheads; 5 mm × 19 mm Abbott Jostent GraftMaster) shifts the

intramural hematoma proximally, creating a new stenosis at
that level (*arrow*).

e   Left carotid angiography, subtracted: Necessary placement of a
second stent (4.5 mm × 9 mm Medtronic Driver) causes further
proximal migration of the intramural hematoma (*arrow*).

f   Left carotid angiography, subtracted: Two additional self-
expanding carotid stents (7–10 mm × 40 mm OptiMed sinus
Carotid Conical RX) must be placed for adequate reconstruction
of the vessel lumen (*arrowheads*).

g   Left carotid angiogram shows the same appearance as **f**, but in
an unsubtracted view. *Arrowheads* indicate the stents.

h   Final diffusion-weighted MRI (b value = 1000) shows only a
small infarction in the head of the left caudate nucleus (*arrow*).

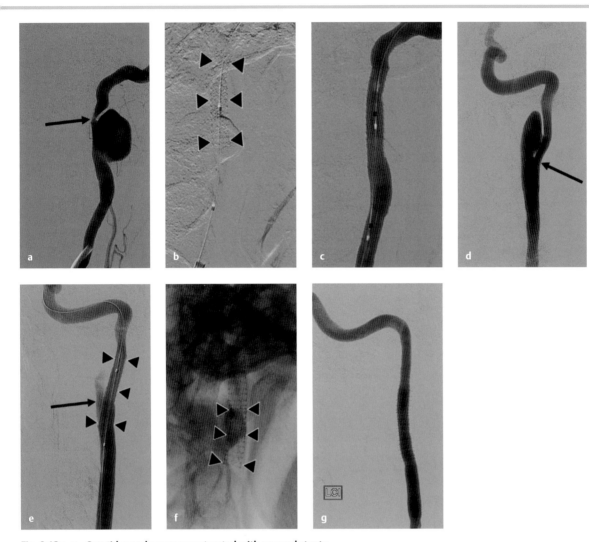

Fig. 8.12a–g Carotid pseudoaneurysms treated with covered stents.

a Right carotid angiogram, unsubtracted, in a 59-year-old woman with a high cervical pseudoaneurysm based on a dissection following thromboendarterectomy. A high-grade stenosis (*arrow*) is noted at the distal end of the pseudoaneurysm.

b Right carotid angiogram, subtracted: The placement of a covered stent (*arrowheads*; 5 mm × 26 mm Abbott Jostent GraftMaster) produces an immediate excellent result.

c Right carotid angiogram, unsubtracted: The aneurysm has been obliterated and the stenosis relieved.

d Left carotid angiogram, unsubtracted, in a 20-year-old man with a similar aneurysm following a spontaneous carotid dissection and associated (but lower-grade) stenosis (*arrow*).

e Left carotid angiogram, unsubtracted: The placement of a covered stent (also a Jostent GraftMaster; *arrowheads*) significantly reduces blood flow into the aneurysm, but residual inflow is still noted at the proximal end of the stent (*arrow*).

f Left carotid angiogram, subtracted: There is the danger of a valve mechanism causing regrowth of the aneurysm. To prevent this, a second covered stent is placed proximally, overlapping the first (*arrowheads*).

g Left carotid angiogram, unsubtracted: The second stent eliminates residual inflow into the aneurysm.

covered stent into position, particularly if the dissection has caused angled elongation or kinking of the affected vessel. Alternatively, an ordinary bare stent may be used (Edgell et al. 2005; Kadkhodayan et al. 2005). The aneurysm can still be coiled through the stent interstices if stent placement alone does not lead to aneurysm occlusion. Coil embolization alone, without stent protection, is generally limited by the configuration of the aneurysm.

If a hemodynamically significant stenosis is present without an aneurysm, it can be treated by the placement of a conventional bare stent, aided if necessary by balloon dilatation. Different stents are used at different locations:

• *Balloon-mounted stents:* These devices should not be used in the cervical carotid artery because of the risk of stent deformation by external compression. They can

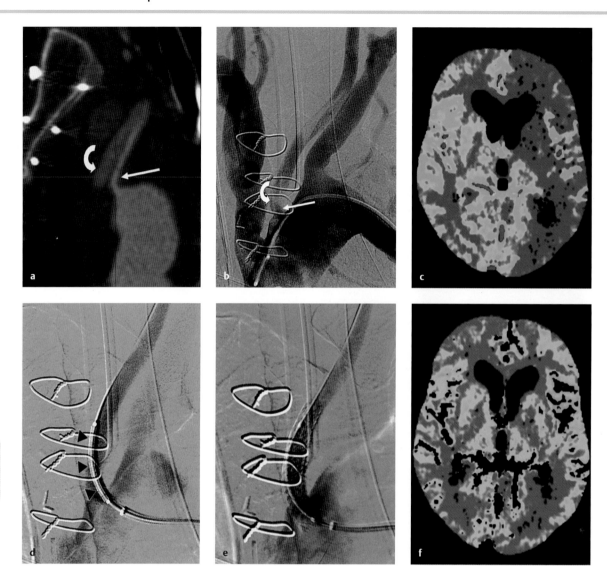

Fig. 8.13a–f　Treatment of a common carotid artery (CCA) dissection following endoluminal prosthetic implantation for a spontaneous type A aortic dissection.

a CTA, sagittal multiplanar reconstruction (MPR): After a brief, uneventful postoperative course following implantation of an aortic prosthesis, the 72-year-old man developed a left hemispheric syndrome with fluctuating right hemiparesis and aphasia. The symptoms were caused by a dissection-induced proximal stenosis of the right CCA (*arrow:* true lumen; *curved arrow:* false lumen).

b Arch aortography: Again, the *arrow* indicates the true lumen and the *curved arrow* the false lumen.

c CTP, color-coded cerebral blood flow map: The stenosis has caused significant reduction of cerebral blood flow.

d Arch aortography: A balloon-mounted stent is introduced (arrowheads; 8 mm × 29 mm Abbott Vascular Omnilink Elite).

e Arch aortography: The false lumen is occluded while the true lumen is restored.

f CTP, color-coded cerebral blood flow map: Normal cerebral blood flow has been restored, accompanied by full resolution of neurologic symptoms.

be used in the proximal portions of the supra-aortic vessels and the vertebral arteries, however (**Fig. 8.13**).

- *Flexible self-expanding stents:* These devices appear to be advantageous in most cases.
- *Multiple stents:* When a stent is used to treat an acute dissection in which fresh intramural hematoma is still narrowing the vessel, the stent angioplasty may "milk" the hematoma proximally or distally along

the vessel wall, thereby moving the stenosis to a new level. It may be necessary in this situation to place multiple stents until a satisfactory result is achieved (see **Figs. 8.10** and **8.11**). Percutaneous transluminal angioplasty alone, without stent protection, is unlikely to be successful because the hematoma will cause the stenosis to recur after the balloon is deflated.

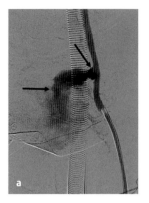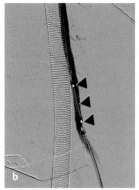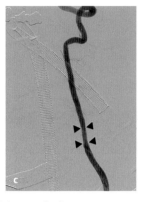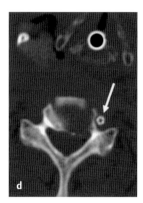

Fig. 8.14a–d Emergency stenting for an intraoperative injury of the vertebral artery.

a A 67-year-old man undergoing cervical decompression surgery sustained an injury of the left vertebral artery with intractable bleeding into the cervical soft tissues (*arrows*).

b A covered stent is introduced (*arrowheads*; 5 mm × 19 mm Jostent GraftMaster).

c Deployment of the covered stent (*arrowheads*) causes immediate arrest of bleeding.

d Posttreatment CT displays the stent morphology (*arrow*) in a transverse foramen on the left side.

The rupture of extradural vessels is rare and usually has a traumatic etiology. It may cause bleeding into the cervical soft tissues (**Fig. 8.14**) or may create an arteriovenous (AV) fistula with the vertebral artery if the vessel has ruptured directly into the perivertebral venous plexus (**Fig. 8.15**). In both cases the rupture can be repaired and the vessel preserved by the placement of a covered stent. Another option is to occlude the vessel if it is well collateralized. A rupture in the cavernous segment of the ICA gives rise to a carotid-cavernous fistula.

In principle, stenoses and aneurysms can also be treated surgically. Surgery would be a second-line choice in most cases, however, due to the high incidence of peri- and postprocedural difficulties and complications (Schievink et al. 1994; Müller et al. 2000). These problems often result from difficult access to the dissection site (below the skull base, V4 segment, proximal supra-aortic vessels). The treatment may also cause cranial nerve injury. Cavernous dissections cannot be treated surgically.

Thrombolytic Therapy

With a dissection leading to vascular occlusion and thrombosis causing an acute ischemic insult within the time window for thrombolysis, the presence of the dissection would not contraindicate thrombolytic therapy. In a retrospective analysis of 1062 patients treated by intravenous thrombolysis, the clinical outcomes in patients with a cervical artery dissection were poorer than in patients without a cervical artery dissection, despite equal numbers of hemorrhagic complications (Engelter et al. 2009). The authors attribute this to the poorer hemodynamics and more frequent tandem occlusions in patients with dissections. This could also explain the results of another study in which endovascular therapy (stent angioplasty

of the dissected ICA and mechanical thrombectomy or intra-arterial thrombolysis of the MCA) had a better success rate than intravenous thrombolysis alone, although only 10 patients were enrolled in that study (Lavallée et al. 2007). Recanalization of the carotid artery and MCA was achieved in all six patients in the endovascular group (vs. 25% in the intravenous rtPA group), and this was reflected in a better clinical outcome (mRS = 0 in 4 patients in the endovascular group, while 3 of 4 patients in the intravenous rtPA group had mRS ≥ 3). Despite limited experience overall, it appears that interventional therapy offers advantages over intravenous thrombolysis.

Patients with dissections in particular could benefit from the development of innovative techniques of thrombus extraction and fragmentation (e.g., using retractable stents and aspiration devices). We believe that thromboembolic occlusions of the ICA, including the carotid T as well as basilar artery occlusions, should be managed by primary interventional therapy (combined if necessary with bridging by intravenous thrombolysis)—analogous to the treatment of thromboembolic occlusions not resulting from a vascular dissection.

Medication for Stent Angioplasty

Periprocedural treatment with dual antiplatelet medications and heparin follows standard practice in patients scheduled for a stent angioplasty. In emergency situations, a glycoprotein IIb/IIIa receptor antagonist can be given instead of oral premedication just prior to the stent angioplasty. If this is considered too risky in a particular case (e.g., treatment of an acutely ruptured intracranial aneurysm), it can be withheld and a loading dose of clopidogrel and aspirin can be initiated after the heparin-protected intervention.

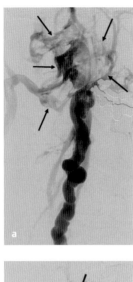
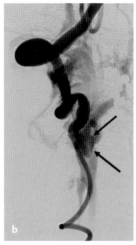
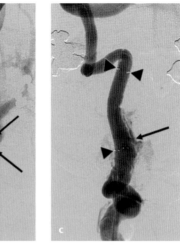
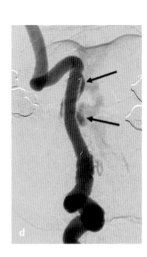

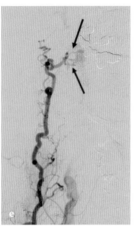
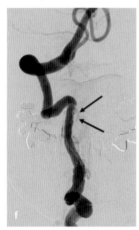
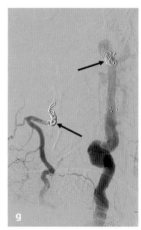

Fig. 8.15a–g   Arteriovenous fistula after rupture of a dissecting vertebral artery aneurysm.

a Vertebral angiogram in a 58-year-old woman with an ~9-month history of pulsatile tinnitus in the right ear. The right vertebral artery displays ectatic changes, and a massive shunt is visible in the perivertebral venous plexus (arrows).

b Vertebral angiogram. Selective injection of the vessel just below the atlas loop reveals the cause of the shunt: a ruptured pseudoaneurysm (*arrows*).

c Vertebral angiogram. Placement of a covered stent (Jostent GraftMaster; *arrowheads*) provides almost complete resolution. Small remnants of the fistula (*arrow*) are still visible at the proximal end of the stent.

d Vertebral angiogram. The fistula remnants occlude spontaneously over the next 4 months. Surprisingly, small vasa vasorum

have opened distal to the stent-supplied vertebral artery segment. These vessels perpetuate the fistula to a small degree (*arrows*) and explain the persistent tinnitus.

e Selective angiogram of the ascending cervical artery reveals additional inflow from small branches of that artery (*arrows*).

f Vertebral angiogram. The ascending cervical artery and fistula vessels from the vertebral artery are finally occluded with coils (*arrows*).

g Contrast injection into the right subclavian artery (visualization of the ascending cervical artery and vertebral artery). *Arrows* indicate the coils.

References

Carotid-T Occlusion

Arnold M, Nedeltchev K, Mattle HP, et al. Intra-arterial thrombolysis in 24 consecutive patients with internal carotid artery T occlusions. J Neurol Neurosurg Psychiatry 2003;74(6):739–742

del Zoppo GJ, Higashida RT, Furlan AJ, Pessin MS, Rowley HA, Gent M. PROACT: a phase II randomized trial of recombinant pro-urokinase by direct arterial delivery in acute middle cerebral artery stroke. PROACT Investigators. Prolyse in Acute Cerebral Thromboembolism. Stroke 1998;29(1):4–11

Eckert B, Kucinski T, Neumaier-Probst E, Fiehler J, Röther J, Zeumer H. Local intra-arterial fibrinolysis in acute hemispheric stroke: effect of occlusion type and fibrinolytic agent on recanalization success and neurological outcome. Cerebrovasc Dis 2003;15(4):258–263

Fesl G, Wiesmann M, Patzig M, et al. Endovascular mechanical recanalisation of acute carotid-T occlusions: a single-center retrospective analysis. Cardiovasc Intervent Radiol 2011;34(2):280–286

Furlan A, Higashida R, Wechsler L, et al. Intra-arterial prourokinase for acute ischemic stroke. The PROACT II study: a randomized controlled trial. Prolyse in Acute Cerebral Thromboembolism. JAMA 1999;282(21):2003–2011

Hacke W, Kaste M, Bluhmki E, et al; ECASS Investigators. Thrombolysis with alteplase 3 to 4.5 hours after acute ischemic stroke. N Engl J Med 2008b;359(13):1317–1329

Jansen O, von Kummer R, Forsting M, Hacke W, Sartor K. Thrombolytic therapy in acute occlusion of the intracranial internal carotid artery bifurcation. AJNR Am J Neuroradiol 1995;16(10):1977–1986

Khatri P, Hill MD, Palesch YY, et al; Interventional Management of Stroke III Investigators. Methodology of the Interventional Management of Stroke III Trial. Int J Stroke 2008;3(2):130–137

Lin R, Vora N, Zaidi S, et al. Mechanical approaches combined with intra-arterial pharmacological therapy are associated with higher recanalization rates than either intervention alone in revascularization of acute carotid terminus occlusion. Stroke 2009;40(6):2092–2097

Mazighi M, Serfaty JM, Labreuche J, et al; RECANALISE investigators. Comparison of intravenous alteplase with a combined intravenous-endovascular approach in patients with stroke and confirmed arterial occlusion (RECANALISE study): a prospective cohort study. Lancet Neurol 2009;8(9):802–809. Correction: Lancet Neurol 2009;8(11):981

National Institute of Neurological Disorders and Stroke rtPA Stroke Study Group. Tissue plasminogen activator for acute ischemic stroke. N Engl J Med 1995;333(24):1581–1587

Penumbra Pivotal Stroke Trial Investigators. The penumbra pivotal stroke trial: safety and effectiveness of a new generation of mechanical devices for clot removal in intracranial large vessel occlusive disease. Stroke 2009;40(8):2761–2768

Rha JH, Saver JL. The impact of recanalization on ischemic stroke outcome: a meta-analysis. Stroke 2007;38(3):967–973

Saqqur M, Uchino K, Demchuk AM, et al; CLOTBUST Investigators. Site of arterial occlusion identified by transcranial Doppler predicts the response to intravenous thrombolysis for stroke. Stroke 2007;38(3):948–954

Shi ZS, Loh Y, Walker G, Duckwiler GR; MERCI and Multi MERCI Investigators. Endovascular thrombectomy for acute ischemic stroke in failed intravenous tissue plasminogen activator versus non-intravenous tissue plasminogen activator patients: revascularization and outcomes stratified by the site of arterial occlusions. Stroke 2010;41(6):1185–1192

Smith WS, Sung G, Starkman S, et al; MERCI Trial Investigators. Safety and efficacy of mechanical embolectomy in acute ischemic stroke: results of the MERCI trial. Stroke 2005;36(7):1432–1438

Smith WS, Sung G, Saver J, et al; Multi MERCI Investigators. Mechanical thrombectomy for acute ischemic stroke: final results of the Multi MERCI trial. Stroke 2008;39(4):1205–1212

Zaidat OO, Suarez JI, Santillan C, et al. Response to intra-arterial and combined intravenous and intra-arterial thrombolytic therapy in patients with distal internal carotid artery occlusion. Stroke 2002;33(7):1821–1826

Occlusion of the Middle Cerebral Artery

Agarwal P, Kumar S, Hariharan S, et al. Hyperdense middle cerebral artery sign: can it be used to select intra-arterial versus intravenous thrombolysis in acute ischemic stroke? Cerebrovasc Dis 2004;17(2–3):182–190

Alexandrov AV, Molina CA, Grotta JC, et al; CLOTBUST Investigators. Ultrasound-enhanced systemic thrombolysis for acute ischemic stroke. N Engl J Med 2004;351(21):2170–2178

Brekenfeld C, Schroth G, Mattle HP, et al. Stent placement in acute cerebral artery occlusion: use of a self-expandable intracranial stent for acute stroke treatment. Stroke 2009;40(3):847–852

Castaño C, Dorado L, Guerrero C, et al. Mechanical thrombectomy with the Solitaire AB device in large artery occlusions of the anterior circulation: a pilot study. Stroke 2010;41(8):1836–1840

del Zoppo GJ, Higashida RT, Furlan AJ, Pessin MS, Rowley HA, Gent M. PROACT: a phase II randomized trial of recombinant pro-urokinase by direct arterial delivery in acute middle cerebral artery stroke. PROACT Investigators. Prolyse in Acute Cerebral Thromboembolism. Stroke 1998;29(1):4–11

Fischer U, Arnold M, Nedeltchev K, et al. NIHSS score and arteriographic findings in acute ischemic stroke. Stroke 2005;36(10):2121–2125

Francis CW, Suchkova VN. Ultrasound and thrombolysis. Vasc Med 2001;6(3):181–187

Furlan A, Higashida R, Wechsler L, et al. Intra-arterial prourokinase for acute ischemic stroke. The PROACT II study: a randomized controlled trial. Prolyse in Acute Cerebral Thromboembolism. JAMA 1999;282(21):2003–2011

Gifford E, Drazin D, Dalfino JC, Nair AK, Yamamoto J, Boulos AS. The effectiveness of microballoon angioplasty in treating middle cerebral artery occlusion beyond the bifurcation. AJNR Am J Neuroradiol 2010;31(8):1541–1548

Gupta R, Yonas H, Gebel J, et al. Reduced pretreatment ipsilateral middle cerebral artery cerebral blood flow is predictive of symptomatic hemorrhage post-intra-arterial thrombolysis in patients with middle cerebral artery occlusion. Stroke 2006;37(10):2526–2530

Hacke W, Zeumer H, Ferbert A, Brückmann H, del Zoppo GJ. Intra-arterial thrombolytic therapy improves outcome in patients with acute vertebrobasilar occlusive disease. Stroke 1988;19(10):1216–1222

Hacke W, Kaste M, Bluhmki E, et al; ECASS Investigators. Thrombolysis with alteplase 3 to 4.5 hours after acute ischemic stroke. N Engl J Med 2008;359(13):1317–1329

IMS II Trial Investigators. The Interventional Management of Stroke (IMS) II Study. Stroke 2007;38(7):2127–2135

II

Jovin TG, Gupta R, Horowitz MB, et al. Pretreatment ipsilateral regional cortical blood flow influences vessel recanalization in intra-arterial thrombolysis for MCA occlusion. AJNR Am J Neuroradiol 2007;28(1):164–167

Jumaa MA, Zhang F, Ruiz-Ares G, et al. Comparison of safety and clinical and radiographic outcomes in endovascular acute stroke therapy for proximal middle cerebral artery occlusion with intubation and general anesthesia versus the nonintubated state. Stroke 2010;41(6):1180–1184

Kelly ME, Furlan AJ, Fiorella D. Recanalization of an acute middle cerebral artery occlusion using a self-expanding, reconstrainable, intracranial microstent as a temporary endovascular bypass. Stroke 2008;39(6):1770–1773

Kim DJ, Kim DI, Byun JS, et al. Simple microwire and microcatheter mechanical thrombolysis with adjuvant intraarterial urokinase for treatment of hyperacute ischemic stroke patients. Acta Radiol 2008;49(3):351–357

Levy EI, Mehta R, Gupta R, et al. Self-expanding stents for recanalization of acute cerebrovascular occlusions. AJNR Am J Neuroradiol 2007;28(5):816–822

Levy EI, Siddiqui AH, Crumlish A, et al. First Food and Drug Administration-approved prospective trial of primary intracranial stenting for acute stroke: SARIS (stent-assisted recanalization in acute ischemic stroke). Stroke 2009;40(11):3552–3556

Mattle HP, Arnold M, Georgiadis D, et al. Comparison of intraarterial and intravenous thrombolysis for ischemic stroke with hyperdense middle cerebral artery sign. Stroke 2008;39(2):379–383

National Institute of Neurological Disorders and Stroke rt-PA Stroke Study Group. Tissue plasminogen activator for acute ischemic stroke. N Engl J Med 1995;333(24):1581–1587

Sauvageau E, Levy EI. Self-expanding stent-assisted middle cerebral artery recanalization: technical note. Neuroradiology 2006;48(6):405–408

Smith WS, Sung G, Starkman S, et al; MERCI Trial Investigators. Safety and efficacy of mechanical embolectomy in acute ischemic stroke: results of the MERCI trial. Stroke 2005;36(7):1432–1438

TIMI Study Group. The Thrombolysis in Myocardial Infarction (TIMI) trial. Phase I findings. N Engl J Med 1985;312(14):932–936

Tokunaga K, Sugiu K, Yoshino K, et al. Percutaneous balloon angioplasty for acute occlusion of intracranial arteries. Neurosurgery 2010;67:189–196, discussion 196–197

Vora NA, Gupta R, Thomas AJ, et al. Factors predicting hemorrhagic complications after multimodal reperfusion therapy for acute ischemic stroke. AJNR Am J Neuroradiol 2007;28(7):1391–1394

Wintermark M, Albers GW, Alexandrov AV, et al; Advanced Neuroimaging for Acute Stroke Treatment Study Group. Acute stroke imaging research roadmap. AJNR Am J Neuroradiol 2008;29(5):e23–e30

Basilar Artery Thrombosis

Arnold M, Nedeltchev K, Schroth G, et al. Clinical and radiological predictors of recanalisation and outcome of 40 patients with acute basilar artery occlusion treated with intra-arterial thrombolysis. J Neurol Neurosurg Psychiatry 2004;75(6):857–862

Brückmann H, Ferbert A, del Zoppo GJ, Hacke W, Zeumer H. Acute vertebral-basilar thrombosis. Angiological-clinical comparison and therapeutic implications. Acta Radiol Suppl 1986;369:38–42

Chopko BW, Kerber C, Wong W, Georgy B. Transcatheter snare removal of acute middle cerebral artery thromboembolism: technical case report. Neurosurgery 2000;46(6):1529–1531

Clarençon F, Blanc R, Gallas S, Hosseini H, Gaston A. Thrombectomy for acute basilar artery occlusion by using double MERCI retriever devices and bilateral temporary vertebral artery flow reversal. Technical note. J Neurosurg 2009;111(1):53–56

Eckert B, Koch C, Thomalla G, Roether J, Zeumer H. Acute basilar artery occlusion treated with combined intravenous Abciximab and intra-arterial tissue plasminogen activator: report of 3 cases. Stroke 2002a;33(5):1424–1427

Eckert B, Kucinski T, Pfeiffer G, Groden C, Zeumer H. Endovascular therapy of acute vertebrobasilar occlusion: early treatment onset as the most important factor. Cerebrovasc Dis 2002b;14(1):42–50

Eckert B, Koch C, Thomalla G, et al. Aggressive therapy with intravenous abciximab and intra-arterial rtPA and additional PTA/stenting improves clinical outcome in acute vertebrobasilar occlusion: combined local fibrinolysis and intravenous abciximab in acute vertebrobasilar stroke treatment (FAST): results of a multicenter study. Stroke 2005;36(6):1160–1165

Ferbert A, Brückmann H, Drummen R. Clinical features of proven basilar artery occlusion. Stroke 1990;21(8):1135–1142

Hacke W, Zeumer H, Ferbert A, Brückmann H, del Zoppo GJ. Intra-arterial thrombolytic therapy improves outcome in patients with acute vertebrobasilar occlusive disease. Stroke 1988;19(10):1216–1222

Liebig T, Reinartz J, Hannes R, Miloslavski E, Henkes H. Comparative in vitro study of five mechanical embolectomy systems: effectiveness of clot removal and risk of distal embolization. Neuroradiology 2008;50(1):43–52

Lindsberg PJ, Soinne L, Tatlisumak T, et al. Long-term outcome after intravenous thrombolysis of basilar artery occlusion. JAMA 2004;292(15):1862–1866

Lindsberg PJ, Mattle HP. Therapy of basilar artery occlusion: a systematic analysis comparing intra-arterial and intravenous thrombolysis. Stroke 2006;37(3):922–928

Mayer TE, Hamann GF, Brueckmann H. Mechanical extraction of a basilar-artery embolus with the use of flow reversal and a microbasket. N Engl J Med 2002;347(10):769–770

Mayer TE, Hamann GF, Schulte-Altedorneburg G, Brückmann H. Treatment of vertebrobasilar occlusion by using a coronary waterjet thrombectomy device: a pilot study. AJNR Am J Neuroradiol 2005;26(6):1389–1394

Meyers PM, Schumacher HC, Higashida RT, et al; American Heart Association. Indications for the performance of

Treatment of Acute Ischemic Stroke

II

intracranial endovascular neurointerventional procedures: a scientific statement from the American Heart Association Council on Cardiovascular Radiology and Intervention, Stroke Council, Council on Cardiovascular Surgery and Anesthesia, Interdisciplinary Council on Peripheral Vascular Disease, and Interdisciplinary Council on Quality of Care and Outcomes Research. Circulation 2009;119(16): 2235–2249

Molina CA. Futile recanalization in mechanical embolectomy trials: a call to improve selection of patients for revascularization. Stroke 2010;41(5):842–843

Nagel S, Schellinger PD, Hartmann M, et al. Therapy of acute basilar artery occlusion: intraarterial thrombolysis alone vs bridging therapy. Stroke 2009;40(1):140–146

Pfefferkorn T, Holtmannspötter M, Schmidt C, et al. Drip, ship, and retrieve: cooperative recanalization therapy in acute basilar artery occlusion. Stroke 2010;41(4):722–726

Schonewille WJ, Wijman CA, Michel P, et al; BASICS study group. Treatment and outcomes of acute basilar artery occlusion in the Basilar Artery International Cooperation Study (BASICS): a prospective registry study. Lancet Neurol 2009;8(8):724–730

Schulte-Altedorneburg G, Brückmann H. Imaging techniques in diagnosis of brainstem infarction. [Article in German] Nervenarzt 2006;77(6):731–743, quiz 744

Schulte-Altedorneburg G, Hamann GF, Mull M, et al. Outcome of acute vertebrobasilar occlusions treated with intra-arterial fibrinolysis in 180 patients. AJNR Am J Neuroradiol 2006;27(10):2042–2047

Schulte-Altedorneburg G, Brückmann H, Hamann GF, et al. Ischemic and hemorrhagic complications after intra-arterial fibrinolysis in vertebrobasilar occlusion. AJNR Am J Neuroradiol 2007a;28(2):378–381

Schulte-Altedorneburg G, Reith W, Brückmann H, Dichgans M, Mayer TE. Thrombolysis of basilar artery occlusion—intra-arterial or intravenous: is there really no difference? Stroke 2007b;38(1):9, author reply 10–11

Schulte-Altedorneburg G, Liebig T, Brückmann H, Jansen O. Treatment of basilar artery occlusion: a prospective randomised therapeutic study is needed. Lancet Neurol 2009;8(12):1084–1085, author reply 1085

Shaltoni HM, Albright KC, Gonzales NR, et al. Is intra-arterial thrombolysis safe after full-dose intravenous recombinant tissue plasminogen activator for acute ischemic stroke? Stroke 2007;38(1):80–84

Straub S, Junghans U, Jovanovic V, Wittsack HJ, Seitz RJ, Siebler M. Systemic thrombolysis with recombinant tissue plasminogen activator and tirofiban in acute middle cerebral artery occlusion. Stroke 2004;35(3):705–709

Yoo AJ, Hakimelahi R, Rost NS, et al. Diffusion-weighted imaging reversibility in the brainstem following successful recanalization of acute basilar artery occlusion. J Neurointervent Surg 2010;2(3):195–197

Zeumer H, Hacke W, Kolmann HL, Poeck K. Local fibrinolysis in basilar artery thrombosis (author's transl). [Article in German] Dtsch Med Wochenschr 1982;107(19):728–731

Zeumer H, Freitag HJ, Zanella F, Thie A, Arning C. Local intra-arterial fibrinolytic therapy in patients with stroke: urokinase versus recombinant tissue plasminogen activator (r-TPA). Neuroradiology 1993;35(2):159–162

Cervical Artery Dissections

Ahn JY, Han IB, Kim TG, et al. Endovascular treatment of intracranial vertebral artery dissections with stent placement or stent-assisted coiling. AJNR Am J Neuroradiol 2006;27(7):1514–1520

Diener HC, Putzki N, Eds. Leitlinien für Diagnostik und Therapie in der Neurologie. 4th ed. Stuttgart: Thieme; 2008

Edgell RC, Abou-Chebl A, Yadav JS. Endovascular management of spontaneous carotid artery dissection. J Vasc Surg 2005;42(5):854–860, discussion 860

Engelter ST, Rutgers MP, Hatz F, et al. Intravenous thrombolysis in stroke attributable to cervical artery dissection. Stroke 2009;40(12):3772–3776

Goyal MS, Derdeyn CP. The diagnosis and management of supraaortic arterial dissections. Curr Opin Neurol 2009;22(1): 80–89

Isokangas JM, Siniluoto T, Tikkakoski T, Kumpulainen T. Endovascular treatment of peripheral aneurysms of the posterior inferior cerebellar artery. AJNR Am J Neuroradiol 2008;29(9):1783–1788

Kadkhodayan Y, Jeck DT, Moran CJ, Derdeyn CP, Cross DT III. Angioplasty and stenting in carotid dissection with or without associated pseudoaneurysm. AJNR Am J Neuroradiol 2005;26(9):2328–2335

Kim Y-K, Schulman S. Cervical artery dissection: pathology, epidemiology and management. Thromb Res 2009;123(6): 810–821

Kim BM, Suh SH, Park SI, et al. Management and clinical outcome of acute basilar artery dissection. AJNR Am J Neuroradiol 2008;29(10):1937–1941

Lavallée PC, Mazighi M, Saint-Maurice J-P, et al. Stent-assisted endovascular thrombolysis versus intravenous thrombolysis in internal carotid artery dissection with tandem internal carotid and middle cerebral artery occlusion. Stroke 2007;38(8):2270–2274

Lylyk P, Miranda C, Ceratto R, et al. Curative endovascular reconstruction of cerebral aneurysms with the pipeline embolization device: the Buenos Aires experience. Neurosurgery 2009;64(4):632–642, discussion 642–643, quiz N6

Mizutani T, Aruga T, Kirino T, Miki Y, Saito I, Tsuchida T. Recurrent subarachnoid hemorrhage from untreated ruptured vertebrobasilar dissecting aneurysms. Neurosurgery 1995;36(5):905–911, discussion 912–913

Müller BT, Luther B, Hort W, Neumann-Haefelin T, Aulich A, Sandmann W. Surgical treatment of 50 carotid dissections: indications and results. J Vasc Surg 2000;31(5):980–988

Park SI, Kim BM, Kim DI, et al. Clinical and angiographic follow-up of stent-only therapy for acute intracranial vertebrobasilar dissecting aneurysms. AJNR Am J Neuroradiol 2009;30(7):1351–1356

II

Pavlisa G, Ozretic D, Murselovic T, Pavlisa G, Rados M. Sole stenting of large and giant intracranial aneurysms with self-expanding intracranial stents—limits and complications. Acta Neurochir (Wien) 2010;152(5):763–769

Peluso JPP, van Rooij WJ, Sluzewski M, Beute GN, Majoie CB. Endovascular treatment of symptomatic intradural vertebral dissecting aneurysms. AJNR Am J Neuroradiol 2008;29(1):102–106

Rabinov JD, Hellinger FR, Morris PP, Ogilvy CS, Putman CM. Endovascular management of vertebrobasilar dissecting aneurysms. AJNR Am J Neuroradiol 2003;24(7):1421–1428

Rohr A, Alfke K, Dörner L, et al. Aneurysmabehandlung der Arteria carotis interna mit gecoverten Stents [Treatment of carotid artery aneurysms with covered stents]. RöFo 2007;179(10):1048–1054

Sacco RL, Adams R, Albers G, et al; American Heart Association; American Stroke Association Council on Stroke; Council on Cardiovascular Radiology and Intervention; American Academy of Neurology. Guidelines for prevention of stroke in patients with ischemic stroke or transient ischemic attack: a statement for healthcare professionals from the American Heart Association/American Stroke Association Council on Stroke: co-sponsored by the Council on Cardiovascular Radiology and Intervention: the American Academy of Neurology affirms the value of this guideline. Stroke 2006;37(2):577–617

Santos-Franco JA, Zenteno M, Lee A. Dissecting aneurysms of the vertebrobasilar system. A comprehensive review on natural history and treatment options. Neurosurg Rev 2008;31(2):131–140, discussion 140

Sasaki O, Ogawa H, Koike T, Koizumi T, Tanaka R. A clinicopathological study of dissecting aneurysms of the intracranial vertebral artery. J Neurosurg 1991;75(6):874–882

Schievink WI, Piepgras DG, McCaffrey TV, Mokri B. Surgical treatment of extracranial internal carotid artery dissecting aneurysms. Neurosurgery 1994;35(5):809–815, discussion 815–816

Shin YS, Kim HS, Kim SY. Stenting for vertebrobasilar dissection: a possible treatment option for nonhemorrhagic vertebrobasilar dissection. Neuroradiology 2007;49(2):149–156

Takagi T, Takayasu M, Suzuki Y, Yoshida J. Prediction of rebleeding from angiographic features in vertebral artery dissecting aneurysms. Neurosurg Rev 2007;30(1):32–38, discussion 38–39

van Rooij WJ, Sluzewski M. Perforator infarction after placement of a pipeline flow-diverting stent for an unruptured A1 aneurysm. AJNR Am J Neuroradiol 2010;31(4):E43–E44

Yasui T, Komiyama M, Nishikawa M, Nakajima H, Kobayashi Y, Inoue T. Fusiform vertebral artery aneurysms as a cause of dissecting aneurysms. Report of two autopsy cases and a review of the literature. J Neurosurg 1999;91(1):139–144

Yi AC, Palmer E, Luh GY, Jacobson JP, Smith DC. Endovascular treatment of carotid and vertebral pseudoaneurysms with covered stents. AJNR Am J Neuroradiol 2008;29(5):983–987

Zenteno MA, Santos-Franco JA, Freitas-Modenesi JM, et al. Use of the sole stenting technique for the management of aneurysms in the posterior circulation in a prospective series of 20 patients. J Neurosurg 2008;108(6):1104–1118

Summary and Recommendations Part II

H. Brueckmann and O. Jansen

The therapeutic options for acute stroke have improved greatly in the past decade as interdisciplinary stroke centers have established a round-the-clock service with stroke units, interventional neuroradiologists, and improved multimodal sectional imaging with telemedicine networks.

An acute cerebrovascular occlusion should be treated as early, rapidly, and effectively as possible, because prompt vascular recanalization can salvage the penumbra of tissue that has already sustained a degree of functional injury but is still structurally intact ("time is brain").

In all studies published to date, successful recanalization and early initiation of treatment have always been the key determinants of a good clinical outcome. Besides the established modalities of intravenous thrombolysis with rtPA and intra-arterial thrombolysis, various catheter-based techniques are now being used for the mechanical recanalization of acute vascular occlusions. At present, intravenous thrombolysis with rtPA is the approved treatment standard during the acute phase of stroke within the first 3 h after symptom onset. The time window for intravenous thrombolysis has even been expanded from 3 h to 4.5 h based on the results of a subgroup analysis in the ECASS III trial. The main advantages of intravenous thrombolysis are its technical simplicity, wide availability, and the capacity for rapid initiation during the acute phase. It does not require a specialized technique or interventional training. Unfortunately, the daily practice of stroke management has revealed the limitations of this therapy, especially in patients with large vessel occlusions, high thrombus burden, and an associated severe neurologic deficit. There has been a rapidly growing willingness among physicians to employ more aggressive and effective treatments in these patients.

Intra-arterial thrombolysis (intra-arterial fibrinolysis) was first used 30 years ago by Hermann Zeumer in the treatment of acute basilar artery thrombosis. This therapy differs from intravenous thrombolysis in that the fibrinolytic agent is injected directly at the thrombus site through a microcatheter. This permits the delivery of a higher local concentration of the agent at a smaller dose, thereby reducing the risk of intracranial hemorrhage. This has made it possible to use an expanded time window for intra-arterial therapy. Intra-arterial thrombolysis has been successfully used in several studies such as the PROACT I and II trials.

With the advent of new mechanical recanalization techniques, cerebrovascular occlusions can now be reopened more quickly and with greater confidence. The therapeutic time window is considerably longer than with classic intravenous and intra-arterial thrombolysis. These techniques can even be used in cases where pharmacologic thrombolysis is contraindicated or primary thrombolytic therapy was unsuccessful.

The time to the start of mechanical recanalization can be bridged by intravenous thrombolysis ("bridging therapy"). Combination therapies that include intra-arterial thrombolysis are also possible and are often used. By combining different treatment strategies, we can shorten the time to treatment in a protocol known as "drip, ship, and retrieve."

Two main principles have led to a breakthrough in mechanical recanalization: aspiration (preferably at the thrombus site) and the placement of a temporary stent. The advantage of temporary stenting is that it quickly reestablishes antegrade flow in the formerly occluded artery while eliminating the need for platelet inhibition (e.g., with tirofiban). It has also been found that retractable stents such as the Solitaire and Trevo devices can be used very successfully for direct thrombus extraction. The modified retriever systems can also achieve good recanalization rates when used with a distal access catheter.

Mechanical thrombectomy techniques yield higher recanalization rates than the thrombolytic therapies. Current registries and studies on the treatment of MCA occlusions, basilar artery occlusions, and particularly carotid-T occlusions are highly promising, especially in terms of clinical outcomes. On the other hand, there is a need for prospective randomized studies that take into account key variables such as the site of the vascular occlusion, the extent of the occlusion, the severity of symptoms before treatment, time to treatment, patient age, etc., so that the value of these techniques can be definitively assessed.

For the future, we expect that the mechanical techniques in particular will undergo further technical refinements. Meanwhile, controlled studies should be done to identify prognostic criteria (e.g., based on imaging, initial clinical findings, or occlusion type) that will aid in selecting patients for recanalization therapy and enable the specific and selective management of acute stroke patients.

In summary, the main therapeutic goal in stroke patients is the rapid recanalization of the underlying vascular occlusion. An array of safe and effective methods are available, ranging from intravenous

II

thrombolysis to modern mechanical recanalization techniques, but these therapies must be applied on a patient-specific basis. Moreover, the race against time does not begin with the treatment of stroke but at the start of the care chain. The recognition of a stroke by the first responder and rapid transport to a hospital will critically influence the further course of the disease. The patient should be taken directly to a stroke center with neuroradiologic access (including teleradiology) and round-the-clock availability of all treatment options including mechanical, catheter-based recanalization techniques.

Treatment of Acute Cerebral Venous Occlusions

9 Treatment of Acute Cerebral Venous Occlusions

T. E. Mayer

Epidemiology

Cerebral venous and sinus thrombosis (CVST) is contributory in 0.5% of all strokes. The incidence is ~4 cases per 1 million population. CVST may occur at any age, but young people and newborns are disproportionately affected. The peak incidence is 30 years of age. Three-fourths of patients are female, due partly to the fact that CVST has a >1:10 000 incidence in the peripartum period (Filippidis et al. 2009).

Etiology, Pathogenesis, and Symptoms

CVST has numerous potential causes. Various prothrombotic states play an essential role. The occlusive process may cause interstitial edema, increased intracranial pressure, or intracerebral hemorrhage as a result of venous congestion, and associated ischemia can lead to intracellular edema and infarction. The clinical presentation may range from an absence of symptoms, headache, nausea, and papilledema to various neurologic deficits, epileptic seizures, and coma.

> **Note**
>
> Deep cerebral venous thrombosis takes a particularly severe course.

Imaging Studies

The diagnosis of CVST relies on CT and CT angiography (CTA) as well as MRI using various weighting schemes and venographic sequences. When MRI is used, it is important to recognize and distinguish the various signal patterns that are associated with thrombi of different ages, organizing tissue, normal pacchionian granulations, and anatomic variants of the dural venous sinuses.

A common feature is that in combination with the new thrombus formation there is some existing dural sinus thrombosis that has progressed to the cerebral veins and therefore become symptomatic. It should also be kept in mind that venous thrombosis may be combined with arteriovenous dural fistula.

Treatment

The gold standards in the treatment of CVST are conservative therapy with intravenous or low-molecular-weight heparin and the symptomatic treatment of increased intracranial pressure and epileptic seizures.

Endovascular Procedures

Various forms of endovascular recanalization therapy have been developed. While they have been used successfully in small series, a definite benefit from these treatments has not yet been proven, due in part to the potential of fibrinolytic agents to intensify bleeding. Nevertheless, appropriate endovascular therapy may be justified for individual case management, especially if disease progresses with medical therapy, initial symptoms are severe, or the occlusion is located at a threatening site (e.g., deep cerebral venous thrombosis). Finally, a decompressive hemicraniectomy should be considered in patients with marked symptoms of increased intracranial pressure due to edema, infarction, or hemorrhage (Coutinho et al. 2009). Combined decompressive neurosurgery and surgical thrombectomy is also reported.

The goal of endovascular therapy is to recanalize the occluded dural sinus or cerebral vein, first to improve tissue perfusion to prevent additional infarction and second to relieve venous congestion, thereby reducing cerebral edema and lowering the risk of intracerebral hemorrhage. Fibrinolytic agents, usually urokinase or rtPA, can be administered by the systemic, local transarterial, or local venous route, the latter ranging from a brief injection to a protracted infusion. Fibrinolytic therapy may be supplemented or replaced by mechanical techniques to dilate the thrombus with a stent or balloon or remove the thrombus using an aspiration or retriever system.

Pharmacologic Thrombectomy

Although systemic fibrinolytic therapy may now be considered obsolete, local intravenous thrombolysis has been performed in the dural sinuses and cerebral veins since 1988. Urokinase is infused for 15 min at a rate of 40 000–750 000 units/h for up to 10 days (or a total rtPA dose of 8–70 mg) by percutaneous venous access or, less commonly, through a burr-hole craniectomy. Case series consisting of one to no more than 20 patients have been reported. Most reports document significant clinical improvement with recanalization rates up to 100%, although deterioration or death from intracranial hemorrhage has occurred in 0–40% of cases (Rahman et al. 2009).

The necessary duration of the thrombolytic infusion probably depends on thrombus age, noting that fresh and old thrombi are frequently combined and may even coexist with arteriovenous dural fistulae in older patients. Infusion duration also depends on the extent of the thrombosis and the thrombus mass. Concomitant heparinization is definitely advised during a continuous, prolonged infusion due to the presence of the indwelling catheter. Otherwise, many groups have discontinued heparinization during thrombolysis.

> **Caution**
>
> Although some groups favor access through the internal jugular vein, transfemoral access appears to be safer. With cervical access, there is a possibility that drainage of the fibrinolytic agent may promote bleeding at the puncture site.

Few reports exist on local transarterial thrombolysis in cerebral venous thrombosis (Liebetrau et al. 2004). This method provides rapid access to the distal venous system by the antegrade route and can also be used in conjunction with local thrombectomy (Chow et al. 2000). Low doses of urokinase (100 000 units/h) and rtPA (5 mg/h per vessel) have been used. Because so few data are available, it remains unclear whether transarterial fibrinolysis promotes intracerebral hemorrhage.

Mechanical Thrombectomy

Because of the duration of infusion required for local intravenous thrombolysis, which may last for days, and to minimize the risk of cerebral hemorrhage, fibrinolysis has been supported or replaced by mechanical endovascular techniques.

AngioJet

Several reports have been published on aspiration thrombectomy (rheolytic thrombectomy) with the AngioJet system in small numbers of patients. A catheter is inserted into the thrombus, and a water jet at the catheter tip creates a vacuum that pulls the thrombus into the catheter, where it is broken into fragments that are evacuated from the body. Good recanalization results have been achieved even with extensive venous thrombosis (**Fig. 9.1**). The small reported case numbers make it difficult to get a clear picture of the true recanalization rate, however. In our experience, older sinus thrombi with supervening fresh venous thrombi are difficult to recanalize, or can be only partially recanalized, with the AngioJet system. This treatment option is also limited by the low availability of these devices for neuroendovascular groups, since this technology is used mainly in cardiology and is not widely utilized even in that specialty.

Penumbra System

Meanwhile, individual case reports have been published on experience with the Penumbra system, a microaspiration catheter with a fragmentation microwire (separator) which was developed for endovascular stroke therapy in the cerebral arterial system (see also the section on the Penumbra System, p. 84). Recanalizations of the dural sinuses have been described using the Penumbra system combined with local fibrinolysis (Kulcsár et al. 2010). The value of this system in cerebral venous thrombosis cannot yet be assessed, however.

Other radiologic aspiration catheters (e.g., Pronto) have also been used.

Retrievers

Balloons for peripheral or coronary angioplasty, usually combined with local fibrinolysis, have been used to displace the thrombus proximally by retraction of the inflated balloon. In one series this method was successfully used in six of eight patients who were treated in up to three sessions (Soleau et al. 2003).

The MERCI Retriever is a coiled microwire device with a very strong geometric memory that is used for clot retrieval in the cerebral arterial system. In one case report this device was successfully combined with local

III

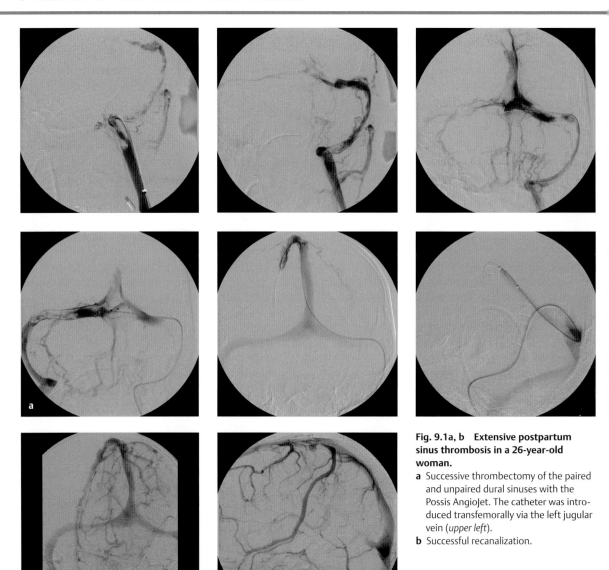

Fig. 9.1a, b Extensive postpartum sinus thrombosis in a 26-year-old woman.

a Successive thrombectomy of the paired and unpaired dural sinuses with the Possis AngioJet. The catheter was introduced transfemorally via the left jugular vein (*upper left*).

b Successful recanalization.

fibrinolysis and coaxial catheter aspiration, while in another case it was described as unsuccessful.

A variety of other retrieval devices are now available and can be combined with aspiration or fibrinolysis.

Angioplasty

Isolated cases have been described in which balloons and stents were used for the dilatation of dural sinus thrombosis and for the treatment of associated arteriovenous dural fistulae, which appear to have an etiologic and pathogenic association with sinus thrombosis. Stenting has also been combined with other mechanical and pharmacologic measures and multiple stents have been used (Formaglio et al. 2010). This treatment also includes platelet inhibition with aspirin and clopidogrel or equivalent agents in addition to heparinization.

Note

The above endovascular therapies have not yet been investigated in randomized trials, and few have been addressed in prospective studies. Nevertheless, the use of combined thrombolytic and mechanical interventions appears to be worthwhile in carefully selected cases.

References

Chow K, Gobin YP, Saver J, Kidwell C, Dong P, Viñuela F. Endovascular treatment of dural sinus thrombosis with rheolytic thrombectomy and intra-arterial thrombolysis. Stroke 2000;31(6):1420–1425

Coutinho JM, Majoie CB, Coert BA, Stam J. Decompressive hemicraniectomy in cerebral sinus thrombosis: consecutive case series and review of the literature. Stroke 2009;40(6): 2233–2235

Filippidis A, Kapsalaki E, Patramani G, Fountas KN. Cerebral venous sinus thrombosis: review of the demographics, pathophysiology, current diagnosis, and treatment. Neurosurg Focus 2009;27(5):E3

Formaglio M, Catenoix H, Tahon F, Mauguière F, Vighetto A, Turjman F. Stenting of a cerebral venous thrombosis. J Neuroradiol 2010;37(3):182–184

Kulcsár Z, Marosfoi M, Berentei Z, Szikora I. Continuous thrombolysis and repeated thrombectomy with the Penumbra System in a child with hemorrhagic sinus thrombosis: technical note. Acta Neurochir (Wien) 2010;152(5):911–916

Liebetrau M, Mayer TE, Bruning R, Opherk C, Hamann GF. Intra-arterial thrombolysis of complete deep cerebral venous thrombosis. Neurology 2004;63(12):2444–2445

Rahman M, Velat GJ, Hoh BL, Mocco J. Direct thrombolysis for cerebral venous sinus thrombosis. Neurosurg Focus 2009;27(5):E7

Soleau SW, Schmidt R, Stevens S, Osborn A, MacDonald JD. Extensive experience with dural sinus thrombosis. Neurosurgery 2003;52(3):534–544, discussion 542–544

Summary and Recommendations Part III

H. Brueckmann and O. Jansen

In dealing with venous occlusions in the cerebral circulation, diagnosis still represents a difficult step in management. Although the recommended treatment standard of full heparinization has been evaluated only in a relatively small population, clinical practice has shown that the great majority of cerebral venous and sinus thromboses can be managed conservatively with full heparinization. More aggressive endovascular therapies should be considered only if conservative therapy is ineffective, the thrombosis progresses, or there is a threat of impending venous infarction (e.g., detection of extensive vasogenic edema without intracerebral hemorrhage). To date, however, experience with available endovascular therapies in CVST has been limited and no systematic case series have been published. When a thrombotic occlusion is present, however, the venous drainage of the brain depends less on the large dural sinuses than on the draining cortical veins and deep cerebral veins, unless dural sinus thrombosis is very extensive. If interventional treatment is deemed necessary, an aspiration procedure would presumably be the most promising approach due to the typically large thrombus mass and may be followed if needed by local thrombolysis. When indicated, the thrombolytic agent should be administered by continuous infusion at a noncritical systemic dose. If cerebral vein thrombosis is combined with old organized thrombosis in the sinuses, recanalization by thrombectomy may be challenging, and stents should be used with caution. If venous infarction and bleeding has already occurred and is detectable by MRI, interventional therapy should be considered only on a highly selective basis or even withheld in favor of surgery.

Treatment of Supra-aortic Extra- and Intracranial Stenoses

10 Equipment: Stents, Filters, and Balloon Systems

M. Holtmannspoetter

Introduction

The techniques for the treatment of intracranial and extracranial stenoses are fundamentally different. The equipment for these techniques is therefore discussed under separate headings.

Technical standards like those used in cerebral angiography also apply in the endovascular treatment of cerebrovascular stenoses (continuous irrigation of the sheath and catheter by pressure infusion, anticoagulation, etc.; Thiex et al. 2010). Elective procedures also require appropriate and timely preparations, including a stock check to make sure that the necessary equipment is available with minimal redundancy, because occasionally items may be inadvertently damaged or contaminated during preparations. Repeating a treatment also poses a repeated risk to the patient—a risk that is not justified by avoidable errors such as the use of faulty or incorrect supplies.

Practical Tip

Checklist (review on previous day, at the latest):
- Long (70–90 cm) reinforced sheath (6–8F)
- Coaxial catheter (6–8F)
- Guidewire (e.g., Terumo 0.035 in [0.89 mm])
- Microwire
- Stent (diameter, length, type—inventory)
- Dilatation balloon (length, diameter)
- Pressure syringe for dilatation
- Premedication: anticoagulant and antiplatelet drugs

Companies that develop and market these products are listed in **Table 10.1**.

A long sheath (70–90 cm), flexible but adequately stiff in its proximal and middle segments, is recommended. This is necessary to ensure a stable position in the aortic arch. A sheath used for treatments in the carotid artery and its branches should extend into the common carotid artery, while a sheath used for treatments of the vertebral and basilar arteries should extend into the subclavian artery. For enhanced stability, sheaths are available that have a braided shaft or are reinforced with coiled wire. The sheath is placed atraumatically at the supra-aortic level by advancing it from the aortic arch into the

target vessel over a coaxial catheter with a hydrophilic-coated standard guidewire (diameter usually 0.035 in [0.89 mm]). The hydrophilic coating on the wire serves to reduce the thrombogenicity of the device and reduce friction within the catheter and along the vessel wall during insertion. To achieve these properties, the wire must be adequately hydrated before use.

Caution

A hydrophilic-coated wire will also slide more easily into smaller arteries than a standard wire. Thus, advancing the coated wire against resistance carries an increased risk of vascular dissection or perforation.

A microwire, usually with a hydrophilic coating, is most often used for the navigation of stents and dilatation balloons. The wire must have good flexibility and should be stable over its entire length. Only the last few centimeters before the atraumatic tip are very soft (diameter 0.014–0.021 in [0.36–0.53 mm], depending on the stent system used).

Materials for the Treatment of Extracranial Stenoses

Self-expanding stents are most commonly used for the treatment of extracranial stenoses in the internal carotid artery, common carotid artery, and the V2 or V3 segment of the vertebral artery. Balloon-expandable stents are used only for rare indications—mainly stenoses affecting the brachiocephalic trunk, the left common carotid artery at its origin from the aortic arch, or the V0 or V1 segment of the vertebral artery. After a self-expanding stent has been placed, a balloon is generally used to dilate the stenosis and appose the stent to the vessel wall. Manufacturers offer various protection systems that are designed to shield the brain from treatment-associated thromboembolism. To date, however, studies have not demonstrated a benefit from the use of embolic protection systems (Barbato et al. 2008),

Table 10.1 Manufacturers of endovascular materials (listed alphabetically)

Manufacturer	Web site	Products
Abbott	http://www.abbottvascular.com/int/index.html	Arterial occlusion system
Acandis	http://www.acandis.com	Intracranial stents
ARROW	http://www.arrowintl-europe.com/webcat/	Sheaths
BALT (Extrusion)	http://www.balt.fr/	Coaxial catheters, microwires, microcatheters, intracranial stents
BARD	http://www.crbard.com	Stents
Boston Scientific	http://www.bostonscientific-international.com/home.bsci	Stents, catheters
Boston Scientific Neurovascular	http://www.stryker.com/en-us/products/ Neurovascularintervention/index.htm	Intracranial stents, microcatheters, microwires, dilatation catheters
Codman & Shurtleff, Inc.,	http://www.depuy.com/about-depuy/ depuy-divisions/codman-and-shurtleff	
Concentric Medical	http://www.concentric-medical.com/home	Guide catheters
Cook medical	http://www.cookmedical.com/home.do	Sheaths
Cordis	http://www.cordis.com/	Guide catheters, stents, dilatation catheters
Covidien	http://www.covidien.com	
Covidien/ev3	http://www.ev3.net	Microcatheters, microwire, intracranial stents
Invatec	http://www.invatec.com	Stents, dilatation catheters, proximal protection system
Krauth Cardiovascular	http://www.cardiovascularbusiness.com	Medical products distributor in Europe
Medtronic	http://www.medtronic.com/	
Microvention	http://www.microvention.com/	Coaxial catheters, microcatheters, microwires
Micrus	http://www.micrusendovascular.com/	Coaxial catheters, microcatheters, microwires
OptiMed	http://www.opti-med.de/home/	Sheaths, stents
Penumbra	http://www.penumbrainc.com/	Coaxial catheters
St. Jude Medical	http://www.sjm.com/	Arterial occlusion system
Stryker	http://www.stryker.com	
Terumo	http://www.terumo-europe.com/	Guidewires

Note: Although not complete, this listing includes most firms that manufacture or distribute products relating to the endovascular treatment of cervical and intracranial arteries supplying the brain. The internet addresses were up-to-date when this book went to press but, like the products themselves, are subject to change over time.

IV

even though they are increasingly used throughout the world, especially in the treatment of internal carotid artery stenoses.

The three main groups of materials—stents, protection systems, and dilatation catheters—are described below with reference to carotid artery stenting.

Stents

Self-Expanding Stents

Both self-expanding and balloon-expandable stent systems are in use. Supra-aortic stenoses of the internal and common carotid arteries are most commonly treated with self-expanding stents—small meshwork tubes made from braided or woven monofilament wires (classic Wallstent; **Fig. 10.1**) or cut from a metal tube with a laser (**Fig. 10.2**). Besides the traditional cobalt-chromium or cobalt-nickel steel, nickel-titanium alloy stents are also widely used. Nickel–titanium alloy (nitinol) has memory properties that increase the radial force of stents made of this material by converting thermal energy (body temperature) to mechanical energy.

Practical Tip

Stents cause variable susceptibility artifacts on MRI, depending on the type of alloy from which the stent is made. This may make it difficult or impossible to evaluate stented vascular segments on MRI follow-up, depending on the type of stent used.

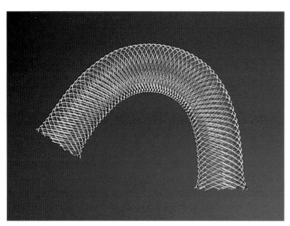

Fig. 10.1 Carotid Wallstent. Example of a woven carotid stent with a closed-cell design (with kind permission of Boston Scientific, Ratingen, Germany).

The stent is secured in an outer sheath or delivery system for insertion and positioning. When the outer sheath is retracted, radial forces cause the stent to self-expand. When released, the previously compressed stent expands and assumes a tapered or cylindrical shape depending on the stent design and vessel configuration. Static and dynamic pressure loads that exceed the radial force exerted by the stent will not cause irreversible stent deformation or stent fracture; this is particularly important at the exposed location of the carotid

bifurcation (Wissgott et al. 2009). Three different types of stent design are available:

- Ring segments with an open-cell design
- Meshworks with a closed-cell design (see **Fig. 10.1**)
- Mixed types in which the outer portions of the stent have an open-cell design while the central portion is a closed-cell meshwork (see **Fig. 10.2**).

The main advantage of open-cell systems is that the stent undergoes very little shortening when deployed (3–7%), whereas a closed-cell stent will shorten by 20–25% (Müller-Hülsbeck et al. 2009). In recent years, stents have been marketed that undergo no shortening because they do not form a closed circle but consist of a rolled nitinol sheet that expands when released within the vessel (**Fig. 10.3**). With a closed-cell design, the struts of the stent completely separate each cell in the scaffold from the adjacent cells. In laser-cut stents, the flexibility of the stent is reduced by a closed-cell design. In woven stents, the struts can move relative to one another; this property maintains relatively high stent flexibility even with a small cell size. The advantage of a closed-cell design is that the meshes making up the scaffold are smaller overall than in an open-cell stent, with the result that stenting places a "tighter" scaffold against the stenosing plaque (Müller-Hülsbeck et al. 2009). In an open-cell stent, the patterned omission of struts creates open connections between adjacent cells. This type of stent has very high flexibility as a rule (Stoeckel et al. 2004). When an open-cell stent is placed along a curved vascular segment, however, the interstices on the outside of the curve tends to widen and may potentially allow plaque material to prolapse into the artery lumen. Meanwhile, the struts along the inside of the curve may bunch together and bulge into the lumen, potentially hampering the later passage of filter systems, dilatation devices, wires, or catheters (Siewiorek et al. 2009).

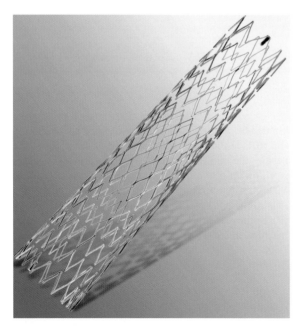

Fig. 10.2 Carotid stent (Cristallo Ideale). Example of a laser-cut nitinol stent with a multisegment design (open cells in the proximal and distal segments, closed cells in the middle segment) (with kind permission of Krauth Cardiovascular GmbH, Hamburg, Germany).

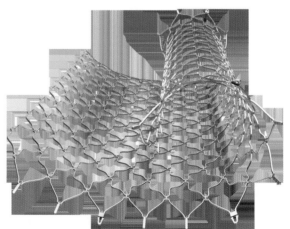

Fig. 10.3 Carotid stent (Adapt Carotid Stent, Boston Scientific). Example of a rolled, laser-cut nitinol stent with a closed-cell design (with kind permission of Boston Scientific, Ratingen, Germany).

Balloon-Expandable Stents

Balloon-expandable stents are generally made of cobalt–chromium alloys and have high shape stability. Owing to their design, these stents can expand without significant shortening but have less elastic recoil than self-expanding stents. If extrinsic pressure loads exceed the specified shape stability of these stents, they cannot self-expand again. Consequently they cannot be used in atherosclerotic stenoses at superficial locations in the cervical soft tissues, such as the carotid bifurcation. Balloon-expandable stents are advantageous for treating proximal stenoses of the brachiocephalic trunk or common carotid artery because they can be positioned more accurately and do not shorten. The use of balloon-mounted coated stents is justified in highly selected cases such as fibrous strictures after radiotherapy, early recurrent stenosis, and proximal vertebral artery stenosis.

The stent is coated with an immunosuppressive or cytostatic-equivalent agent: paclitaxel or sirolimus. A meta-analysis has confirmed the superiority of the sirolimus-eluting stent over paclitaxel-coated stents, finding that the risk of restenosis associated with sirolimus was only about half that of paclitaxel-coated stents (Schömig et al. 2007). Work has begun on the development of self-absorbing and nonmetallic stents as well as antibody-coated "healing" stents, which may make it possible to reduce the need for antiplatelet drugs and may also permit a wider range of treatment options, including surgical endarterectomy in the event of recurrent stenosis (Palmaz 2004).

Dilatation Catheters

Primary self-expanding stents are used in the treatment of carotid stenoses at typical locations (common carotid artery and brachiocephalic trunk). The purpose of a dilatation balloon is to widen the stenotic segment, if necessary by breaking a calcified plaque, and to appose the stent to the vessel wall. The dilatation catheters in current use generally have guidance "by wire" (also called a monorail or rapid-exchange system), which allows the balloon catheter to be positioned without the need for additional time-consuming exchange maneuvers over a long exchange wire (**Fig. 10.4**).

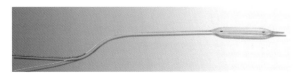

Fig. 10.4 Dilatation catheter. Example of a by-the-wire dilatation catheter, in which only the distal portion of the micro guidewire runs inside the system. This makes it easier to exchange the stent delivery system for the dilation catheter over the same microwire without having to use an exchange wire. This type of system is also called a rapid-exchange or monorail system (with kind permission of Krauth Cardiovascular GmbH, Hamburg, Germany).

Also, the balloons are noncompliant and are inflated by pressure manometer with a 50:50 mixture of contrast medium and saline solution. The delivery pressure is adjusted to a diameter that matches the measured normal vessel diameter without stenosis and will precisely appose the stent to the vessel wall.

> **Note**
>
> To prevent dissection outside the stent-protected vascular segment, the length of the balloon should not exceed the length of the stent.

Protection Systems

Embolic protection systems have been available for two decades and are used almost exclusively in the treatment of carotid stenosis. The purpose of these systems is to prevent atherosclerotic plaque material from embolizing to distal arterial branches during the intervention. Distal filter systems as well as proximal and distal balloon occlusion systems have been developed for this purpose (**Figs. 10.5** and **10.6**).

Filter Systems

Varied as the technical design and handling of current filter systems are, a common feature of all systems is that they must be advanced distally through the stenosis. The purpose of the filter is to capture any plaque particles that may be dislodged from the vessel wall and travel downstream. Basically the device should keep any debris from embolizing past the filter pores or mesh, while still allowing unrestricted blood flow. The filter pore size ranges from 65 to 200 μm to ensure that even the smallest particles will be trapped. Just as important as pore size is the ability of the filter to conform to the vessel lumen and fully cover its cross-section. Any debris dislodged by the intervention will be removed through a retrieval sheath or coaxial catheter along with the filter system (see **Fig. 10.5**). Filter deployment, filter friction against the distal vascular segment, and filter retrieval naturally add to the potential complications of the procedure.

Distal and Proximal Balloon Occlusion Systems

Several types of balloon occlusion system are available:
- *Distal balloon systems:* These systems temporarily occlude blood flow in the internal carotid artery to prevent the distal embolization of any plaque particles

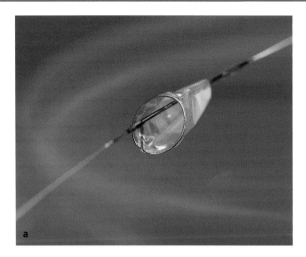

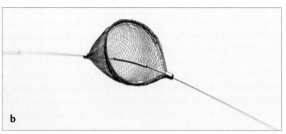

Fig. 10.5a,b Distal protection systems.
a FilterWire EZ embolic protection system (with kind permission of Boston Scientific, Ratingen, Germany).
b Spider FX embolic protection device (with kind permission of ev3 GmbH, Bonn, Germany).

dislodged during stent release and expansion. Suction is applied to the coaxial catheter to remove these potential emboli from the artery before the balloon is deflated and antegrade flow is restored.

- *Proximal balloon systems:* In proximal balloon occlusion systems, a balloon is mounted at the tip of the guide catheter. When the balloon is inflated in the common carotid artery, simultaneous occlusion of the external carotid artery also prevents possible antegrade collateral flow to the internal carotid artery via the external carotid artery.

- *Combined systems:* A combined system has two balloons—a small distal balloon inflated in the external carotid artery plus a larger proximal balloon inflated in the common carotid artery (see **Fig. 10.6**). This prevents both antegrade and retrograde collateral flow via the external carotid artery.

> **Caution**
>
> In assessing the need for filter protection, it should be kept in mind that the distal filter systems are more likely to induce vasospasms. Also, complications may occur when the system is retrieved through the deployed stent (material retention in the stent, etc.). One disadvantage of proximal filter systems is that, during the period of carotid occlusion, ipsilateral bypass flow cannot occur through the external carotid branches and no residual flow can occur across the stenosis. As a result, proximal protection is especially risky in the presence of a contralateral occlusion or contralateral high-grade stenosis.

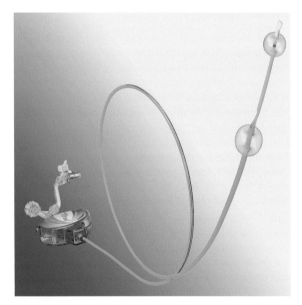

Fig. 10.6 Proximal protection system. Proximal protection system with two occlusion balloons. The smaller distal balloon is placed over a guidewire in the external carotid artery, and the larger proximal balloon is positioned below the carotid bifurcation after the guidewire is withdrawn. The carotid stent, and later the dilatation catheter, can be advanced through the side opening in the catheter shaft of the protection system just distal to the large proximal occluding balloon (with kind permission of Krauth Cardiovascular GmbH, Hamburg, Germany).

Materials for the Treatment of Intracranial Stenoses

The same materials are used for the treatment of stenoses in the anterior and posterior circulations. In contrast to extracranial stenoses, filter systems are *not* used in the treatment of intracranial stenoses. As with extracranial stenoses, the coaxial guide catheter should be advanced as close to the stenosis as possible. It is helpful to use longer and more flexible coaxial catheters, because of the greater distance and intervening curves (atlas loop, carotid siphon; **Fig. 10.7**). However, more flexible catheters

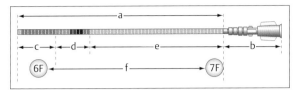

Fig. 10.7a–f Chaperon 2 guide catheter (MicroVention). Diagram illustrates the design of a modern coaxial catheter, which is optimized for distal placement in the petrous or cavernous segment of the internal carotid artery or in the vertebral artery distal to the atlas loop (with kind permission of MicroVention GmbH, Düsseldorf, Germany).

a Useful length

b Connector for hemostatic valve

c Very flexible but kink-resistant catheter end with radiopaque marker at the tip

d Transition zone between the very flexible catheter end and the reinforced catheter shaft, providing a smooth transition to the soft tip

e Reinforced catheter shaft allows for stable proximal placement

f Catheter outer diameter tapers from 7F at the proximal end to 6F at the distal end

are more difficult to maneuver through the aortic arch, and so the passage of the aortic arch is achieved by using a diagnostic catheter with an appropriate tip shape. Subsequently the diagnostic catheter is exchanged for a flexible catheter with suitable properties for distal access via an exchange wire or after advancing the sheath into the supra-aortic vessel. Alternatively, immediate triaxial access can be obtained with a long, more steerable inner catheter inside the flexible distal access catheter. Flexible, atraumatic microwires with a 0.014-in [0.36-mm] diameter are particularly useful for the navigation of stent systems.

Stents

Two main types of stents are currently used in the treatment of intracranial stenoses: balloon-expandable and self-expanding.

Balloon-Expandable Stents

Balloon-mounted stents (**Fig. 10.8**) can be navigated into the stenosis over a microwire. The necessary stent diameter must be accurately determined.

> **Caution**
>
> Never use an oversized balloon-expandable stent. Intracranial arteries are similar to coronary arteries in their caliber but have much thinner walls. An oversized stent would pose a high risk of vessel rupture.

Undersizing the stent by 0.25 mm will generally provide adequate safety.

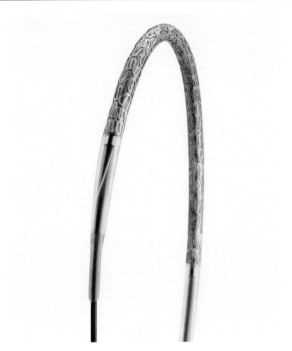

Fig. 10.8 Balloon-expandable intracranial stent (Pharos vitesse, Micrus, Johnson & Johnson Codman). A balloon-mounted open-cell stent with micro guidewire is shown (with kind permission of Johnson & Johnson Medical Codman, Norderstedt, Germany). The balloon and stent are not yet deployed. The balloon-mounted stent has been bent sharply to demonstrate its flexibility.

IV

Self-Expanding Stents

Self-expanding stents (**Fig. 10.9**) are advanced into the stenosis through a microcatheter with an inner diameter of 0.021–0.027 in (0.53–0.69 mm), depending on the type of stent used. Also, self-expanding stents that were formerly used to treat wide-necked aneurysms in the remodeling technique are currently used for the treatment of atherosclerotic stenoses (see **Fig. 10.9a**). As in the extracranial vessels, intracranial stents may have an open- or closed-cell design. One disadvantage of self-expanding stents is that stent deployment and dilatation are done as consecutive steps. Following stent release, postdilatation or stent apposition either requires a microwire exchange maneuver with a 300-cm microwire to insert the dilatation catheter, or the stenosis must be recrossed with a microwire and dilatation catheter while the stent is in place (see **Fig. 10.9b**).

Dilatation Catheters

There are a few situations in which dilatation catheters may still be considered for the primary treatment of a stenosis, especially if the lumen of the stenosed segment is too small or borderline. This situation is occasionally

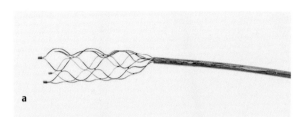

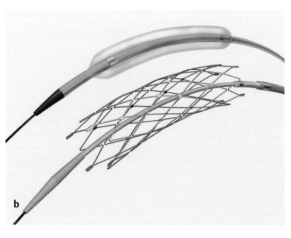

Fig. 10.9a,b Self-expanding intracranial stents.
a Example of a partially released, laser-cut rolled nitinol stent with a closed-cell design (Solitaire FR, with kind permission of Covidien/ev3 GmbH, Bonn, Germany).
b View of a deployed Wingspan stent (open-cell design with matching dilatation catheter). The stent delivery system is shown at the center of the stent lumen. Pictured above it is a Gateway dilatation balloon which, unlike the Submarine (see **Fig. 10.4**), is an "over-the-wire" device in which the micro guidewire runs inside the dilatation catheter over the full length of the system (Wingspan Stent System with Gateway PTA Balloon Catheter, with kind permission of Stryker, Neurovascular Division, Duisburg, Germany).

encountered in the main trunk of the middle cerebral artery, for example. The indication for stent placement should be viewed very critically if the vessel diameter is significantly less than 2 mm.

References

Barbato JE, Dillavou E, Horowitz MB, et al. A randomized trial of carotid artery stenting with and without cerebral protection. J Vasc Surg 2008;47(4):760–765

Müller-Hülsbeck S, Schäfer PJ, Charalambous N, Schaffner SR, Heller M, Jahnke T. Comparison of carotid stents: an in-vitro experiment focusing on stent design. J Endovasc Ther 2009;16(2):168–177

Palmaz JC. Intravascular stents in the last and the next 10 years. J Endovasc Ther 2004;11(Suppl 2):II200–II206

Schömig A, Dibra A, Windecker S, et al. A meta-analysis of 16 randomized trials of sirolimus-eluting stents versus paclitaxel-eluting stents in patients with coronary artery disease. J Am Coll Cardiol 2007;50(14):1373–1380

Siewiorek GM, Finol EA, Wholey MH. Clinical significance and technical assessment of stent cell geometry in carotid artery stenting. J Endovasc Ther 2009;16(2):178–188

Stoeckel D, Pelton A, Duerig T. Self-expanding nitinol stents: material and design considerations. Eur Radiol 2004;14(2):292–301

Thiex R, Norbash AM, Frerichs KU. The safety of dedicated-team catheter-based diagnostic cerebral angiography in the era of advanced noninvasive imaging. AJNR Am J Neuroradiol 2010;31(2):230–234

Wissgott C, Schmidt W, Behrens P, Schmitz KP, Andresen R. Performance characteristics of self-expanding peripheral nitinol stents. [Article in German] Rofo 2009;181(6):579–586

11 Extracranial Carotid Stenoses

M. Tietke and O. Jansen

Introduction

The interventional treatment of atherosclerotic stenoses of the common carotid artery (CCA) and internal carotid artery (ICA) began in the late 1970s and early 1980s, consisting initially of conventional percutaneous transluminal balloon angioplasty. One of the first reports on this treatment was published by Kerber et al. (1980). The number of publications on this subject grew steadily thereafter, with most authors reporting good clinical outcomes (Bockenheimer and Mathias 1983; Tievsky et al. 1983; Wiggli and Gratzl 1983; Tsai et al. 1986). A high rate of restenosis was a serious initial problem, however (Diethrich et al. 1995). Carotid artery stenting was first performed in 1989 to reappose an intimal flap caused by percutaneous transluminal balloon angioplasty. The first report of a carotid stenosis treated by stent angioplasty was published in 1995. It involved the treatment of a recurrent stenosis following thromboendarterectomy (Mathias et al. 2001). When stent angioplasty was found to decrease restenosis rates and yield better long-term results, it began to replace conventional percutaneous transluminal balloon angioplasty in the interventional treatment of carotid stenosis. The results of the Carotid and Vertebral Artery Transluminal Angioplasty Study (CAVATAS) I trial (CAVATAS Investigators 2001) in particular were instrumental in showing the superiority of stent-assisted percutaneous transluminal balloon angioplasty over conventional percutaneous transluminal balloon angioplasty. Since then, stent-assisted percutaneous transluminal balloon angioplasty has become the endovascular procedure of first choice for carotid stenosis. Standard techniques have been devised, and researchers have developed a range of new self-expanding stents designed for specific types of stenosis.

Embolic protection systems were introduced in the late 1990s in the belief that they could reduce the risk of peri-interventional embolization. A variety of systems have been developed over the years, with distal filter systems becoming the most popular. Various publications in subsequent years sought to document the protective effect of these systems over unprotected stenting (Reimers et al. 2001; Castriota et al. 2002; Cremonesi et al. 2003).

The interventional treatment of carotid stenosis requires only a small inguinal stab incision, as opposed to a longer cervical incision. The latter carries a risk of lower cranial nerve injury and creates a larger wound area. This may be particularly objectionable in female patients and is often cited as a reason for favoring an interventional technique. The procedure times for interventional and surgical treatment are comparable (~1 h). Interventions are generally performed under local anesthesia, whereas surgical treatment usually requires general endotracheal anesthesia. One problem in previous randomized studies comparing surgical carotid endarterectomy with interventional carotid artery stenting has been the demonstrably higher incidence of minor strokes associated with interventional treatment. There is considerable evidence, however, that proper stent selection, sound interventional technique, and adequate operator experience can reduce the complication rate of carotid stenting to a level that makes it competitive with surgery. There is still considerable debate as to the value of using protection systems in interventional procedures, but the analysis of data from large randomized prospective trials (SPACE I, EVA 3S, and ICSS; see below) indicates advantages for unprotected stenting.

Indications

Study Results

The results of the ECST (European Carotid Surgery Trial; European Carotid Surgery Trialists' Collaborative Group 1998) and NASCET (North American Carotid Endarterectomy Trial; Barnett et al. 1998) trials have shown that surgical treatment can significantly reduce the risk of stroke in patients with a symptomatic high-grade carotid artery stenosis (NASCET: > 50%). A subanalysis of NASCET data on asymptomatic contralateral ICA stenoses in patients symptomatic for the other side showed that the risk of stroke from the asymptomatic stenosis was significantly reduced only in cases where the degree of stenosis (NASCET) was less than 60% (Inzitari et al. 2000). The ECST trial studied a total of 3024 patients at 97 centers from 12 European countries and one Australian center during the period 1981–1994. Of that total, 1811 patients were randomly assigned to the surgical arm and 1213 to the control arm, in which surgical treatment was avoided for as long as possible. The study found that the Kaplan–Meier estimate of the frequency of a major stroke or death at 3 years was 26.5% in the control arm vs. 14.5% in the surgical arm in patients with > 80% carotid stenosis (ECST). The authors conclude that surgical treatment is indicated for patients with symptomatic carotid stenosis > 80% (ECST). This corresponds to a ~65% stenosis by the NASCET criteria.

The NASCET trial, conducted at 106 American centers from 1987 to 1996, randomly assigned 2226 patients with symptomatic carotid stenosis to a medical arm (1118 patients) and a surgical arm (1108 patients). Two groups were formed based on the degree of initial stenosis: one group with < 50% stenosis (NASCET) and a second group with 50–69% stenosis (NASCET). After 5 years, the rate of ipsilateral stroke in the group with 50–69% stenosis (NASCET) was 15.7% in patients treated surgically vs. 22.7% in patients treated medically. In the group with < 50% stenosis (NASCET), no statistically significant difference was found at 5 years between the surgically and medically treated patients (Barnett et al. 1998; European Carotid Surgery Trialists' Collaborative Group 1998).

> ### Note
>
> Based on these study findings, treatment is currently recommended for patients with symptomatic carotid stenosis > 50% (NASCET), but only if the complication rate associated with the treatment is < 6% at the institution in question.

Thus far, data on degree of stenosis have been based on the NASCET method of measurement, in which the residual lumen within the stenosis is measured in relation to the closest unaffected distal vascular segment with parallel walls. This method is employed in digital subtraction angiography (DSA), CT angiography (CTA), and MR angiography (MRA). By contrast, the ECST method is based on a Doppler ultrasound technique in which the original diameter of the vessel lumen is determined at the affected site and the stenosis is measured relative to the original lumen. This cannot be done in the NASCET method, which is based on angiographic measurements (**Fig. 11.1**).

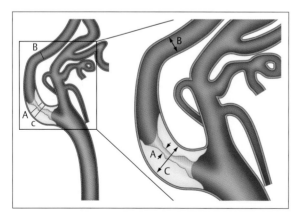

Fig. 11.1 The ECST and NASCET methods for determining degree of stenosis.
(A/C) × 100 = degree of stenosis (%) by the ECST method
(A/B) × 100 = degree of stenosis (%) by the NASCET method

The following formula can be used to convert between the measurements:

ECST stenosis (%) = 0.6 × NASCET stenosis (%) + 40%

Patients with asymptomatic carotid stenoses have a significantly lower risk of stroke. Even so, it may generally be assumed that the age-independent 5-year risk is < 10% (Halliday et al. 2004), and that the stroke risk for women is almost 2.5% lower than that for men. The ACST (Asymptomatic Carotid Surgery Trial) trial compared surgical and medical treatment in patients with asymptomatic carotid stenosis and found that surgical treatment provided a significant benefit in terms of risk reduction only if the complication rate of the treatment was < 3%. This seems reasonable until we consider that the corresponding number needed to treat to prevent one stroke is 53!

Wholey et al. (2003) published the results of a registry (Multi-Centre World Carotid Registry) reviewing the results of carotid stenting regardless of the exact procedure used (including the use of protection devices). In a total of 6734 stent placements, they found a 30-day complication rate of 5.8% for ipsilateral strokes.

Garg et al. (2009) took a somewhat more differentiated approach in a review of 134 publications from 1995 to 2007 that met the authors' inclusion criteria. A pooled analysis of these 134 publications showed that carotid stenting was associated with a relative risk of 0.62 (95% confidence interval [CI] 0.54–0.72) for ipsilateral stroke. A subgroup analysis revealed a significant benefit from protected stenting in symptomatic patients (relative risk [RR] 0.67; 95% CI 0.52–0.56) and asymptomatic patients (RR 0.61; 95% CI 0.41–0.90; $p < 0.05$).

In the late 1990s, various prospective randomized multicenter studies were planned to compare stent angioplasty of the carotid artery with conventional carotid endarterectomy. The EVA-3S trial (Endarterectomy vs. Angioplasty in Patients with Symptomatic Severe Carotid Stenosis), which began in 2000 and was conducted at 30 centers in France, was stopped early in 2005 after the enrollment of 527 symptomatic patients for "reasons of both safety and futility" in showing equality between interventional and surgical treatment. The initial degree of stenosis necessary for enrollment was 60–99% (NASCET). The complication rate for stroke and death was 3.9% (95% CI 2.0–7.2) after carotid endarterectomy and 9.6% (95% CI 6.4–14.0) after carotid stent angioplasty (Mas et al. 2006).

SPACE I (Stent-Protected Percutaneous Angioplasty of the Carotid Artery vs. Endarterectomy) was a more rigorously designed and conducted trial involving 35 centers in Germany, Austria, and Switzerland. The results published in 2006 could not demonstrate noninferiority of stent angioplasty compared with surgical treatment. Between 2001 and 2006, a total of 1200 symptomatic patients with an initial stenosis of at least 50% (NASCET) or

70% (ECST) were randomly assigned to an interventional arm (605 patients) and a surgical arm (595 patients). The final analysis encompassed 599 patients in the stent arm and 584 patients in the carotid endarterectomy arm. The primary endpoint of ipsilateral stroke or death was reached in 6.84% of the patients with carotid artery stenting and 6.34% of the patients with carotid endarterectomy (Ringleb et al. 2006).

The ICSS (International Carotid Stenting Study) did not yield a positive result (Ederle et al. 2010). The trial enrolled 1713 patients at 50 European, Australian, New Zealand, and Canadian academic centers between 2001 and 2008. Seven hundred fifty-one (88%) of 853 patients in the stent arm and 760 (89%) of 857 patients in the surgical arm were finally treated and evaluated. The incidence of stroke, death, or myocardial infarction between randomization and 120 days was 8.5% after carotid stent angioplasty and 5.2% after carotid endarterectomy (72 vs. 44 events; hazard ratio = 1.69; 95% CI 1.16–2.45; $p = 0.006$; Ederle et al. 2010).

> **Note**
>
> Previous subanalyses of randomized prospective studies show benefits for unprotected stenting with regard to periprocedural complication rate, and the ICSS MRI subgroup exhibited fewer postinterventional DWI lesions with unprotected stenting (Jansen et al. 2009; Bonati et al. 2010).

Although the differences between the procedures related chiefly to minor strokes in all the studies, it was obvious that stent angioplasty was increasingly called into question as a treatment for carotid artery stenosis. For this reason, the results of the CREST study (Carotid Revascularization Endarterectomy vs. Stenting Trial), still in progress at that time, were awaited with great interest. The CREST study enrolled 2502 symptomatic and asymptomatic patients at 108 centers in the U.S. and Canada from 2000 to 2008. The initial degree of stenosis had to be > 50% (NASCET) or > 70% (ECST) at time of enrollment. The 4-year rate of stroke or death was 6.4% with stenting and 4.7% with endarterectomy. When the patients were divided into symptomatic and asymptomatic groups, the respective rates were 8.0 vs. 6.4% and 4.5 vs. 2.7% in the stent and surgical arms. The rates for specific periprocedural end points were as follows: 0.7 vs. 0.3% for death, 4.1 vs. 2.3% for stroke, and 1.1 vs. 2.3% for myocardial infarction in the interventional and surgical arms. Thus, while carotid stenting was associated with a slightly higher risk of strokes (mostly minor), more myocardial infarctions were observed in the surgical arm. Overall, the authors of the CREST study concluded that the composite risk profiles were comparable in the groups undergoing carotid stenting and carotid endarterectomy (Brott et al. 2010). Previous study data also indicate a tendency for younger patients to benefit more from stenting while older patients benefit more from surgery.

Meier et al. (2010) performed a meta-analysis of the results from 11 studies comparing carotid endarterectomy and carotid artery stenting. For the primary composite endpoint of the risk of periprocedural stroke or death, the meta-analysis shows a significantly better result for carotid endarterectomy than carotid stent angioplasty (OR 0.67; 95% CI 0.47–0.95). This result related chiefly to a lower risk of strokes with carotid endarterectomy than with carotid artery stenting (OR 0.65; 95% CI 0.43–1.00; $p = 0.049$). The difference was driven mainly by the occurrence of minor (nondisabling) strokes. As in the CREST trial, surgical treatment was associated with a significantly higher risk of myocardial infarction than interventional treatment (OR 2.69; 95% CI 1.06–6.79; $p = 0.036$). Moreover, the data showed for the first time that the risk of lower cranial nerve injury or cervical nerve injury was significantly higher after carotid endarterectomy. The confidence intervals of the results are very broad, however. This highlights the heterogeneity of the results from different studies and the small case numbers, which do not provide a basis for drawing reliable conclusions (Meier et al. 2010).

> **Note**
>
> In summary, the results to date show that even the large, multinational multicenter studies have not provided adequate case numbers in order to draw evidence-based conclusions for or against the interventional or operative treatment of carotid stenosis.

IV

Clear Indications for Stenting

Despite the lack of definitive statistical evidence, there are initial situations that would definitely favor carotid artery stenting over carotid endarterectomy. For example, stenting is preferable in cases where a stenosed ICA is poorly collateralized by a deficient circle of Willis. This type of case could also be described as an "isolated" carotid artery. Moreover, carotid endarterectomy would be difficult or impossible to perform in patients with a high carotid bifurcation located at a poorly accessible site behind the mandibular angle. The same applies to other surgically inaccessible stenoses of the proximal CCA and distal ICA. Also, tandem stenoses consisting of a bifurcation stenosis plus a stenosis of the proximal CCA or distal ICA would not be surgically treatable in most cases. Recurrent stenosis after carotid endarterectomy, radiogenic stenosis, and carotid stenosis following a neck dissection (generally combined with radiation) would also contraindicate surgery. An occlusion of the contralateral ICA or a high-grade stenosis is associated with a significant increase in perioperative morbidity (see also NASCET study, earlier). Another important consideration is comorbid conditions, especially preexisting cardiac and cardiovascular diseases, which would tend to favor carotid artery stenting because of the increased risks involved in general anesthesia.

Materials

In principle, carotid stent angioplasty can be performed with or without the use of protection systems.

Protection Systems

Embolic protection systems are available in various designs. The most widely used devices are net-type filters, and the most popular device of this kind is the FilterWire EX (Boston Scientific, Natick, MA, USA). It is a small filter (< 3.5F) mounted on a 0.014-in (0.36-mm) microwire. With a pore size of 80 μm, the filter permits antegrade blood flow while preventing the distal embolization of debris. The design is characterized by an eccentrically placed filter with a "fish-mouth" opening. A radiopaque nitinol framework provides for stability and adequate visibility on radiographs. Other protection systems based on the distal filter concept are AccuNet, AngioGuard, Emboshield, Interceptor PLUS, NeuroShield, SPIDER, and Rubicon.

Another concept is the balloon occlusion system, which may be of the distal or proximal occlusion type. Proximal balloon occlusion systems are further subdivided into devices that interrupt flow and devices that produce retrograde flow via an inguinal arteriovenous shunt. A proximal balloon occlusion system should be considered only for a very high-grade ulcerating stenosis with a high-risk MRI profile or pronounced kinking just past the stenosis to avoid unprotected crossing of the stenosis. Examples of proximal balloon protection systems are the Parodi and MO.MA systems and the Kachel balloon. Distal balloon protection systems are illustrated by the PercuSurge, Guardwire Plus, and Tri Activ System.

> **Note**
>
> Basic disadvantages of distal protection systems are the unprotected crossing of the stenosis with the protection device as well as incomplete protection against small emboli, which has been demonstrated in various studies. Proximal systems avoid these problems but require large-gauge inguinal access (up to 10F).

Carotid Stents

The available carotid stents can be classified as having either an open- or closed-cell design. In a closed design, all the cells in the stent are interconnected with one another to form a structure similar to a knitted stocking. In an open design, there are gaps in the latticework that give the stent greater flexibility. One drawback of the open-cell design is that the omission of struts may increase the risk of embolization during postdilatation, especially in elongated vessels. By contrast, some closed stent designs have extremely small cells that offer better embolic protection by fixing the plaque against the vessel wall, but these stents have a tendency to straighten an elongated vessel and may cause kinking of the vessel at the distal end of the device.

The best-known stent for the treatment of atherosclerotic carotid stenosis is the Carotid Wallstent (Boston Scientific Corp., Natick, MA, USA). It has a closed-cell design composed of braided wires made of a cobalt-chromium-iron-nickel-molybdenum alloy (commonly known as Elgiloy or Conichrome) and has the smallest pore size available on the market (1.08 mm^2). Other frequently used carotid artery stents are listed below:

- Acculink (Guidant Corporation, Santa Clara, CA): laser-cut nitinol stent with open-cell design.
- OptiMed Sinus-Carotid (Conical) RX (OptiMed, Ettlingen, Germany): nickel–titanium alloy stent with open-cell design. One model has a tapered shape conforming to the caliber change at the CCA–ICA junction.
- Precise (Cordis Endovascular, Warren, NJ, USA).
- Cristallo ideale (Invatec, Roncadelle, Italy): nitinol hybrid stent with a closed-cell design in the central part to prevent embolism and an open-cell design in the distal and proximal sections for better conformability.
- NexStent (Boston Scientific Corp., Natick, MA, USA): This stent does not have a closed tubular shape like other stents but consists of a rolled nitinol sheet with a closed-cell design and a pore size of ~4 mm^2. It is claimed that this rolled design enables the stent to conform to a range of vessel diameters (4–9 mm).

> **Practical Tip**
>
> When placing stents with an open-cell design, it may be advantageous to use a protection system. A closed-cell stent with a small cell size will generally provide adequate embolic protection and can be safely used without an extra protection system (Jansen et al. 2009).

Technical Approach

Diagnostic Studies, Informed Consent, and Medication

Ideally, carotid artery stenting should be preceded by MRI of the brain parenchyma and intra- and extracranial vessels. If MRI is omitted due to contraindications such as cardiac pacemakers, other implants, or foreign bodies, cranial CT (which may include perfusion imaging) and CTA should be done instead. Doppler ultrasound scanning of the arteries supplying the brain is a desirable adjunct.

Following an interdisciplinary evaluation and general patient selection process for carotid stenosis treatment, informed consent should be obtained. This should include disclosure of the usual angiographic risks such as allergies to local anesthetic and contrast medium, risk of stroke and arterial dissection, and the potential for an inguinal hematoma requiring treatment. Disclosure also includes a potential risk of intracerebral hemorrhage that may require emergency surgery and may result in death. Patients should understand that in-stent restenosis may develop and may necessitate reintervention.

The standard pre- and postinterventional drug regimen includes dual antiplatelet therapy with aspirin and clopidogrel. In elective cases, oral treatment with 100 mg aspirin and 75 mg clopidogrel once daily should be started at least 3 days before stent placement. If treatment is more urgent and needs to be scheduled the next day or the same day, a loading dose of 4×75 mg clopidogrel should be given 1 day before stent placement, or 8×75 mg on the day of the procedure (Patti et al. 2005; Schillinger et al. 2006). If sufficient aspirin premedication has not been given, the additional administration of 500 mg aspirin is required. Following the stent procedure, medication is continued with 100 mg aspirin and 75 mg clopidogrel taken orally once a day for 6 weeks. After this the patient is placed on aspirin only, and this is continued for at least 6 months after the intervention. By that time the stent should be overgrown by intimal cells and will no longer cause activation of blood platelets or the coagulation cascade.

Heparinization based on activated clotting time (ACT) is done in immediate preparation for carotid stent angioplasty. A weight-adjusted intravenous heparin bolus should increase the ACT to 250–350 s, depending on the baseline value.

An increasingly common and effective practice before stent angioplasty is to test platelet function by whole-blood aggregometry and determine in-vitro bleeding time to identify patients who are low or nonresponders to antiplatelet therapy and make necessary medical adjustments to prevent thrombotic complications. According to the cardiologic literature, up to 30% of patients fall within this category of low or nonresponders (Steinhubl et al. 2002; Geisler and Gawaz 2008; Krötz et al. 2008). There is growing evidence, moreover, that concomitant use of the proton pump inhibitor omeprazole reduces the efficacy of clopidogrel, since omeprazole is also metabolized by CYP2C19. Another proton pump inhibitor, pantoprazole, does not interfere with clopidogrel.

Based on the unfavorable pharmacokinetic properties of previously available platelet aggregation inhibitors and the nonresponder problem, there is room for further progress in the development of antiplatelet drugs. One promising development in the field of platelet aggregation inhibitors is prasugrel, which has demonstrated several advantages compared with clopidogrel in the cardiology literature (Wiviott et al. 2007, 2011). In particular, there is a significantly lower proportion of nonresponders. On the other hand, more intracranial hemorrhages were found in a subgroup with previous brain infarctions, and in carotid artery stenting many patients belong to this particular subgroup. So it is still an individual decision; a global recommendation to change the pharmacologic regimen from clopidogrel to prasugrel cannot be given as yet.

Patient Preparations and Technique

While the procedure is being explained to the patient, the pulses should be taken, giving particular attention to the vascular access route so that, if a procedural change is needed, it can be organized before the patient is on the angiography table. The patient should also be assessed for cooperativeness and for any preexisting conditions such as spinal deformities or disorders that would make it difficult for them to lie still on a hard surface for a prolonged period. If the patient in unable to cooperate sufficiently, the procedure will have to be performed under general endotracheal anesthesia, and appropriate preparations should be made. Patients with a contralateral ICA occlusion, filiform stenosis, and/or severe arterial hypertension will require intra-arterial blood pressure monitoring, and the cannula should be placed as an in-patient procedure. If an inguinal approach is planned, the groin area is also shaved on an in-patient basis. If the patient desires it, a bladder catheter can be placed, on the ward, on the day of the intervention. Wearing an examination gown, the patient is taken to the angiography suite and positioned on the angiography table. At that point the ECG leads are placed, and either a blood pressure cuff is applied or the intra-arterial blood pressure line is connected to the monitor. An oxygen saturation clip is applied, and a large-bore IV line is inserted, if this has not previously been done.

Inguinal Approach

Atropine (1 mL = 0.5 mg) is administered by subcutaneous injection (caution: glaucoma). Meticulous aseptic preparation and draping of the skin come next, followed by right inguinal local anesthesia with mepivacaine (3%, 5 mL). A cutaneous stab incision is made with a slender

IV

pointed scalpel, and a large-gauge access needle is inserted into the right common femoral artery ~2 finger-widths below the inguinal ligament. A sheath guidewire is introduced, and a short 5F sheath is placed within the artery. An arterial blood sample is taken for determination of ACT. The initial sheath is then exchanged for a 90-cm (e.g., metal-reinforced) 6F Arrow sheath, which is passed into the distal aorta and connected to 0.5-L saline pressure irrigation with 1000IU heparin and 2mg nimodipine added to 1L saline solution. A 125-cm 5F multipurpose catheter or 6F Sidewinder Supertorque catheter is introduced next, depending on the anatomy of the aortic arch and the origins of the supra-aortic vessels (which ideally have already been evaluated by previous CTA or MRA). The catheter is threaded into the aortic arch over a 0.035-in (0.89-mm) Terumo wire, and the sheath is passed over the catheter into the proximal descending aorta. The catheter is then advanced into the CCA on the treatment side, and the sheath is carefully advanced into the distal CCA.

Transbrachial Approach

Transbrachial access can be established in patients with high-grade stenoses or occlusions of the aorta or iliac vessels or extensive soft plaques in the aortic arch and markedly elongated supra-aortic branches. The selected arm is strapped to a padded board, and the course of the brachial artery is drawn on the skin with a marking pen. This is followed by meticulous skin preparation and draping of the patient's body and arm using additional self-adhesive drapes. Local anesthesia is administered, and a large-gauge hollow needle is inserted into the brachial artery through a stab incision in the skin.

> **Practical Tip**
>
> If this is unsuccessful, the initial puncture can be done with a small cannula on a saline-filled syringe while gentle suction is applied. The thin cannula is removed, and the large hollow needle is introduced in the same direction and at the same angle. (This technique can also be used in the femoral artery.)

Next, as in the inguinal approach, a 5F sheath is carefully introduced over a short wire. Some blood should be drawn from the sheath tubing at this point to confirm intra-arterial placement and obtain a sample for ACT determination. The sheath is exchanged for a pressure-irrigated 90-cm metal-reinforced 6F Arrow sheath, and a 5F multipurpose catheter or 125-cm 6F Sidewinder Supertorque catheter is threaded into the brachiocephalic trunk or aorta over a 0.035-in (0.89-mm) wire. For treatment of a right ICA stenosis, the catheter is advanced

cephalad from the trunk of the CCA. For treatment of a left ICA stenosis, first the aorta and then the left CCA are catheterized via the right or left arm, depending on the elongation and takeoff angle of the vessels from the aortic arch. The treatment vessel is visualized, and the sheath is carefully advanced into the distal CCA. The rest of the procedure is comparable to the inguinal technique.

> **Practical Tip**
>
> If the sheath is not stable enough for advancement, pass the 0.035-in (0.89-mm) guidewire as far into the external carotid artery (ECA) as possible. A lateral roadmap is helpful at this stage. A posteroanterior (PA) projection with a large field of view (FOV) allows the aortic arch to be surveyed along with the other vessels during the procedure.

From 3000 to 5000IU of heparin is administered by IV injection, depending on the patient's body weight and initially measured clotting time, and the ACT is determined again ~10min later. The target ACT is between 250 and 350s. During the waiting interval, the stenosis is imaged in 2–4 planes and an intracranial run is obtained by injection of the CCA to document pretreatment flow status. When the ACT target value is reached, the stenosis is crossed with a 0.014-in (0.36-mm) microwire and the distal wire tip is placed in the midpetrous portion of the carotid artery.

> **Note**
>
> The tighter the stenosis, the less curved the microwire tip should be to allow for problem-free lesion crossing while still allowing adequate maneuverability of the microwire.

If a very high-grade stenosis cannot be crossed initially, it is helpful to introduce a microcatheter over a long exchange microwire and pass it directly into the carotid stump so that the stenosis can be scrutinized at high magnification with a small FOV. Then the long microwire is advanced through the microcatheter to the stenosis to provide additional stability for lesion crossing. Once the stenosis has been crossed, a predilatation balloon 2–3mm in diameter is introduced and the stenosis is moderately predilated. Incremental balloon sizes may be used if necessary to allow problem-free passage of the stent through the stenosis. Primary stent placement may be possible in lower-grade stenoses. On the whole, we have found predilatation to be helpful in a very large percentage of cases.

In patients with an occlusion or high-grade stenosis of the contralateral carotid artery, it is important to work swiftly to avoid hemodynamic complications. A supra-bulbar stenosis can often be treated with a shorter, 5-mm diameter stent placed entirely within the ICA (**Fig. 11.2**). With a proximal stenosis involving the origin of the ICA, we recommend stenting from the ICA into the CCA with

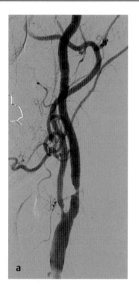 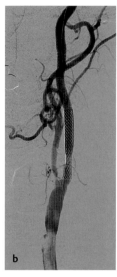 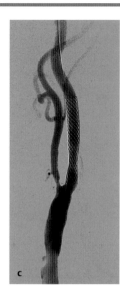

Fig. 11.2a–c Stenosis of the left ICA (50% NASCET). Angiographic images. Note: A high carotid bulb stenosis can be treated with a smaller stent placed entirely in the ICA.
a Before treatment.
b After stent placement.
c After final percutaneous transluminal balloon angioplasty.

a 7-mm × 30-mm or even a 9-mm × 40-mm stent, depending on individual anatomy (**Fig. 11.3**). Angiograms are obtained after predilatation and after stent deployment, and the patient is tested clinically. For postdilatation, the balloon is positioned proximal to the stent and 1 mL (0.5 mg) of atropine is administered intravenously, barring contraindications. As the heart rate rises, the balloon is advanced into the stenosis and postdilatation is performed. The balloon is then withdrawn from the former stenosis site, leaving the microwire in its original position with the tip in the petrous segment of the ICA. The wire tip should be visible in at least one plane at all times during the procedure. A final angiographic run is taken of the angioplasty result, and clinical neurologic testing is performed. If both appear normal, the balloon and microwire are removed and a final intracranial run is taken to document the absence of embolic complications and altered intracranial flow status (see **Fig. 11.3d,e**). Next the sheath is pulled back into the distal descending aorta and removed over a long wire. An arterial closure device (we use AngioSeal 6F) is introduced over the wire. Finally a light pressure dressing is applied, and at least 12 h bed rest is prescribed. The patient is transferred to the stroke unit for 24 h of observation. Patients who have had a purely elective stent angioplasty without complications may be discharged the following day.

Practical Tip

The primary insertion of a Sidewinder catheter is advised in patients with a bicarotid trunk or a markedly elongated left CCA. If the aortic arch is extremely elongated or if access is difficult for other reasons, we recommend brachial artery access via the ipsilateral arm.

Stent Selection

Closed small-cell stents can be used without difficulty in cases where the ICA arises at a small angle at the carotid bifurcation. A stent with a closed-cell design can often be used even with a slightly elongated ICA, although there are cases in which an open-cell stent should be used because of its greater conformability. This will slightly increase the risk of periprocedural embolization, however, so it may be helpful to add a protection filter—keeping in mind that protection systems lengthen the procedure time, increase the complexity of the procedure, and have an inherent complication risk because they may induce vasospasms. For these reasons, protection systems are used only in highly exceptional cases at our institution and we can treat the majority of cases with closed-cell systems.

Postprocedure Care

Circulation in the leg is assessed immediately after dressing placement and again on arrival at the stroke unit. Additional assessments are initially made at hourly intervals. After 24 h, the interventionalist inspects the access site after removal of the dressing. In patients considered at risk for hyperperfusion syndrome, invasive blood pressure monitoring and rigorous pharmacologic blood pressure control are maintained for at least 3 days.

Doppler ultrasound scanning is performed the day after treatment to establish a baseline for future follow-ups, which are scheduled initially at 3-month intervals and later at 6-month intervals.

IV

Treatment of Supra-aortic Extra- and Intracranial Stenoses

IV

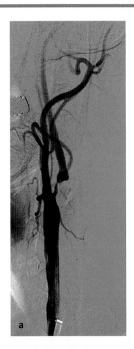

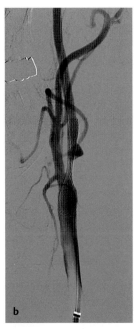

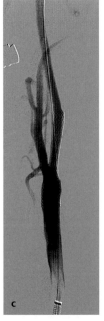

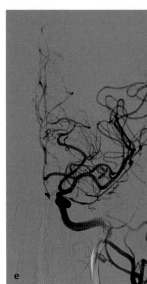

Fig. 11.3a–e Filiform stenosis of the left ICA. With a proximal stenosis, the stent should extend from the ICA into the CCA to prevent restenosis proximal to the stent.
a Before treatment.
b After stent placement.
c After final percutaneous transluminal balloon angioplasty.
d Intracranial angiography of the left ICA before stent placement.
e Intracranial angiography of the left ICA after stent angioplasty with final percutaneous transluminal balloon angioplasty. Note particularly the change of flow pattern in the anterior cerebral artery (ACA) territory in the final angiogram after stent angioplasty. In **d** the vessel was still supplied by nonopacified blood from the opposite side. In **e**, opacified blood is entering the ACA and indicates the initial change in flow. Note also the different filling dynamics of the external and internal carotid arteries in the two images.

Special Case of an ICA Pseudo-occlusion

The treatment of a pseudo-occlusion requires good preparation, especially in the preinterventional phase. On the day before the intervention, a cannula should be placed for intra-arterial blood pressure monitoring. The diagnostic work-up should include an initial assessment of the collateral circulation. If an angiographic run with contrast injection into the CCA shows an occlusion of the ICA, a microcatheter run may reveal the presence of a filiform stenosis.

Lesion crossing and predilatation should be done swiftly to ensure the fastest possible flow restoration, because

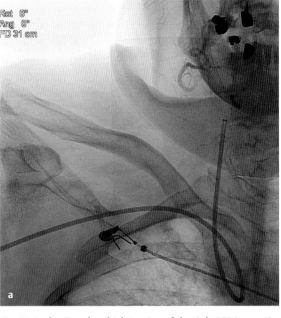
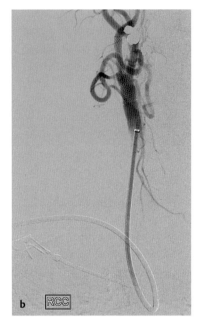

Fig. 11.4a, b Transbrachial stenting of the right ICA in a patient with severe peripheral arterial occlusive disease, coronary heart disease, and multiple stenoses of the supra-aortic vessels.
Final angiograms after stent implantation and postdilatation in a pseudo-occlusion of the proximal right ICA.
a Unsubtracted view.
b Subtracted view.

even the microwire is often sufficient to occlude the stenosis. As soon as the stent has been placed and postdilatation completed (**Fig. 11.4**), the blood pressure should be lowered to ~110 mmHg systolic due to the increased risk of hyperperfusion syndrome and intracranial hemorrhage, especially in patients with a contralateral occlusion or high-grade stenosis. This is why surveillance in the intensive care unit (ICU) with close blood pressure monitoring should be maintained for several days after the procedure. In selected cases, one may even consider performing the dilatation in two stages and scheduling the final luminal reconstruction for a future date (e.g., 6 weeks later) to avoid hyperperfusion injury. To date, however, there have been no substantive studies on this technique.

Potential Complications

- *Vascular dissections:* If a dissection occurs along the inguinal access route, the approach should be switched to the opposite side before insertion of the Arrow sheath. A transbrachial approach may be considered if necessary. If a dissection occurs during catheterization of the CCA, it should be assessed for its significance and possible progression and may require treatment with an additional stent. With CCA dissections that do not require interventional treatment, it is sufficient to continue heparinization for 24h after the procedure and monitor the dissection with ultrasound or MRA. In all cases an effort should be made to complete the actual stenosis treatment and manage any endovascular complications that arise.

- *Vasospasms:* If a carotid vasospasm occurs, the sheath should be pulled back at once. Generally this maneuver will be sufficient to relieve the spasm. If the spasm persists, irrigation through the sheath can be increased. The nimodipine in the irrigating solution will usually be sufficient to relieve the spasticity. If the vasospasm still persists, a more concentrated nimodipine solution should be infused through the carotid sheath until the spasm relaxes.

- *Stroke:* Various studies have shown that the great majority of periprocedural strokes are minor. But if a significant neurologic deficit should occur and angiography shows a visible thrombus, the occlusion should be recanalized at once by mechanical and/or pharmacologic means.

- *Occlusion of the residual lumen in a pseudo-occlusion:* In rare cases this may occur when crossing is attempted with a microwire but the stenosis cannot be crossed. In this case the treatment attempt should be terminated and the occlusion subsequently evaluated by ultrasound and/or MRA. These occlusions are clinically asymptomatic in nearly all cases. The situation does not become hazardous until secondary recanalization occurs, which then becomes an indication for reintervention or operative treatment.

- *Inguinal hematoma:* If a secondary inguinal hematoma develops, the affected area should be cooled and treated with heparin-containing (or comparable) ointments, depending on the extent of the hematoma. Large hematomas and retroperitoneal spread would require surgical evacuation. A large false aneurysm should also be treated. Ultrasound-guided fibrin injection into the aneurysm is generally sufficient to coagulate the blood in the false lumen. If this is not sufficient, vascular surgery is indicated.

- *Angio-Seal migration:* In rare cases, intravascular migration of the Angio-Seal anchor may occur, causing ischemic symptoms to develop in the lower limb. This problem is managed by interventional or surgical retrieval of the anchor. If the anchor has caused local stenosis at the original insertion site, interventional or surgical treatment may also be necessary depending on the degree of stenosis.

- *Restenosis:* Hemodynamically significant restenosis (> 70% ECST) is observed in 5–10% of cases, generally occurring during the first 18 months after the intervention (**Fig. 11.5**). Because carotid stenosis is an emboligenic rather than hemodynamic process in the great majority of cases, these recurrent stenoses are almost always asymptomatic. Treatment is indicated if the stenosis recurs very soon after the intervention and is progressive or hemodynamically significant. We manage these cases by simple angioplasty with a drug-eluting balloon. The latest generation of balloons require inflation times of only 30 s (up to 3 times). Even so, this iatrogenic occlusion of the ICA requires close clinical monitoring. This can be done by having the patient perform a simple manual task during the balloon occlusion (e.g., squeezing a rubber toy). Re-stenting is almost never necessary, but corresponding pharmacologic preparation is still advised so that stenting could be done in case of an emergency (dissection) or failed angioplasty. Re-restenosis may occur, especially in patients who have developed a postirradiation stenosis. The technical procedure in these cases is the same as for an initial restenosis.

Authors' Results

In a review of the carotid stent angioplasties performed at our institution from January 2003 to June 2009, we found an overall complication rate of 4.19% in a total of 358 unprotected stent angioplasties. Among these complications were 3 deaths, 5 cases of hyperperfusion syndrome (including 1 death from secondary intracranial hemorrhage), 1 asymptomatic subarachnoid hemorrhage, and 7 ischemic strokes. Most of the complications occurred in patients who were initially symptomatic. This patient group (73% of all patients) had a complication rate of 5.3% (14 of 261 patients). Complications occurred in just 1% of patients who were initially asymptomatic (1 of 97 patients). If we disregard complications unrelated to the procedure, the overall complication rate for the mixed cohort of symptomatic and asymptomatic patients was only 3.35%.

Peri-interventional complications arose in 3 of the 358 patients (0.8%). Since in theory these are the only complications that could have been prevented by a

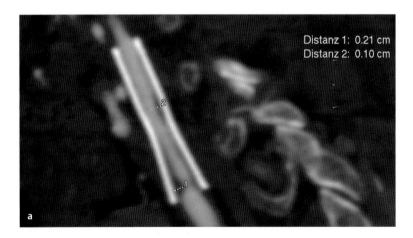
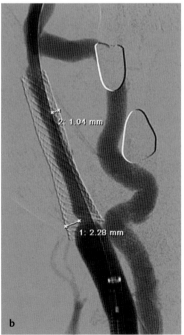

Fig. 11.5a, b   In-stent restenosis. Good metric correlation of CTA findings with the gold standard of DSA. This means that when restenosis is suspected by Doppler ultrasound, CTA can determine the degree of restenosis in many cases without having to repeat conventional angiography.
a Maximum intensity projection (MIP) from CT angiography. Scale: centimeters.
b Correlative DSA. Scale: millimeters.

protection system, our data document the high success rate of unprotected stenting.

All patients but one who suffered a hyperperfusion syndrome had an initial ICA stenosis > 90%. That one patient, who had a 50–70% stenosis, was the only one who did not develop a subsequent intracerebral hemorrhage. The only fatal intracerebral hemorrhage due to hyperperfusion syndrome occurred in the only woman in this group, who also had an occlusion of the contralateral ICA.

Caution

Very high-grade stenoses of the ICA, possibly accompanied by a contralateral ICA occlusion, are considered a predisposing factor for hyperperfusion syndrome. Rigorous medical control and invasive arterial blood pressure monitoring are strongly advised in these patients.

Long-term Doppler ultrasound follow-up in our population revealed > 50% restenosis (ECST) in 12.3% of the patients. These cases could be broken down into 5.3% of patients with 50–70% restenosis and 7% with > 70% in-stent restenosis (ECST). The higher-grade in-stent restenosis remained detectable for an average period of ~10 months (Tietke et al. 2010).

Summary

Ideally, the indication for treating atherosclerotic and nonatherosclerotic stenoses of the CCA and/or ICA should be based on detailed clinical, laboratory, and radiologic studies reviewed in an interdisciplinary conference. The recently published results of the CREST trial show an approximate equivalence between surgical and interventional therapy. Interventional treatment has a higher association with minor strokes, while endarterectomy has a higher association with myocardial infarctions.

The treatment of carotid artery stenosis is indicated in patients with:

- symptomatic stenoses > 50% (NASCET)
- asymptomatic stenoses > 60% (NASCET)

Interventional treatment is consistently preferred over surgical treatment for the following indications:

- Recurrent stenosis after thromboendarterectomy and radiogenic stenosis
- "Isolated" carotid artery (deficient circle of Willis)
- Tandem stenoses and surgically inaccessible stenoses
- Contralateral carotid occlusion
- Cardiac comorbidity

The successful performance of interventional therapy requires an experienced interventionalist and a demonstrably low complication rate in patients with symptomatic stenoses (< 6%) and asymptomatic stenoses (< 3%). The complication rates should be recorded and tracked in an external quality registry.

Randomized multicenter studies have shown that with an expert interventionalist using the proper technique and materials, the stent angioplasty of carotid stenosis is an acceptable alternative to surgery and can be offered to patients as a treatment for their vascular disease at appropriate centers. On the other hand, stent angioplasty is definitely not a treatment that can be performed without supervision at an inexperienced facility; otherwise the benefits of this treatment for patients relative to pharmacologic therapy would be lost.

References

Barnett HJM, Taylor DW, Eliasziw M, et al; North American Symptomatic Carotid Endarterectomy Trial Collaborators. Benefit of carotid endarterectomy in patients with symptomatic moderate or severe stenosis. N Engl J Med 1998;339(20):1415–1425

Bockenheimer SAM, Mathias K. Percutaneous transluminal angioplasty in arteriosclerotic internal carotid artery stenosis. AJNR Am J Neuroradiol 1983;4(3):791–792

Bonati LH, Jongen LM, Haller S, et al; ICSS-MRI study group. New ischaemic brain lesions on MRI after stenting or endarterectomy for symptomatic carotid stenosis: a substudy of the International Carotid Stenting Study (ICSS). Lancet Neurol 2010;9(4):353–362 Correction: Lancet Neurol 2010;9(4):345

Brott TG, Hobson RW II, Howard G, et al; CREST Investigators. Stenting versus endarterectomy for treatment of carotid-artery stenosis. N Engl J Med 2010;363(1):11–23

Castriota F, Cremonesi A, Manetti R, et al. Impact of cerebral protection devices on early outcome of carotid stenting. J Endovasc Ther 2002;9(6):786–792

CAVATAS Investigators. Endovascular versus surgical treatment in patients with carotid stenosis in the Carotid and Vertebral Artery Transluminal Angioplasty Study (CAVATAS): a randomised trial. Lancet 2001;357(9270):1729–1737

Cremonesi A, Manetti R, Setacci F, Setacci C, Castriota F. Protected carotid stenting: clinical advantages and complications of embolic protection devices in 442 consecutive patients. Stroke 2003;34(8):1936–1941

Diethrich EB, Gordon MH, Lopez-Galarza LA, Rodriguez-Lopez JA, Casses F. Intraluminal Palmaz stent implantation for treatment of recurrent carotid artery occlusive disease: a plan for the future. J Interv Cardiol 1995;8(3):213–218

European Carotid Surgery Trialists' Collaborative Group. Randomised trial of endarterectomy for recently symptomatic carotid stenosis: final results of the MRC European Carotid Surgery Trial (ECST). Lancet 1998;351(9113):1379–1387

Garg N, Karagiorgos N, Pisimisis GT, et al. Cerebral protection devices reduce periprocedural strokes during carotid angioplasty and stenting: a systematic review of the current literature. J Endovasc Ther 2009;16(4):412–427

IV

Geisler T, Gawaz M. Resistance to antiplatelet substances—a real clinical problem. [Article in German] Herz 2008;33(4): 260–268

Halliday A, Mansfield A, Marro J, et al; MRC Asymptomatic Carotid Surgery Trial (ACST) Collaborative Group. Prevention of disabling and fatal strokes by successful carotid endarterectomy in patients without recent neurological symptoms: randomised controlled trial. Lancet 2004;363(9420):1491–1502

Ederle J, Dobson J, Featherstone RL, et al; International Carotid Stenting Study investigators. Carotid artery stenting compared with endarterectomy in patients with symptomatic carotid stenosis (International Carotid Stenting Study): an interim analysis of a randomised controlled trial. Lancet 2010;375(9719):985–997

Inzitari D, Eliasziw M, Gates P, et al; North American Symptomatic Carotid Endarterectomy Trial Collaborators. The causes and risk of stroke in patients with asymptomatic internal-carotid-artery stenosis. N Engl J Med 2000;342(23):1693–1700

Jansen O, Fiehler J, Hartmann M, Brückmann H for the SPACE investigators. Protection or nonprotection in carotid stent angioplasty: the influence of interventional techniques on outcome data from the SPACE Trial. Stroke 2009;40(3):841–846

Kerber CW, Cromwell LD, Loehden OL. Catheter dilatation of proximal carotid stenosis during distal bifurcation endarterectomy. AJNR Am J Neuroradiol 1980;1(4):348–349

Krötz F, Sohn HY, Klauss V. Antiplatelet drugs in cardiological practice: established strategies and new developments. Vasc Health Risk Manag 2008;4(3):637–645

Mas JL, Chatellier G, Beyssen B, et al; EVA-3S Investigators. Endarterectomy versus stenting in patients with symptomatic severe carotid stenosis. N Engl J Med 2006;355(16):1660–1671

Mathias K, Jäger H, Hennigs S, Gissler HM. Endoluminal treatment of internal carotid artery stenosis. World J Surg 2001;25(3):328–334, discussion 334–336

Meier P, Knapp G, Tamhane U, Chaturvedi S, Gurm HS. Short term and intermediate term comparison of endarterectomy versus stenting for carotid artery stenosis: systematic review and meta-analysis of randomised controlled clinical trials. BMJ 2010;340:c467

Patti G, Colonna G, Pasceri V, Pepe LL, Montinaro A, Di Sciascio G. Randomized trial of high loading dose of clopidogrel for reduction of periprocedural myocardial infarction in patients undergoing coronary intervention: results from the ARMYDA-2 (Antiplatelet therapy for Reduction of MYocardial Damage during Angioplasty) study. Circulation 2005; 111(16):2099–2106

Reimers B, Corvaja N, Moshiri S, et al. Cerebral protection with filter devices during carotid artery stenting. Circulation 2001;104(1):12–15

Ringleb PA, Allenberg J, Brückmann H, et al; SPACE Collaborative Group. 30 day results from the SPACE trial of stent-protected angioplasty versus carotid endarterectomy in symptomatic patients: a randomised non-inferiority trial. Lancet 2006;368(9543):1239–1247

Schillinger M, Karnik R, Kerschner K, et al; Writing Committee of the Arbeitsgruppe für Interventionelle Kardiologie der Österreichischen Kardiologischen Gesellschaft Karotisintervention. Positionspapier. J Kardiol 2006;13:356–363

Steinhubl SR, Berger PB, Mann JT III, et al; CREDO Investigators. Clopidogrel for the Reduction of Events During Observation. Early and sustained dual oral antiplatelet therapy following percutaneous coronary intervention: a randomized controlled trial. JAMA 2002;288(19):2411–2420

Tietke MW, Kerby T, Alfke K, et al. Complication rate in unprotected carotid artery stenting with closed-cell stents. Neuroradiology 2010;52(7):611–618

Tievsky AL, Druy EM, Mardiat JG. Transluminal angioplasty in postsurgical stenosis of the extracranial carotid artery. AJNR Am J Neuroradiol 1983;4(3):800–802

Tsai FY, Matovich V, Hieshima G, et al. Percutaneous transluminal angioplasty of the carotid artery. AJNR Am J Neuroradiol 1986;7(2):349–358

Wholey MH, Jarmolowski CR, Wholey M, Eles GR. Carotid artery stent placement—ready for prime time? J Vasc Interv Radiol 2003;14(1):1–10

Wiggli U, Gratzl O. Transluminal angioplasty of stenotic carotid arteries: case reports and protocol. AJNR Am J Neuroradiol 1983;4(3):793–795

Wiviott SD, Braunwald E, McCabe CH, et al. Prasugrel versus clopidogrel in patients with acute coronary syndromes. N Engl J Med 2007;357(20):2001–2015

Wiviott SD, Desai N, Murphy SA, et al. The TIMI Study Group. Efficacy and safety of intensive antiplatelet therapy with prasugrel from TRITON-TIMI 38 in a core clinical cohort defined by worldwide regulatory agencies. Am J Cardiol 2011;108(7):905–911

12 Intracranial Stenoses

W. Kurre

Introduction

Worldwide, intracranial atherosclerotic stenoses are the most frequent cause of strokes in general. This epidemiologic significance is due primarily to the high prevalence of intracranial stenoses in Asia. In Europe and North America, by contrast, only 6–10% of all stroke patients are found to have a narrowing of intracranial vessels (Sacco et al. 1995; Weimar et al. 2006). Nevertheless, the high overall incidence of stroke, at 182 per 100 000 population, results in a significant number of affected individuals in Europe and North America too, and it is important to find an optimum treatment for these patients.

Drug therapy with aspirin alone has an overall risk of stroke recurrence of ~12% per year for all patients and up to 20% for individuals with high-grade stenoses. The recently published results of the SAMMPRIS trial proved that intensified conservative treatment effectively reduced recurrences to 12% in the latter "high-risk" subgroup also (Chimowitz et al. 2011).

For patients experiencing new ischemic events despite an optimized drug regimen, alternative treatment options are warranted. The EC/IC Bypass Study found that surgical revascularization with an extra- or intracranial bypass did not improve the prognosis (EC/IC Bypass Study Group 1985). Approximately 10 years after publication of the negative results of that study, initial case reports were published on intracranial angioplasty. Since then, the endovascular treatment of intracranial stenoses has been increasingly practiced and is now offered as a treatment option at almost all interventional neuroradiologic centers. High technical success rates are being achieved through the further development of the available materials.

This chapter reviews the circumstances in which the modern endovascular treatment of intracranial stenosis can be of clinical benefit in selected patients using appropriate techniques.

Patient Selection

The interventional endovascular treatment of a symptomatic intracranial stenosis is a secondary prophylactic procedure done to minimize the risk of repeated stroke events. It must be demonstrated that the overall cumulative risk, consisting of strokes occurring as procedural complications plus recurrent strokes after technically successful stent therapy, is significantly less than the spontaneous risk with medical treatment alone.

The WASID (Warfarin-Aspirin Symptomatic Intracranial Disease) trial tested and compared the efficacy of aspirin and warfarin in the secondary prophylaxis of symptomatic stenoses. Besides the fact that anticoagulants provided no benefit over antiplatelet drugs, it was found that the 1-year cumulative risk of recurrent stroke was 12% despite medical therapy (Chimowitz et al. 2005). A subgroup analysis of the same trial showed that patients with a high-grade intracranial stenosis had an almost 20% risk of a subsequent cerebral ischemia (Kasner et al. 2006).

Analyses of published single- and multicenter case series on intracranial stenting indicated a procedural morbidity and mortality ranging from 7.7 to 9.5% (Cruz-Flores and Diamond 2006; Gröschel et al. 2009). The estimated risk of recurrent stroke after successful treatment is as high as 5.1% (Levy et al. 2007).

The first device developed and approved for interventional treatment of intracranial atherosclerotic disease was the Wingspan stent system (Boston Scientific, San Leandro, CA, USA). From approval studies and subsequent registries a 1-year stroke risk of 15% was assumed for patients treated with Wingspan. Based on the results of the WASID trial and registry data, a randomized trial (SAMMPRIS) was initiated to test "best medical treatment" vs. Wingspan stent angioplasty in patients with high-grade (> 70%) symptomatic stenoses assuming an absolute risk reduction of 5% in the endovascular treatment arm. For this trial noninvasive management was intensified with a dual antiplatelet regimen during the first 3 months, rigorous control of all vascular risk factors, and lifestyle modification. Unexpected high procedure-related complication rates in the endovascular arm and astonishingly few recurrent strokes under medical treatment alone led to early termination of the trial. The 30-day morbidity and mortality was as high as 14.7% with endovascular treatment and 5.8% with medical treatment. Details of the procedure-related adverse events have not yet been published and the follow-up of enrolled patients is not complete, so a final judgment is not possible at the moment. However, until more details are released, a risk-benefit analysis would prohibit the uncritical use of intracranial angioplasty. Interventions should be reserved for selected patients who do not respond adequately to medical treatment.

An analysis of the data from the GESICA (Grupo de Estudio de la Sobrevida en la Insuficiencia Cardiac en

Treatment of Supra-aortic Extra- and Intracranial Stenoses

IV

Argentina) trial identified clinically significant hemodynamic stenosis as a risk factor for stroke recurrence (Mazighi et al. 2006). Hemodynamic compromise can be an argument for early treatment because this factor is not influenced sufficiently, or not rapidly enough, by antithrombotic treatment. In addition, these patients were probably not randomized to a large extent in the SAMMPRIS trial due to a high probability of new ischemic events during the randomization process.

Note

- The interventional treatment of symptomatic intracranial stenoses may be considered in cases of failed secondary medical prophylaxis.
- First-line interventional treatment of high-grade symptomatic intracranial stenoses may be offered to patients with hemodynamically relevant luminal narrowing under the humanitarian device exemption.
- The interventional treatment of asymptomatic intracranial stenoses cannot be recommended on the basis of current risk-benefit considerations.
- The interventional treatment of intracranial stenoses should only be done in specialized centers with high expertise in endovascular management of atherosclerotic disease, to keep complication rates as low as possible.

Informed Consent

As in any surgical or interventional procedure, the patient must provide informed consent. This process should allow adequate time for reflection and should include the disclosure of general and specific procedural risks, alternative therapies, and special patient instructions regarding drug administration and follow-up.

The most important aspect of informed consent, and the most relevant for the patient, is the disclosure of acute complication rates. Based on a systematic analysis of published case series and the results of the SAMMPRIS trial, the procedure-related stroke or death rate lies between 7.7 and 14.7%. Apart from these average numbers, all operators are obliged to assess their institutional morbidity and mortality rates, especially in the light of the SAMMPRIS results. These highly significant events overshadow any potential angiographic complications relating to vascular access or contrast administration, but the latter risks are still important and should also be disclosed.

Only a few stents and balloon catheters have been approved for the treatment of intracranial stenoses. In theory, there are many more materials with properties that would make them suitable for use in the intracranial circulation. The individual vascular anatomy of the patient as well as complications may necessitate the use of unapproved materials, and patients as well as local boards

should be informed about the use of off-label products according to national regulations.

As for patient instructions after the procedure, the need for compliance with medication should be emphasized. This is necessary to prevent acute thrombotic occlusion after stent placement with possible ischemic complications. In addition to medication compliance, regular follow-up examinations are recommended because up to 30% of patients develop restenosis.

Practical Tip

Points to remember during the informed consent procedure:
- Humanitarian device exemption in patients with failure of medical treatment or hemodynamically relevant stenoses
- Procedure-related stroke and death rate is 7.7–14.7%; institutional complication rates should also be assessed and communicated
- Off-label use of angioplasty materials may be necessary
- Restenosis rates are up to 30%
- Compliance with antiplatelet therapy must be emphasized

Planning, Preparations, and Techniques

Scheduling the Procedure

Once a patient has been selected for the interventional treatment of an intracranial stenosis, the optimum timing of the procedure needs to be considered. In the WASID trial, the subsequent stroke risk was significantly greater for patients enrolled less than 17 days after the acute transient ischemic attack (TIA) or stroke than for patients enrolled later (Kasner et al. 2006). Thus, the risk of recurrent stroke appears to be particularly high a short time after clinical presentation. This is an argument for early intervention in symptomatic patients, analogous to the management of extracranial stenoses. On the other hand, case series have shown a higher complication rate in patients treated during the acute phase up to 10 days after the initial event; this suggests that timing the intervention too early may affect the outcome just as adversely as a delay in treatment (Nahab et al. 2009). Possible explanations for higher complication rates in the acute phase are persistent thrombi, the instability of atherosclerotic plaques, and the risk of hemorrhage in large subacute infarctions. A pragmatic solution would be to schedule treatment at the start of the second week after the acute event. For high-grade hemodynamically significant stenosis presenting with progressive stroke, an expectant approach would of course be inadvisable and immediate action would be indicated.

Antiplatelet and Anticoagulant Therapy

Dual antiplatelet therapy with aspirin (100 mg/day) and clopidogrel (75 mg/day) has proven essential in preparing patients for the stenting of supra-aortic arterial vessels. Inadequate platelet inhibition increases the risk of stent thrombosis and thromboembolic events. For planned procedures, clopidogrel should be started 1 week before the intervention at 75 mg/day, as pharmacokinetically it requires several days for optimum effect. Alternatively, a higher loading dose may be administered the day before the procedure. A 600-mg oral dose of clopidogrel will produce adequate platelet inhibition after 4 h in most patients (Hochholzer et al. 2005). Aspirin, on the other hand, acts immediately after gastrointestinal absorption, so dosing may be started on the day before the intervention. Even if simple balloon angioplasty without a stent is planned, premedication with aspirin and clopidogrel is still recommended so that stent placement can be done safely in the event of an acute change of treatment plan or in an emergency (rescue stenting).

Caution

With the increasing use of intracranial stents, there has been growing interest in the problem of clopidogrel resistance. The efficacy of clopidogrel is subject to large interindividual variations, and up to half of patients have been classified as "low responders" in different studies (Prabhakaran et al. 2008).

The main reason for this is that clopidogrel is converted to its active form in the liver, and several enzymes of the cytochrome P450 group are involved in this process. The low activity of clopidogrel in certain patients may be genetically determined or may result from interactions with other substances that compete for cytochrome P450 enzymes.

Laboratory tests are available for testing the efficacy of platelet inhibition and are increasingly used in interventional neuroradiology when stenting is scheduled. Unfortunately there is still a lack of definitive studies that can clinically validate the various tests and define accurate cutoff values. Laboratory tests do not offer absolute protection, however, and there are known cases of clinical non-responders who have developed stent thrombosis despite laboratory evidence of effective platelet inhibition. If clopidogrel resistance is found, doubling the dose will improve platelet inhibition in some cases. The platelet inhibitor prasugrel may be considered as an alternative. This drug has been studied in large numbers of cardiology patients and appears to be highly effective in preventing stent thrombosis. It should be added, however, that prasugrel therapy in patients with cerebral ischemic events was associated with an increased rate of incidents of major bleeding (Wiviott et al. 2007). It is still unclear whether the use of prasugrel will provide a net benefit in patients with symptomatic intracranial stenoses causing cerebral ischemia.

Platelet inhibition is supplemented by intraprocedural intravenous heparin to prevent catheter thrombosis. The intravenous administration of 80–100 IU of heparin/kg body weight is generally sufficient. Anticoagulation should be checked by measuring the activated clotting time during angiography. The goal is to double the baseline value. It is unnecessary to continue heparinization after the procedure.

Anesthesia

Intracranial angioplasty requires careful catheterization of the peripheral cerebral vessels and accurate placement of the angioplasty material. General endotracheal anesthesia has proven effective for preventing patient movements during the procedure. There have also been case descriptions of intracranial stenting under regional anesthesia, but the great majority of interventions are performed under general anesthesia for the reasons noted above. Another advantage of treatment under general anesthesia is that it allows for swifter and more targeted action in the event of a complication.

IV

Practical Tip

Special attention should be given to controlling arterial pressure during the procedure. A hemodynamically significant stenosis that has not yet been treated requires mild hypertension to ensure adequate cerebral blood flow. Immediately after vasodilatation, however, the arterial blood pressure should be returned to normotensive values to prevent a hyperperfusion syndrome.

Arterial Access and Guide Catheter

Arterial access to the target lesion is generally challenging as a result of vascular elongation, atherosclerotic wall lesions, and the occasional presence of more proximal stenoses in patients selected for intracranial angioplasty. The success of the procedure, in which the angioplasty material must be delivered far into the peripheral portion of the cerebral vasculature, depends critically on stable arterial access. Most materials used for stent angioplasty require at least a 6F guide catheter. This "minimal" delivery system is recommended only for stenoses in relatively straight vascular segments in the intra- and extracranial circulation, as it provides only moderate proximal support. For treating intracranial stenoses in the anterior circulation, it is better to use a more stable 7F delivery catheter. In more difficult cases, an extra-long sheath or a combination of an extra-long sheath and guide catheter can be used as a coaxial system. Guide catheters with a flexible tip, known as distal access catheters, have also become available in recent years. They have an inner lumen that is large enough to accommodate angioplasty materials. The soft endpiece can be advanced far distally and even maneuvered through tortuous vessels without obstructing flow. When combined with a more proximally placed rigid sheath, this type of catheter system is a useful aid to successful completion of the procedure (**Fig. 12.1**).

The vertebral arteries have small lumina that will tolerate only a small-caliber guide catheter. Proximal support can be provided by a long sheath that is left in the subclavian artery. With very difficult access conditions in the posterior circulation, an ipsilateral transbrachial approach may also yield the desired result.

The tip of the guide catheter should be positioned as far distally as possible to permit an adequate forward push. A guide catheter in the vertebral arteries should ideally be positioned below the atlas loop, and in the anterior circulation in the distal internal carotid artery (ICA) at the start of the petrous segment. Guide catheters with a flexible tip can also be placed more distally, depending on local anatomy. Optimum distal positioning depends on local vascular anatomy, however, and cannot always be achieved. In these cases the catheter should remain at a more proximal site to protect the vessel, prevent vasospasms, and maintain antegrade blood flow.

Following acceptable placement of the delivery system, survey runs should be taken in two standard projections. They should also be acquired if diagnostic angiography was performed before the procedure to allow pre- and postinterventional comparison. Otherwise it may be difficult to distinguish pre-existing vascular occlusions from procedure-related emboli. Three-dimensional (3D) rotational angiography may be helpful in locating the working projection and selecting the right materials. It is particularly useful for determining vascular diameter and lesion length. While absolutely precise measurements cannot be taken from 3D reconstructions, high-quality rotational angiography with careful windowing can be an effective aid to orientation.

> ### Practical Tip
>
> The working projection should be selected to provide an optimum clear projection of the stenosis. High magnification facilitates precise, atraumatic lesion crossing. The tip of the guidewire should be visible in at least one plane so that any uncontrolled movement can be promptly recognized and stopped.

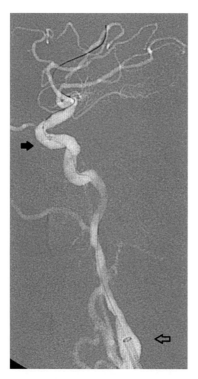

Fig. 12.1 Optimum stable distal access. The tip of a long sheath is within the carotid bulb (*open arrow*). A flexible-tip guide catheter has been passed through the sheath and advanced into the cavernous segment of the ICA (*black arrow*). This significantly shortens the intracranial vascular segments that need to be crossed to treat a stenosis of the middle cerebral artery (with kind permission of Dr. B. Turowski, Düsseldorf, Germany).

Tips on Material Selection

The goal of intracranial angioplasty is to achieve permanent enlargement of the narrowed vessel lumen at the lowest possible risk. The question of whether this goal is best served by balloon angioplasty alone or by the placement of a self-expanding or balloon-expandable stent cannot presently be answered on a sound scientific basis. The selection of materials is based in large part on the personal experience and habits of the operator. However, some objective statements relating purely to the technical conduct of the procedure can be made:

- A *balloon* for percutaneous transluminal angioplasty is much more flexible than a stent delivery system and can reach stenoses located at peripheral sites. Even more proximal stenoses that are located past elongated vascular segments can be crossed more easily with a balloon catheter. One disadvantage of angioplasty without a stent is that it cannot stabilize any dissections that may occur. Balloon-mounted stents are relatively easy to handle and allow for swift and sure completion of the procedure. But since both the balloon and stent are mounted on the delivery catheter, the system is considerably more rigid and more difficult to maneuver through curved vessels. Thus, a balloon-mounted stent is best suited for short, easily accessible stenoses located at a relatively proximal (often extradural) site.

- The use of *self-expanding stents* generally requires pre-dilatation, making it necessary to perform an exchange maneuver and lengthening the procedure time. One advantage of self-expanding stents is that, depending on the system used, it may be easier to negotiate vascular curves than it is with a balloon-mounted stent. Thus, a self-expanding stent is best suited for longer stenoses located at a distal (intradural) site that is more difficult to access. Another advantage of self-expanding stents is their ability to conform to different vascular calibers. A self-expanding stent should be used if the area bridged by the device is characterized by marked caliber variations proximal and distal to the lesion. Self-expanding stents also conform better to curved vascular segments.

The selection of approved materials for the intracranial angioplasty of atherosclerotic stenoses is small. Materials approved for the European market (CE-certified) are listed in **Table 12.1**. Given the limited selection, operators have very little latitude if they limit themselves entirely to the materials specifically approved for this indication.

Note

If stents originally designed for treating aneurysms or cardiologic stents and balloon catheters are used, the patient should be advised of this off-label use during informed consent.

Balloon Angioplasty

Only a few balloons are approved for intracranial angioplasty, so materials designed for the treatment of coronary arteries are most commonly used. Most interventionists

Table 12.1 Intracranial angioplasty materials certified for the European market (CE) for that indication

Material	Name	Manufacturer
Balloon for percutaneous transluminal angioplasty	Gateway	Boston Scientific Corporation
Balloon-expandable stents	Pharos Vitesse	Micrus Endovascular
Self-expanding stents	Wingspan	Boston Scientific Corporation
	Leo plus	Balt Extrusion

prefer monorail systems owing to their ease of use. Commercially available balloons should be used, with 0.014-in (0.36-mm) guidewires with a hydrophilic coating. Direct insertion of the wire–balloon assembly is often possible. If passage through the intracranial vessels and stenosis proves difficult, the lesion can be crossed initially with a microcatheter.

After careful crossing of the target lesion, the balloon catheter is introduced over a long exchange wire after removal of the microcatheter. Very high-grade stenoses require incremental dilatation, starting with an undersized balloon followed by percutaneous transluminal angioplasty with a larger-diameter balloon.

Caution

When sizing the balloon, do not exceed the anticipated normal size of the vessel. It is better to undersize by ~10%.

The balloon for percutaneous transluminal angioplasty should be inflated slowly and gently so that it will expand uniformly and the vessel wall can adapt.

Balloon angioplasty is often followed by the appearance of a visible intimal flap, which may occasionally be occlusive. For this reason the guidewire should remain in place across the lesion for several minutes after the angioplasty and should be removed only after a final angiogram has confirmed unrestricted flow. If an extra-long exchange wire is used from the start, it provides a higher degree of safety because if complications arise, microcatheters for stent placement can be delivered across the stenosis without losing access to the vascular segment. An example of a balloon angioplasty is shown in **Fig. 12.2**.

Stent Angioplasty

Balloon-Expandable Stents

The use of balloon-mounted stents allows for direct stent placement in favorable cases, resulting in a shorter procedure time. This presumes, however, that the stent–balloon assembly can be passed through the proximal vessels and across the stenosis without difficulty. Because the stiffness of the system increases markedly with increasing stent length, the balloon-expandable stent should be as short as possible. The minimum necessary length can be accurately measured with rotational 3D angiography. If tortuosity proximal to the stenosis makes delivery difficult, it may be possible to introduce a second, parallel 0.014-in (0.36-mm) guidewire to serve as a guide. Another possibility is to try inserting a microcatheter–guidewire combination first and then exchange it for the stent.

The feasibility of primary stent placement across a high-grade stenosis depends greatly on the outer diameter of the

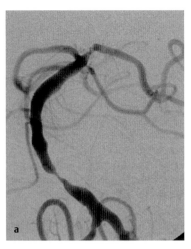 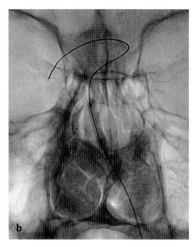 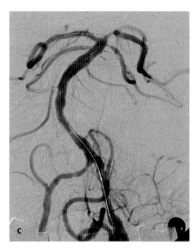

Fig. 12.2a–c   Balloon angioplasty of a high-grade basilar artery stenosis.

a Angiogram demonstrates a high-grade basilar artery stenosis.
b Percutaneous transluminal angioplasty. The lesion is crossed and dilated with a 3-mm balloon.

c Final angiogram after balloon withdrawal with guidewire still in place shows normal basilar artery perfusion with no visible intimal dissection.

system. A low profile of the constrained stent will increase the chances for successful primary placement. If direct placement is not possible, the stent should never be forced into position as this could damage the vessel wall. Stent placement should be preceded in these cases by percutaneous transluminal angioplasty with an undersized balloon.

As in a simple angioplasty, the balloon should be inflated slowly during stent deployment. After the balloon is deflated, expansion of the stent can be assessed fluoroscopically. If stent expansion is incomplete, a second dilatation can be done immediately. Otherwise the balloon is pulled back several centimeters and the wire is left in place while a postdeployment angiogram is obtained. The stent may require repeated "modeling" to the vessel wall in some cases. After the angioplasty is completed, the guidewire may be removed once patency of the treated vessel and distal branches has been confirmed. **Figure 12.3** shows an example of a tandem stenosis treated with balloon-expandable stents.

Self-Expanding Stents

Self-expanding stent systems usually require predilatation with an undersized balloon. The technique is basically the same as for balloon angioplasty without a stent, and the same recommendations apply. A long exchange wire should be used initially so that when percutaneous transluminal angioplasty is completed, the balloon can be exchanged for the stent delivery catheter. With the microcatheter placed distal to the stenosis, the stent is advanced to a position just proximal to the catheter tip. The microcatheter is then withdrawn to the deployment position, and the distal end of the stent is released by advancing the stent pusher or microwire. Further stent

release is accomplished by pulling on the catheter, pushing the microwire or pusher, or a combination of both maneuvers depending on system type and local anatomy. Some systems even allow repositioning of an imperfectly placed stent, as long as the stent has not been completely unconstrained.

Following complete stent deployment, a final angiographic run is performed to assess the stent position and the patency of distal vessels. **Figure 12.4** illustrates an intracranial stenosis treated with a self-expanding stent.

Management of Complications

Cervical artery dissections are not uncommon, especially under difficult access conditions. Intimal flaps that do not cause significant flow obstruction in the dependent vascular territory may be left untreated. The dual antiplatelet therapy given after stent implantation is generally sufficient to minimize the risk of thromboembolic events. On the other hand, a hemodynamically significant dissection-induced stenosis of the cervical arteries should be treated by stenting. Traditional carotid stents can be used in the cervical portion of the ICA. Stenoses in the vertebral arteries or distal ICA can be treated with self-expanding stents suitable for intracranial use. Self-expanding stents should exert a radial force sufficient to reappose the intimal flap and restore antegrade flow. If a complete vascular occlusion occurs and there is adequate collateral flow from the other cerebrovascular territories, it is safe in some cases to leave the occlusion untreated.

Bleeding from an injured intracranial vessel is a life-threatening complication that is also more difficult to manage. It may result from perforation by a guidewire or local vascular injury at the angioplasty site.

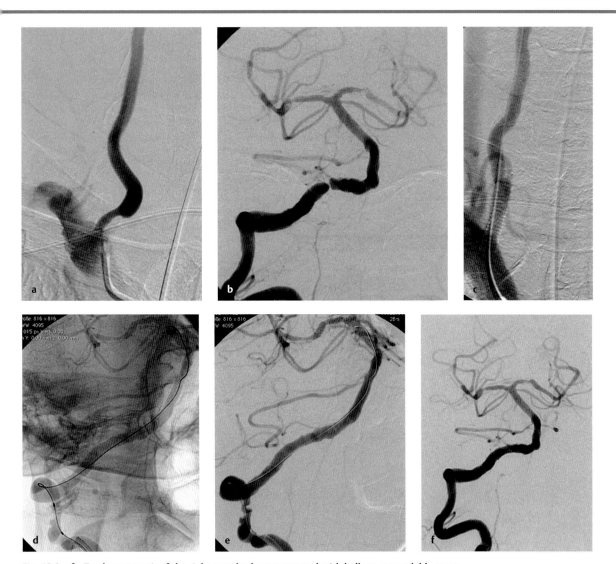

Fig. 12.3a–f **Tandem stenosis of the right vertebral artery treated with balloon-expandable stents.**

a Diagnostic angiogram shows moderate proximal stenosis of the right vertebral artery.

b High-grade luminal narrowing is noted in the V4 segment.

c To gain access to the intracranial stenosis, the V0 stenosis is treated first with a balloon-expandable stent.

d,e Next the V4 stenosis is dilated with a 4-mm × 8-mm balloon-expandable stent.

f Final run documents good restoration of the vessel lumen.

Practical Tip

Recommended immediate measures for intracranial bleeding: (1) locoregional inflation of an angioplasty balloon to interrupt the blood flow and (2) antagonism of periprocedural heparin. Several minutes of balloon inflation will provide effective hemostasis in favorable cases.

If the bleeding is not controlled by repeated balloon inflations, covered stent implantation may be considered as a last resort, at least for proximal vascular ruptures, if the affected segment is not too tortuous. Perforations of small peripheral vessels by wire manipulation are generally treatable by balloon inflation.

Thrombus formation on the stent during the procedure, or even complete stent thrombosis, can be managed by the regional administration of thrombolytic agents, accepting a certain risk of intracerebral hemorrhage in patients with large, pre-existing subacute infarcts. When mechanical recanalization systems are used, it is best to employ techniques that pose little risk of dislocating the newly implanted stent. One option would be to use an aspiration system. Also, percutaneous transluminal

IV

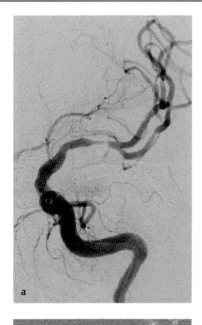

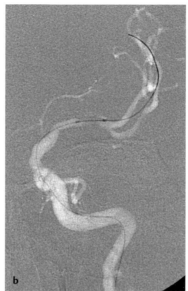

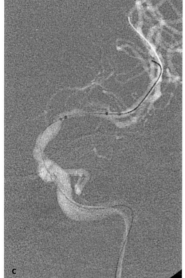

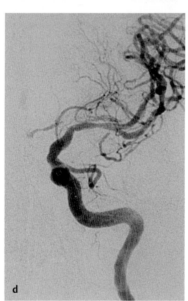

Fig. 12.4a–d M1 stenosis treated with a self-expanding stent (with kind permission of Dr. B. Turowski, Düsseldorf, Germany).

a Symptomatic high-grade stenosis in the M1 segment of the MCA.

b The stenosis is predilated with a 2-mm balloon for percutaneous transluminal angioplasty.

c The microcatheter is pulled back to initiate stent release. The distal stent markers are visible in the upper M2 branch.

d Final angiogram after complete stent deployment. There is no residual stenosis.

angioplasty of the thrombus may help to restore flow distal to the stent.

Postinterventional Management

Patients should be kept under continuous surveillance in an intensive care unit (ICU), stroke unit, or intermediate care unit for at least 24 h after the procedure. Blood pressure and other vital signs are closely monitored and neurologic status is regularly assessed. If an acute deterioration of clinical neurologic status is noted, imaging should be performed without delay. Noncontrast CT is adequate for exclusion of

hemorrhage. If the underlying cause is ischemic rather than hemorrhagic, MRI can give more discriminating information on the etiology of the blood flow reduction than CT. MRI is the preferred modality in settings where it is available and the patient can tolerate the examination.

The quality of information supplied by noninvasive vascular imaging depends on the angioplasty materials that were used. If simple balloon dilatation was performed, CTA (CT angiography) or MRI can accurately assess the patency of the treated vascular segment. If a stent has been placed, the quality of the study may vary greatly depending on the stent design and the alloy composition of the implanted material. Ultrasound techniques may be helpful but will not yield reliable information in all cases. If the patency of a stent is still in doubt following a noninvasive diagnostic

Causes of Postinterventional Bleeding

- *Reperfusion hemorrhage:* This is a potential complication after successful revascularization, especially in patients with poorly collateralized high-grade stenoses. The pathophysiology of this phenomenon is not yet fully understood but is probably based on impaired auto-regulation due to chronic ischemia. Blood flow can no longer adapt to sudden expansion of the vessel, leading to seizures, edema, or the most severe manifestation of reperfusion, cerebral hemorrhage. Reperfusion hemorrhage occurs in ~1% of all cases (Kurre et al. 2010). It is difficult to define a subgroup at high risk for this side effect. Studies on extracranial carotid angioplasty identified high-grade stenosis, hypertension, and advanced age as risk factors for reperfusion hemorrhage (Abou-Chebl et al. 2004; Kaku et al. 2004). Although these risk factors were not consistently reproducible in other studies and a direct application of findings to intracranial stenoses is not a scientifically valid approach, blood pressure should still be monitored after the procedure so that a hemorrhage-promoting rise in blood pressure can be promptly treated. Ideally this goal is achieved by continuous monitoring and facilities for the intravenous administration of antihypertensive drugs. Reperfusion hemorrhage is most common during the first 1–3 days but in rare cases may occur at a later time.
- *Guidewire injury:* Bleeding may also result from a guidewire-induced vascular injury that was unnoticed during the procedure. Guidewire perforations may lead to a subarachnoid or parenchymal hemorrhage, depending on their location. When bleeding is localized to the area formerly occupied by the guidewire tip, it may reasonably be attributed to a guidewire injury. However, this lesion may be difficult or impossible to distinguish from a reperfusion hemorrhage in any given case.
- *Bleeding in a pre-existing infarction:* This cause of postprocedural hemorrhage should be considered when bleeding is confined to the ischemically damaged tissue area.

The main treatment options for an intracerebral hemorrhage are conservative therapy and surgical evacuation. The decision depends on the extent of the mass. In the case of a subarachnoid hemorrhage, the placement of an external ventricular drain depends on the volume of the blood collection and the progression of ventricular size. Treatment also includes standard conservative measures that are traditionally used in the management of subarachnoid hemorrhage.

Causes of Postinterventional Ischemia

Cerebral ischemia may also have a variety of causes. A new clinical deficit with disseminated infarctions in various territories noted immediately after the procedure is attributable to embolism from the aortic arch. This phenomenon is particularly common in patients with generalized atherosclerosis, though it is not always clinically apparent. Embolic occlusions of large arteries supplying the brain can be treated by mechanical recanalization.

Occlusions of perforating arteries may be manifested immediately or several hours after the procedure. Gradual clinical deterioration may occur. No specific treatment option is available for procedure-related occlusions of perforating arteries.

The differential diagnosis should include acute stent thrombosis and cervical artery dissection. Both are managed by interventional recanalization.

Practical Tip

After the intervention:
- Continuous monitoring of vital signs and neurologic status for the first 24 h
- Blood pressure monitoring (invasive monitoring may be used in high-risk patients) with pressures adjusted to normotensive or slightly hypotensive range

Neurologic deterioration may have the following vascular causes:
- Reperfusion syndrome or reperfusion hemorrhage
- Stent thrombosis
- Thromboembolism
- Occlusion of perforating arteries
- Dissection of cervical arteries

After vital signs have stabilized:
- Immediate CT with CTA or MRI with MR angiography (MRA) if neurologic deterioration occurs
- Adjunctive Doppler or duplex ultrasound scans if needed
- With suspected stent thrombosis or embolic occlusion of major arteries: angiography with equipment ready for an interventional procedure

procedure, angiography should be performed with standby equipment ready for an interventional procedure. The patency of the cervical arteries should also be assessed, since a procedure-related dissection may have gone unnoticed but may secondarily induce new ischemic symptoms.

Follow-Up Care

Antiplatelet Therapy

Note

Besides controlling cardiovascular risk factors in atherosclerosis patients, special emphasis should be placed on compliance with antiplatelet therapy following intracranial stenting.

IV

One reason for ineffectual drug therapy may be a lack of patient compliance. Another reason may be the restrictive prescribing policy of the next attending physician. Scheduled surgical or dental procedures may also prompt the discontinuation of antiplatelet drugs. The importance of continuing dual antiplatelet therapy at home should be emphasized in the closing interview with the patient and should be stated explicitly on the discharge instruction sheet. The question of how long to continue dual antiplatelet therapy has not yet been specifically resolved for intracranial stenosis. Drawing on data in the cardiology literature, combined therapy with aspirin and clopidogrel should be continued for 3–6 months, after which monotherapy is maintained for life.

Recurrent Stenosis

A problem that has not yet been adequately resolved in intracranial angioplasty is the high incidence of recurrent stenosis. Depending on the publication, significant luminal narrowing recurs in up to 30% of all cases, and approximately one-third of all patients with restenosis will develop new ischemic symptoms (Levy et al. 2007). The risk appears to be particularly high in younger patients with stenoses in the anterior circulation (Turk et al. 2008). In cardiology, the use of drug-eluting stents that inhibit intimal proliferation has brought dramatic progress in lowering restenosis rates. Some investigators have resorted to the off-label use of cardiologic drug-eluting stents, or balloons in combination with stents, in the cerebral vasculature. Results of this appear promising and will hopefully lead to the development and approval of devices intended for the intracranial vasculature (Abou-Chebl et al. 2005; Gupta et al. 2006; Steinfort et al. 2007; Vajda et al. 2012).

Practical Tip

Given the problem of restenosis, it makes sense to offer treated patients a structured follow-up program. The ultrasound evaluation of intracranial vessels after stent placement is possible in selected cases but is not always feasible. Diagnostic catheter angiography (DCA) permits a more accurate evaluation of the stented segment but carries the usual angiographic risks. If doubt exists, however, preference should be given to catheter angiography as the more reliable study.

When restenosis has been diagnosed, it must be decided whether reintervention is justified. Symptomatic restenosis should definitely be treated. Asymptomatic restenosis is a more difficult issue because there are no known predictors for estimating the future risk of ischemic events in the absence of further treatment. Moreover,

there have been some reports on the regression of purported restenosis in response to dual antiplatelet therapy. Consequently, moderate asymptomatic restenoses should be managed by conservative treatment and follow-up. In the case of a high-grade asymptomatic restenosis, the decision for further treatment can be made only on an individual basis. Factors that influence the decision are patient age, intracranial collateral supply, and the estimated individual risk of intervention based on the location and accessibility of the stenosis.

If reintervention is indicated, in-stent restenosis can be treated by percutaneous transluminal angioplasty, which has an average procedural risk of ~3%. The risk that a treated restenosis will recur is ~50% (Fiorella et al. 2009). If percutaneous transluminal angioplasty was performed initially, the reintervention may consist of stent placement. The use of drug-eluting balloons may improve the long-term results of the reintervention in theory, but this is mere speculation based on anecdotal reports rather than documented data.

Summary

In summary, balloon angioplasty and stenting for the treatment of intracranial stenosis can be offered to selected patients with recurrent symptoms under medical treatment and in case of hemodynamic compromise.

Given the inherent treatment risk, intracranial stent procedures should only be offered in specialized units with a high level of operator experience.

References

Abou-Chebl A, Yadav JS, Reginelli JP, Bajzer C, Bhatt D, Krieger DW. Intracranial hemorrhage and hyperperfusion syndrome following carotid artery stenting: risk factors, prevention, and treatment. J Am Coll Cardiol 2004;43(9):1596–1601

Abou-Chebl A, Bashir Q, Yadav JS. Drug-eluting stents for the treatment of intracranial atherosclerosis: initial experience and midterm angiographic follow-up. Stroke 2005;36(12): e165–e168

Chimowitz MI, Lynn MJ, Derdeyn CP, et al; SAMMPRIS Trial Investigators. Stenting versus aggressive medical therapy for intracranial arterial stenosis. N Engl J Med 2011;365(11):993–1003

Chimowitz MI, Lynn MJ, Howlett-Smith H, et al; Warfarin-Aspirin Symptomatic Intracranial Disease Trial Investigators. Comparison of warfarin and aspirin for symptomatic intracranial arterial stenosis. N Engl J Med 2005;352(13):1305–1316

Cruz-Flores S, Diamond AL. Angioplasty for intracranial stenosis. Cochrane Database Syst Rev 2006;19(3):CD004133

EC/IC Bypass Study Group. Failure of extracranial-intracranial arterial bypass to reduce the risk of ischemic stroke.

Results of an international randomized trial. N Engl J Med 1985;313(19):1191–1200

Fiorella DJ, Levy EI, Turk AS, et al. Target lesion revascularization after wingspan: assessment of safety and durability. Stroke 2009;40(1):106–110

Gröschel K, Schnaudigel S, Pilgram SM, Wasser K, Kastrup A. A systematic review on outcome after stenting for intracranial atherosclerosis. Stroke 2009;40(5):e340–e347

Gupta R, Al-Ali F, Thomas AJ, et al. Safety, feasibility, and short-term follow-up of drug-eluting stent placement in the intracranial and extracranial circulation. Stroke 2006;37(10): 2562–2566

Hochholzer W, Trenk D, Frundi D, et al. Time dependence of platelet inhibition after a 600-mg loading dose of clopidogrel in a large, unselected cohort of candidates for percutaneous coronary intervention. Circulation 2005;111(20): 2560–2564

Kaku Y, Yoshimura SI, Kokuzawa J. Factors predictive of cerebral hyperperfusion after carotid angioplasty and stent placement. AJNR Am J Neuroradiol 2004;25(8):1403–1408

Kasner SE, Chimowitz MI, Lynn MJ, et al; Warfarin Aspirin Symptomatic Intracranial Disease Trial Investigators. Predictors of ischemic stroke in the territory of a symptomatic intracranial arterial stenosis. Circulation 2006;113(4):555–563

Kurre W, Berkefeld J, Brassel F, et al; INTRASTENT Study Group. In-hospital complication rates after stent treatment of 388 symptomatic intracranial stenoses: results from the INTRASTENT multicentric registry. Stroke 2010;41(3):494–498

Levy EI, Turk AS, Albuquerque FC, et al. Wingspan in-stent restenosis and thrombosis: incidence, clinical presentation, and management. Neurosurgery 2007;61(3):644–650, discussion 650–651

Mazighi M, Tanasescu R, Ducrocq X, et al. Prospective study of symptomatic atherothrombotic intracranial stenoses: the GESICA study. Neurology 2006;66(8):1187–1191

Nahab F, Lynn MJ, Kasner SE, et al; NIH Multicenter Wingspan Intracranial Stent Registry Study Group. Risk factors associated with major cerebrovascular complications after intracranial stenting. Neurology 2009;72(23):2014–2019

Prabhakaran S, Wells KR, Lee VH, Flaherty CA, Lopes DK. Prevalence and risk factors for aspirin and clopidogrel resistance in cerebrovascular stenting. AJNR Am J Neuroradiol 2008;29(2):281–285

Sacco RL, Kargman DE, Gu Q, Zamanillo MC. Race-ethnicity and determinants of intracranial atherosclerotic cerebral infarction. The Northern Manhattan Stroke Study. Stroke 1995;26(1):14–20

Steinfort B, Ng PP, Faulder K, et al. Midterm outcomes of paclitaxel-eluting stents for the treatment of intracranial posterior circulation stenoses. J Neurosurg 2007;106(2):222–225

Turk AS, Levy EI, Albuquerque FC, et al. Influence of patient age and stenosis location on wingspan in-stent restenosis. AJNR Am J Neuroradiol 2008;29(1):23–27

Vajda Z, Aguilar M, Göhringer T, Horváth-Rizea D, Bäzner H, Henkes H. Treatment of Intracranial Atherosclerotic Disease with a Balloon-Expandable Paclitaxel Eluting Stent: Procedural Safety, Efficacy and Mid-Term Patency. Clin Neuroradiol 2012 Jan 18. [Epub ahead of print]

Weimar C, Goertler M, Harms L, Diener HC. Distribution and outcome of symptomatic stenoses and occlusions in patients with acute cerebral ischemia. Arch Neurol 2006;63(9):1287–1291

Wiviott SD, Braunwald E, McCabe CH, et al; TRITON-TIMI 38 Investigators. Prasugrel versus clopidogrel in patients with acute coronary syndromes. N Engl J Med 2007;357(20):2001–2015

IV

13   Subclavian Steal Syndrome
A. Berlis

Introduction

The phenomenon of retrograde blood flow in the vertebral artery relating to an occlusion of the subclavian artery was first described by Contorni in 1960 (Contorni 1960). The term "subclavian steal" was introduced by Fisher (1961), in an editorial comment on the publication by Reivich et al. (1961). Reivich was the first to describe the neurologic symptoms associated with the subclavian steal phenomenon.

Etiology and Clinical Presentation

The subclavian steal syndrome is a relatively common vascular disorder, with prevalence data in the literature ranging from 0.6 to 6.4%. A 2010 study published by Labropoulus et al. stated a prevalence of 5.4%. Duplex scans of the carotid arteries were performed in 7881 patients over a 6-year period (Labropoulus et al. 2010). It was found that a blood pressure differential of > 20 mmHg between the right and left arms had a high correlation with subclavian steal syndrome. The authors found that subclavian steal was detectable in 77% of patients ($n = 254$) with a pressure differential of 20–30 mmHg (4.2% of all patients), in 90% of patients ($n = 90$) with a differential of 31–40 mmHg, and in 100% of patients ($n = 85$) with a differential of > 41 mmHg.

> **Note**
>
> Interestingly, it is relatively rare for a detected subclavian steal syndrome to produce clinical symptoms.

It is not surprising to find that as the blood pressure differential rises, symptoms become more prevalent. Labropoulus et al. (2010) found that only 1.38% of patients with a pressure differential of 20–30 mmHg had a symptomatic subclavian steal syndrome, whereas 38.5% of patients with a pressure differential > 50 mmHg were symptomatic.

The classic manifestations of subclavian steal syndrome are symptoms of vertebrobasilar ischemia such as dizziness and ataxia. Not infrequently, hemispheric symptoms are also found in patients with the syndrome.

Atherosclerosis is the most frequent cause of subclavian artery occlusion or stenosis and has an incidence of ~17%. Because atherosclerosis tends to be generalized, associated vascular diseases in the anterior circulation are common and are generally responsible for symptoms. In patients with subclavian steal syndrome and additional vascular diseases in the anterior circulation, Hennerici et al. (1988) found that the 36% incidence of neurologic symptoms fell to 5% following the treatment of anterior circulation disease. Though over two decades old, these figures reflect current epidemiologic data, and clinical symptoms should be very carefully evaluated with regard to their origin before a patient is selected for treatment.

> **Note**
>
> The severity of symptoms should also be considered as a factor in patient selection.

This is emphasized by the study of Labropoulos et al. (2010), who treated only 1.4% of their patients, corresponding to 18.4% of all symptomatic patients.

Besides subclavian steal syndrome, an occlusion or high-grade stenosis of the subclavian artery can also lead to angina pectoris with rest and exercise ischemia of the arm or thromboembolism to the arm. Angina pectoris symptoms occur in patients with an internal mammary artery bypass (coronary subclavian steal syndrome). Flow reversal in the bypass graft may occur in the setting of subclavian stenosis or occlusion. Rarely, finger ischemia has also been described as a result of decreased blood flow during exercise (e.g., hand-over-head activities) or thromboemboli from the stenosis. Moreover, arm ischemia may result from a combination of subclavian stenosis and arteriovenous shunts created for hemodialysis, or it may develop in patients with an axillofemoral bypass. There is even a published report of a 74-year-old man with a subclavian stenosis that diverted blood from the anterior spinal artery; this patient presented clinically with bilateral arm weakness (Rughani et al. 2008).

Published reports consistently indicate a left-sided predominance. In the epidemiologic study by Labropoulus et al. (2010), the left subclavian artery was affected in 82% of cases; 46% of patients were men 42–86 years old, with an average age of 61 years.

Indications

Subclavian steal syndrome is not uncommon and is increasingly detected even in asymptomatic patients owing to the widespread use of imaging studies such as duplex sonography, CTA, and MR angiography (MRA). This makes it all the more important to take a discriminating approach to patient selection and not base treatment decisions solely on morphologic findings. The classic clinical manifestations of subclavian steal syndrome include drop attacks, vertigo, and ataxia. Other possible signs are arm ischemia at rest and during exercise or rare symptoms such as angina pectoris in patients who have had bypass surgery (see above).

Treatment

Operative Treatment

Operative treatment may consist of an axilloaxillary or carotid–axillary bypass or transposing the subclavian artery to the common carotid artery. Perioperative mortality is low, at 0–0.8%, and stroke rates range from 0.5 to 5%. The patency rates published in the 1990s literature are 92–95% at 5 years and 83–85% at 8–10 years.

Endovascular Treatment

Despite excellent surgical results, the treatment of subclavian steal syndrome during the past decade has been trending toward percutaneous endovascular techniques. Sixt et al. (2009) reported technical success rates of 100% for stenoses and 86% for occlusions. Endovascular treatment is associated with a high procedural success rate, low periprocedural mortality, and good short- and long-term patency rates of 70–90%. Two patients in the 2009 study had periprocedural complications with a pseudoaneurysm at the access site, which was successfully treated by ultrasound-guided compression. Ischemic problems did not occur.

Imaging Studies

The cornerstone for successful endovascular therapy is a complete angiographic survey of the supra-aortic vessels to define the true extent of the subclavian steal and the potentially complex collateral pathways. Frequent collateral routes are the occipital artery anastomosis between the external carotid artery and vertebral artery, thyroid artery anastomoses, and intersegmental anastomoses that form rope-ladder connections between the two vertebral arteries. Once the hemodynamics are known, the treatment procedure can be planned and the procedural risk can be assessed.

Technique

Endovascular treatment may consist of percutaneous balloon angioplasty alone or balloon angioplasty plus stenting. The stent may be of the self-expanding or balloon-expandable type.

> **Caution**
>
> Self-expanding stents may be disadvantageous for a short circumferential stenosis because the deployed stent may slip to a position that is proximal or distal to the stenosis.

This can be prevented by predilating the stenosis or using a longer self-expanding stent that extends past the stenosis into an adjacent vessel. Another option is the direct placement of a balloon-expandable stent (**Figs. 13.1** and **13.2**). One advantage of this method is that stent length can be more accurately tailored to vessel morphology and a shorter stent can be used. Because the vessel will generally have the same approximate diameter proximal and distal to the stenosis, a cylindrical stent will be used more often than a tapered model.

The stenosis can be accessed through the femoral or brachial artery. The transbrachial approach is better for subclavian and innominate occlusions since the vascular stump is generally easier to catheterize via the brachial artery than from the aortic arch, where the ostium may no longer be visible. Access to a high-grade stenosis depends on aortic arch anatomy and whether the direct placement of a guide catheter, stent, and/or angioplasty balloon is technically feasible. Again, this is usually easier with a transbrachial approach owing to the straight course of the subclavian artery, which provides stable interventional access.

> **Practical Tip**
>
> The brachial artery is usually difficult to palpate in the presence of a proximal stenosis or occlusion and therefore difficult to puncture. Identification can be aided by scanning with a sterile-packaged Doppler probe. When a stenosis is present, another technique is to pass a wire across the stenosis from the aortic arch and advance it into the brachial artery for localization. An important consideration in the transbrachial approach is maintaining adequate blood flow to the arm and hand before, during, and after the intervention. This is aided, for example, by monitoring oxygen saturation with a finger-clip sensor.

IV

Treatment of Supra-aortic Extra- and Intracranial Stenoses

IV

Platelet Inhibition and Anticoagulation

Anticoagulation and platelet inhibition are essential components of endovascular therapy, crucial for preventing periprocedural in-stent thrombosis and longer-term in-stent stenosis. Antiplatelet therapy and efficacy testing are the same as in periprocedural dual antiplatelet therapy and lifelong monotherapy after the stenting of carotid or intracranial stenoses (see also Chapter 12). A typical regimen consists of 75 mg clopidogrel (once in the morning) taken for a limited period and 100 mg aspirin (once in the evening) maintained for life. Because response is sometimes poor, especially to clopidogrel, alternative agents such as prasugrel are increasingly being used. In the future, it is likely that new agents such as ticagrelor will offer advantages as reversible antiplatelet drugs, especially in the management of periprocedural complications. Anticoagulation during the procedure serves mainly to prevent thromboembolus formation on wires and embolus ejection from flushed catheters.

Follow-up Care

The endovascular procedure is immediately followed by a clinical neurologic examination and duplex scanning

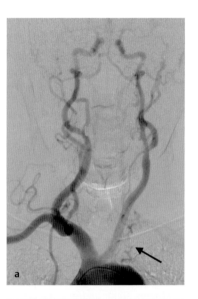
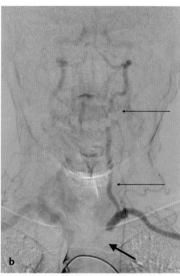
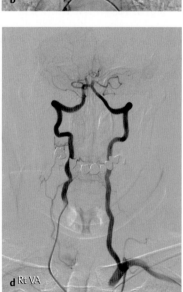

Fig. 13.1a–j A 64-year-old woman with a subclavian occlusion who presented with dizziness and falling toward the left side caused by a steal effect from the basilar artery territory with diminished blood flow.

a Injection of the aortic arch with a pressure syringe demonstrates an occlusion of the left subclavian artery (*thick arrow*).

b Second injection of the aortic arch shortly thereafter shows retrograde flow in the left vertebral artery (*thin arrows*) and opacification of the left subclavian artery distal to the occlusion (*thick arrow*).

c Selective injection of the vertebral artery (**c, d**) shows that the steal effect has caused nonfilling of the basilar artery, with almost all blood flow diverted to the left subclavian artery.

d Same view as in **c** later in the run.

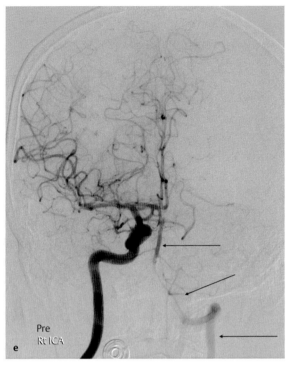

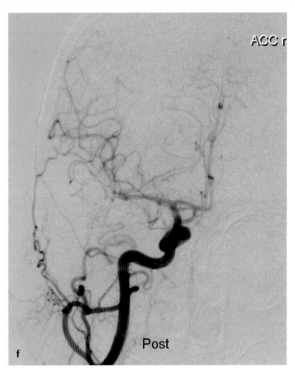

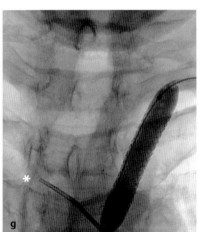

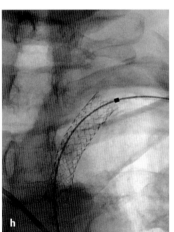

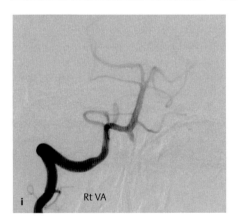

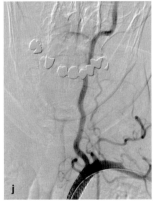

Fig. 13.1e–j *(continued)*

e Angiogram of the right internal carotid artery (ICA) before recanalization. The basilar artery receives retrograde flow from the right ICA via the posterior communicating artery and also contributes to retrograde filling of the left vertebral artery (*arrows*).

f Post-treatment angiogram shows hemodynamic reversal with nonvisualization of the basilar artery after successful recanalization of the proximal left subclavian artery.

g The occlusion is recanalized with an 8-mm × 38-mm balloon-mounted stent delivered through a short 6F stent placed in the left basilar artery. A diagnostic catheter configured for the vertebral artery (5F, *asterisk*) has been passed into the aortic arch through the right femoral artery. The balloon, filled with a mixture of contrast medium and saline, overlaps the ends of the stent and straightens the vascular segment during balloon inflation.

h Same view as in **g**. The stent extends only a few millimeters into the aortic arch.

i Completion angiogram of the right vertebral artery demonstrates antegrade flow in the basilar artery.

j Completion angiogram. The left subclavian artery is again perfused by antegrade flow, which ensures antegrade flow in the left vertebral artery and basilar artery. The clinical symptoms of dizziness and falling resolved completely after treatment.

IV

IV

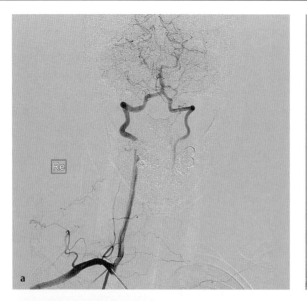

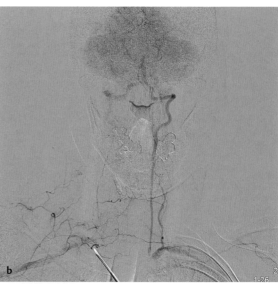

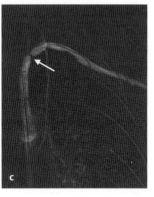

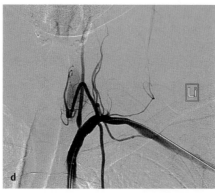

Fig. 13.2a–d **A 50-year-old woman with stage IIb peripheral arterial occlusive disease and a symptomatic high-grade stenosis of the left subclavian artery presented with claudication. She had no neurologic symptoms typical of a subclavian steal syndrome.**

a Right subclavian angiogram shows retrograde filling of the left vertebral artery. The steal effect is only moderate at this stage. This still allows retrograde filling of the basilar artery and explains the absence of typical symptoms such as dizziness and drop attacks.

b Same view somewhat later shows moderate opacification of the left subclavian artery.

c For treatment of the underlying stenosis, a guide catheter is introduced through the femoral artery and positioned in the subclavian artery. A 6-mm × 25-mm balloon-mounted stent is then introduced through the catheter. Because the stenosis is just proximal to the ostium of the left vertebral artery, it was overstented (*arrow*).

d Final angiogram demonstrates antegrade flow in the left subclavian artery and left vertebral artery, which shows a proximal stenosis.

of the neck and shoulder vessels. Follow-up visits may be scheduled at 3, 6, and 12 months, depending on initial findings and clinical complaints. If no changes are found, the follow-up interval can be lengthened to 12 months.

References

Contorni L. The vertebro-vertebral collateral circulation in obliteration of the subclavian artery at its origin. [Article in Italian] Minerva Chir 1960;15:268–271

Fisher CM. A new vascular syndrome—the subclavian steal. N Engl J Med 1961;265:912–913

Hennerici M, Klemm C, Rautenberg W. The subclavian steal phenomenon: a common vascular disorder with rare neurologic deficits. Neurology 1988;38(5):669–673

Labropoulos N, Nandivada P, Bekelis K. Prevalence and impact of the subclavian steal syndrome. Ann Surg 2010;252(1):166–170

Reivich M, Holling HE, Roberts B, Toole JF. Reversal of blood flow through the vertebral artery and its effect on cerebral circulation. N Engl J Med 1961;265:878–885

Rughani AI, Visioni A, Hamill RW, Tranmer BI. Subclavian artery stenosis causing transient bilateral brachial diplegia: an unusual cause of anterior spinal artery syndrome. J Neurosurg Spine 2008;9(2):191–195

Sixt S, Rastan A, Schwarzwälder U, et al. Results after balloon angioplasty or stenting of atherosclerotic subclavian artery obstruction. Catheter Cardiovasc Interv 2009;73(3):395–403

14 Proximal Vertebral Artery Stenosis

N. Lummel and H. Brueckmann

Anatomy

The vertebral artery can be divided anatomically into four segments (V1–V4). Some authors additionally designate the origin of the vertebral artery from the subclavian artery as V0.

- V1 segment: extends from the origin of the vertebral artery from the subclavian artery to the site where the vertebral artery enters the transverse foramen, generally at the level of the C6 vertebra
- V2 segment: ascends through the transverse foramina (from C6 to C1)
- V3 segment: extends from above the transverse foramen at C1 to the entrance into the dura at the level of the foramen magnum
- V4 segment: intradural segment of the vertebral artery extending to its junction with the opposite vertebral artery to form the basilar artery

The vertebral artery has an average diameter of 3–5 mm. Asymmetry between the right and left arteries is common. Approximately 50% of the population have a dominant left vertebral artery, 25% have a dominant right vertebral artery, and 25% have arteries of equal diameter. Up to 15% of the population constitutionally have only one vertebral artery.

Usually, the vertebral artery is the first branch arising from the proximal subclavian artery. A left vertebral artery arising directly from the aortic arch between the origin of the left common carotid artery and the left subclavian artery is the most common variant (4–5% of the population) (Koenigsberg et al. 2003). Other rare anatomic variations are a direct origin of the vertebral artery from the aortic arch distal to the left subclavian artery, an origin from the subclavian artery distal of the thyrocervical trunk, an origin of the right vertebral artery from the right common carotid artery, or a duplication of the vertebral artery, which may involve any of the arterial segments.

Likewise, the localization of the vertebral artery's origin from the subclavian artery is variable. The vertebral artery arises from the superior aspect of the subclavian artery in approximately half the population and from the posterior aspect in the remaining half. In a small percentage of cases the vertebral artery arises from the inferior aspect of the subclavian artery.

The vertebral artery is frequently elongated and tortuous, especially in its V0/V1 segment. Equally to the anterior circulation, this phenomenon correlates with the patient's age and the presence of arterial hypertension.

Etiology of Stenosis

Atherosclerotic stenoses of the extracranial vertebral artery are common. The incidence in the general population is not exactly known, but in patients with cardiovascular diseases they have been found at autopsy in 25–40% (Wityk et al. 1998). The origin of the vertebral artery (V0/V1) is considered a site of predilection for atherosclerotic stenosis. Plaques often begin in the subclavian artery and extend into the proximal vertebral artery. In correlation to the anterior circulation, histologies of the atherosclerotic lesion in the proximal vertebral artery are diverse (fatty deposits, fibrous plaques, calcified or complicated lesions) (Castaigne et al. 1973). Ulcerations within the atherosclerotic plaques are less common in the proximal vertebral artery than in the intradural vertebral artery or internal carotid artery.

Risk factors for atherosclerotic stenosis of the extracranial vertebral artery correspond to the known risk factors for cardiovascular disease such as arterial hypertension, diabetes mellitus, age, and smoking. Here too, males are predominantly affected by a 2:1 ratio (Zaytsev et al. 2006).

Other causes of proximal vertebral artery stenosis such as fibromuscular dysplasia, aortoarteritis, radiotherapy, and dissection are rare. An involvement of the V1 segment is evident in 23% of patients with a vertebral artery dissection (Wityk et al. 1998). However, dissections rarely originate at the ostium.

Approximately one-fifth of all ischemic cerebral strokes occur in the vertebrobasilar territory. Hemodynamically significant proximal vertebral artery stenosis is found in 20% of patients with vertebrobasilar ischemia. In 9% of patients, no cause other than a proximal vertebral artery stenosis can be found for the ischemic event, although the stenosis should be well tolerated considering the anatomic conditions with possible compensatory collateral flow of the contralateral vertebral. Three possible mechanisms could account for posterior circulation ischemia in patients with a vertebral artery stenosis:

- Artery-to-artery embolism (considered the most frequent cause)
- Hemodynamic insufficiency
- Occlusion of the vertebral artery

IV

> **Note**
>
> Contrary to the long-held belief that transient ischemic attacks in the vertebrobasilar territory have a more benign course than in the internal carotid artery (ICA) territory, it has been found that the opposite is true: Transient ischemic attacks and ischemia in the vertebrobasilar system have a poor prognosis with a 5-year risk of stroke of 22–35%, especially in the acute phase (Wehman et al. 2004). The mortality of ischemic events is also markedly higher in the vertebrobasilar territory (20–30%) than in the anterior circulation. Hence, the diagnosis and management of vertebral artery stenosis play an important role in stroke patients.

Diagnosis

Unlike carotid artery stenosis, valid criteria for the grading of vertebral artery stenosis have not yet been established. Randomized studies have shown that the risk of stroke and benefit of vascular surgery or endovascular therapy depends on the degree of carotid artery stenosis (> 70%). It is still unclear whether there is a similar threshold for proximal vertebral artery stenosis beyond which the risk of stroke rises markedly, and the potential benefit from interventional treatment is evident. Furthermore, the considerably smaller lumen of the vertebral artery compared with the carotid artery makes it more difficult to evaluate the degree of vertebral artery stenosis. For these reasons a simple classification for proximal vertebral artery stenosis is commonly used: either "present" (50–99%) or "not present" (< 50%). Occasionally, the stenosis is further classified as "none" (< 50%), "moderate" (50–69%), or "high-grade" (70–99%).

Invasive Studies

Digital Subtraction Angiography

Digital subtraction angiography (DSA) is still considered the gold standard for the diagnosis of proximal vertebral artery stenosis despite the ~1% risk of iatrogenic periprocedural stroke.

Noninvasive Studies

Noninvasive imaging modalities for the diagnosis of proximal vertebral artery stenosis are ultrasound (Doppler and duplex scanning), CT angiography (CTA), and MR angiography (MRA). Due to the smaller vessel lumen and lesion localization, imaging of proximal vertebral artery stenosis is technically more challenging than for carotid stenosis. The above-mentioned imaging modalities offer different logistic advantages and disadvantages.

Doppler and Duplex Ultrasound

Ultrasound is a noninvasive, cost-effective, widely available modality that has an established track record in the evaluation of vascular stenosis (carotid, renal, femoral arteries). In contrast to the anterior circulation, where the cutoff values are exactly defined in 10% increments for carotid artery stenosis (Widder and Görtler 2004), proximal vertebral artery stenoses are graded on the basis of approximate values. Peak systolic velocity (PSV) is considered the most sensitive parameter. The following cutoff values are used (Hua et al. 2009):
- For < 50% stenosis: PSV > 85 cm/s
- For 50–69% stenosis: PSV > 140 cm/s
- For 70–99% stenosis: PSV > 210 cm/s

Evaluation of the proximal vertebral artery using ultrasound is frequently limited by the anatomic conditions and, due to the method, is operator-dependent. Moderate flow disturbances at the vertebral artery origin are frequent nonpathologic findings, as the vessel usually arises at a right angle. Hence, luminal narrowing can only be directly evaluated when the vessel is normo- or hyperplastic and the vessel walls are clearly delineated. Doppler and duplex sonography thus have lower sensitivity and specificity than CTA and contrast-enhanced MRA.

CT Angiography

CTA is generally regarded as a valid method for the evaluation of proximal vertebral artery stenosis. As shoulders are located at the same level as the vertebral artery origin, artifacts commonly occur, but can be eliminated by increasing the tube current (210 mA). One advantage of CTA over conventional angiography is that postprocessing allows the vessel to be evaluated in all planes in three-dimensional (3D) renderings. On the other hand, calcified plaques can lead to overestimation of stenosis when plaques are superimposed on the contrast-filled vessel lumen, especially in maximum intensity projection (MIP) reconstructions (Farrés et al. 1996). Furthermore, the technique involves the known disadvantages of CT (radiation exposure and use of iodinated, possibly nephrotoxic, contrast medium).

MR Angiography

Two different methods are available for MRA of the cervical vessels: noncontrast-enhanced time-of-flight (TOF) MRA and contrast-enhanced MRA. TOF MRA provides a flow-dependent view of vessels and thus yields information on flow characteristics. The proximal vertebral artery is often elongated or tortuous and thus shows decreased signal intensity due to saturation and/or dephasing of spins. For this reason, TOF MRA is not the method of choice for evaluating vertebral artery stenosis. Contrast-enhanced MRA, on the other hand, has proved to be a valid method, equivalent to CTA, for evaluating proximal vertebral artery stenosis. As in CTA, images can be reconstructed in all planes and rendered in 3D views. Contrast-enhanced MRA can also supply information on the plaques causing the stenosis. Disadvantages are current MRI-associated problems such as cost efficiency, contraindications in patients with metal implants (e.g., cardiac pacemakers), and claustrophobia.

Treatment

Three main options are available for the treatment of proximal vertebral artery stenosis:
- Conservative medical therapy
- Surgical treatment
- Endovascular treatment by percutaneous transluminal angioplasty or stenting

The medical treatment options for proximal vertebral artery stenosis consist of antiplatelet and anticoagulant drugs. The goal of medical therapy is to prevent embolism. Drugs cannot improve the decreased blood flow that results from a hemodynamically significant stenosis (Spetzler et al. 1987). The efficacy of antiplatelet drugs in the vertebrobasilar system has not been systematically investigated so far, but a protective effect similar to that in the carotid system can be assumed. The effect of anticoagulant therapy on proximal vertebral artery stenosis has also not been investigated in clinical trials, but it carries a significant additional risk of hemorrhage, especially in patients with underlying atherosclerotic disease (Sandercock et al. 2003).

It is very rare for proximal vertebral artery stenosis to be treated surgically, because of the difficulty of surgical access (Crawley et al. 1998). Three vascular surgical techniques are available for vertebral artery reconstruction:
- Detaching the vertebral artery distal to the stenosis and reimplanting it in the ipsilateral carotid or subclavian artery
- Endarterectomy
- Patch grafting

Overall perioperative morbidity and mortality are relatively high (~20% of patients; Phatouros et al. 2000).

The following complications have been described (Kline and Berguer 1993): Horner syndrome (15% of patients), lymphocele (4%), recurrent laryngeal nerve palsy (2%), thrombosis (1%), chylothorax (0.5%), and death (up to 4%). Secondary patency rates in these (few) patients were 95% at 5 years and 91% at 10 years.

The endovascular treatment options for proximal vertebral artery stenosis are balloon dilatation (percutaneous transluminal angioplasty) and/or stent placement. High restenosis rates (10–75%) have been reported with balloon dilatation (Crawley et al. 1998). Therefore, the current endovascular options for proximal vertebral artery stenosis are balloon angioplasty plus stenting or primary stent placement. The latter method employs balloon-mounted stents and coated or uncoated coronary stents. The intervention usually has a high technical success rate and provides good initial clinical results. Again, however, the main limiting factor is a high rate of restenosis of ~30% (0–67%) (Vajda et al. 2009).

Indications

The indications for treatment of proximal vertebral artery stenosis are still controversial, as data from large randomized studies are lacking. Medical therapy is still considered the first-line treatment. Today the indication for endovascular treatment is acknowledged in symptomatic patients with proximal vertebral artery stenosis refractory to drug therapy, despite the known limitations of endovascular techniques. Factors that also influence patient selection are degree of stenosis, the angiographic morphology of the stenosis (e.g., ulceration), the collateral supply, patient age (Mukherjee and Pineda 2007), and the presence of bilateral vertebral artery stenosis or unilateral stenosis coexisting with contralateral vertebral artery hypoplasia (Brückmann et al. 1986).

Asymptomatic patients are almost always managed with drug therapy. Proximal vertebral artery stenosis showing short-term progression may be an indication for endovascular therapy in selected cases even in asymptomatic patients.

Endovascular Therapy

According to stenting of carotid stenosis (see Treatment, p. 103), vertebral artery stenting should be preceded by dual antiplatelet therapy, e.g., 100 mg aspirin + 4 × 75 mg clopidogrel the day before the intervention and platelet aggregometry (Multiplate) performed on the day of the intervention.

Activated clotting time (ACT) should be measured at the start of the intervention to monitor the efficacy of anticoagulation. The patient receives a weight-adjusted

IV

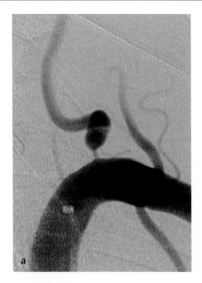
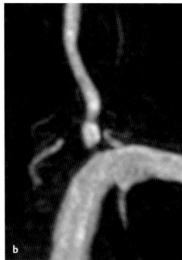
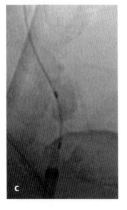
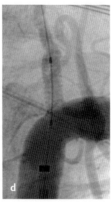
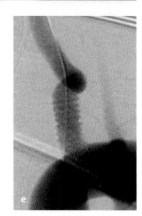

Fig. 14.1a–e   Filiform stenosis of the proximal left vertebral artery.
a Pretreatment DSA.
b Pretreatment MRA.
c The stenosis is crossed with a Choice PT wire, then predilated with a 2.5-mm Maverick balloon inflated to 14 atm. A TAXUS 5.0 stent (coated) is deployed and dilated to the nominal pressure of 9 atm.
d DSA (without contrast) after stent placement confirms expansion of the proximal vertebral artery stenosis.
e Subtracted view after stent placement.

bolus of unfractionated heparin (60 U/kg body weight) to achieve a target ACT twice the baseline value or > 250 s. Further ACT determinations are also recommended over time. When the ACT reaches a value of > 250 s, the stenosis can be crossed with the wire.

Practical Tip

We recommend that the procedure is performed under general endotracheal anesthesia, especially in patients with bilateral vertebral artery stenosis, because dilatation and stenting may briefly occlude the vessel, causing a transient brainstem insult and respiratory arrest in some patients.

Balloon predilatation may be used at the discretion of the interventionist. It is advantageous, as it facilitates the subsequent passage of a balloon-mounted stent. The balloon selected for percutaneous transluminal angioplasty should not be too large, as an oversized balloon would increase the risk of perforation or dissection. Stenting may be performed with balloon-mounted stents like those used in the treatment of intracranial stenoses or with coated (**Fig. 14.1**) or uncoated coronary stents. The type of stent used should be adapted to the individual anatomy. The optimal stent diameter is determined by measuring the caliber of the unaffected proximal V1 segment.

Note

The stent should completely cover the origin of the vertebral artery. As a result, the stent will often protrude 1–2 mm into the subclavian artery. Balloon-mounted stents are easier to secure in that position than self-expanding stents.

An embolic protection system is not normally used in the stenting of a proximal vertebral artery stenosis.

A complete neurologic examination should be performed before and after the intervention, and neurologic surveillance should be maintained for at least 24 h after the procedure. We also recommend blood pressure monitoring and any necessary peri- and postinterventional treatment for arterial hypertension (optimal blood pressure range is 110–130/75–80 mmHg) to minimize the risk of hyperperfusion hemorrhage.

To reduce the risk of recurrent stenosis, patients who have undergone vertebral artery stenting should take aspirin daily for life. They should also take clopidogrel for 3 months if an uncoated stent was used and for 12 months if a coated stent was used. Follow-up examinations, preferably by ultrasonography, should be scheduled at regular intervals (3 days, 6 weeks, and 12 months after the intervention).

Complications

The following complications may arise during the endovascular treatment of proximal vertebral artery stenosis: dissection, perforation, perforator occlusion, or plaque displacement leading to embolic cerebral ischemia. In ~22% of patients, MRI will demonstrate new, small, clinically silent ischemic areas caused by microemboli released during the intervention. The endovascular treatment of proximal vertebral artery stenosis has an overall mortality rate of 0.3%. The incidence of periprocedural neurologic complications reported in the literature is 1–5%. Late (intermediate-term) strokes due to an infarction in the vertebrobasilar territory are rare (< 1% of patients; Mukherjee and Pineda 2007). The incidence of early thrombosis after stenting can be greatly reduced by the use of potent antiplatelet drugs such as clopidogrel, ticlopidine (caution: causes a change in blood cell counts) or prasugrel (Schömig et al. 1996).

The main problem in the endovascular treatment of proximal vertebral artery stenosis is restenosis due to neointimal hyperplasia (**Fig. 14.2**). Attempts to lower the restenosis rate after stenting by intraluminal brachytherapy (Albiero et al. 2000) have not become established in clinical use. While coated stents have significantly lowered restenosis rates in coronary arteries compared with traditional stents (Regar et al. 2002), these devices have not significantly reduced restenosis rates after stenting of proximal vertebral artery stenosis according to current data (Lugmayr et al. 2004).

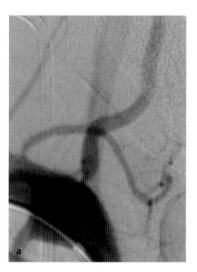
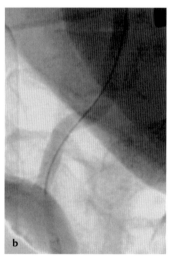
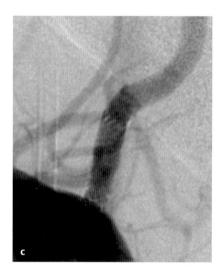
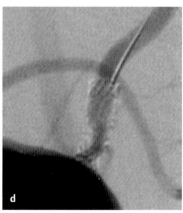
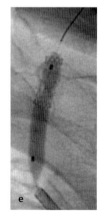

Fig. 14.2a–e   Short, high-grade stenosis of the proximal right vertebral artery.
a Preinterventional view.
b The stenosis is crossed with a Synchro 14 wire. A Pharos stent (3.5 mm × 13 mm) is placed across the stenosis and expanded by dilating the delivery balloon.
c Postinterventional view confirms expansion of the proximal stenosis.
d Follow-up image at 11 months reveals a short, high-grade in-stent stenosis.
e A coated In.Pact Falcon balloon (3.5 mm × 20 mm) is introduced over a Synchro 14 wire, advanced into the stent lumen, and dilated.

IV

Treatment of Supra-aortic Extra- and Intracranial Stenoses

IV

References

Albiero R, Nishida T, Adamian M, et al. Edge restenosis after implantation of high activity (32)P radioactive beta-emitting stents. Circulation 2000;101(21):2454–2457

Brückmann H, Ringelstein EB, Buchner H, Zeumer H. Percutaneous transluminal angioplasty of the vertebral artery. A therapeutic alternative to operative reconstruction of proximal vertebral artery stenoses. J Neurol 1986;233(6):336–339

Castaigne P, Lhermitte F, Gautier JC, et al. Arterial occlusions in the vertebro-basilar system. A study of 44 patients with postmortem data. Brain 1973;96(1):133–154

Crawley F, Brown MM, Clifton AG. Angioplasty and stenting in the carotid and vertebral arteries. Postgrad Med J 1998;74(867):7–10

Farrés MT, Grabenwöger F, Magometschnig H, Trattnig S, Heimberger K, Lammer J. Spiral CT angiography: study of stenoses and calcification at the origin of the vertebral artery. Neuroradiology 1996;38(8):738–743

Hua Y, Meng XF, Jia LY, et al. Color Doppler imaging evaluation of proximal vertebral artery stenosis. AJR Am J Roentgenol 2009;193(5):1434–1438

Kline RA, Berguer R. Vertebral artery reconstruction. Ann Vasc Surg 1993;7(5):497–501

Koenigsberg RA, Pereira L, Nair B, McCormick D, Schwartzman R. Unusual vertebral artery origins: examples and related pathology. Catheter Cardiovasc Interv 2003;59(2):244–250

Lugmayr H, Kastner M, Fröhler W, Meindl S, Zisch R. Sirolimus-eluting stents for the treatment of symptomatic extracranial vertebral artery stenoses: early experience and 6-month follow-up. [Article in German] Rofo 2004;176(10):1431–1435

Mukherjee D, Pineda G. Extracranial vertebral artery intervention. J Interv Cardiol 2007;20(6):409–416

Phatouros CC, Higashida RT, Malek AM, et al. Endovascular treatment of noncarotid extracranial cerebrovascular disease. Neurosurg Clin N Am 2000;11(2):331–350

Regar E, Serruys PW, Bode C, et al; RAVEL Study Group. Angiographic findings of the multicenter Randomized Study With the Sirolimus-Eluting Bx Velocity Balloon-Expandable Stent (RAVEL): sirolimus-eluting stents inhibit restenosis irrespective of the vessel size. Circulation 2002;106(15):1949–1956

Sandercock P, Mielke O, Liu M, Counsell C. Anticoagulants for preventing recurrence following presumed non-cardioembolic ischaemic stroke or transient ischaemic attack. Cochrane Database Syst Rev 2003;(1):CD 000248

Schömig A, Neumann FJ, Kastrati A, et al. A randomized comparison of antiplatelet and anticoagulant therapy after the placement of coronary-artery stents. N Engl J Med 1996;334(17):1084–1089

Spetzler RF, Hadley MN, Martin NA, Hopkins LN, Carter LP, Budny J. Vertebrobasilar insufficiency. Part 1: Microsurgical treatment of extracranial vertebrobasilar disease. J Neurosurg 1987;66(5):648–661

Vajda Z, Miloslavski E, Güthe T, et al. Treatment of stenoses of vertebral artery origin using short drug-eluting coronary stents: improved follow-up results. AJNR Am J Neuroradiol 2009;30(9):1653–1656

Wehman JC, Hanel RA, Guidot CA, Guterman LR, Hopkins LN. Atherosclerotic occlusive extracranial vertebral artery disease: indications for intervention, endovascular techniques, short-term and long-term results. J Interv Cardiol 2004;17(4):219–232

Widder B, Görtler M. Doppler- und Duplexsonographie der hirnversorgenden Arterien. 6th ed. Berlin: Springer; 2004: 168

Wityk RJ, Chang HM, Rosengart A, et al. Proximal extracranial vertebral artery disease in the New England Medical Center Posterior Circulation Registry. Arch Neurol 1998;55(4):470–478

Zaytsev AY, Stoyda AY, Smirnov VE, et al. Endovascular treatment of supra-aortic extracranial stenoses in patients with vertebrobasilar insufficiency symptoms. Cardiovasc Intervent Radiol 2006;29(5):731–738

15 Proximal Stenosis of Supra-aortic Vessels

J. Berkefeld

Epidemiology and Risk of Stroke

Much less attention has been paid to proximal supra-aortic stenoses than to the more common stenoses of the carotid bifurcation. This is partly because atherosclerotic plaques in the brachiocephalic trunk, proximal common carotid artery, and subclavian artery are less common than bifurcation stenoses. Moreover, the supra-aortic stenoses are probably less often embolic and are less likely to cause neurologic symptoms. Based on epidemiologic estimates, subclavian stenosis is present in 2% of the population and in 7% of patients in medical institutions. Smoking, hypertension, hypercholesterolemia, and the presence of peripheral arterial occlusive disease are considered the main risk factors (Shadman et al. 2004). According to recent data, proximal stenoses cause ~5% of severe life-threatening strokes and thus play a minor role compared with the more dangerous carotid and proximal vertebral artery stenoses (Mazighi et al. 2009). Although the risk of stroke is relatively low, subclavian stenosis has been identified as a risk factor for significantly increased mortality from cardiovascular disease (Aboyans et al. 2007).

Besides embolic ischemia, subclavian or innominate stenosis also gives rise to steal phenomena such as flow reversal in the vertebral artery and flow diversion to the arm, which may cause hemodynamic problems in the posterior circulation during exercise (see Chapter 13). The stroke risk in patients with steal phenomena is not precisely known. Based on observations in older case series, transient ischemia is relatively common although strokes appear to be rare (Moran et al. 1988).

Atherosclerosis is by far the most dominant cause of proximal stenoses and rare aneurysmal vascular dilatations. Nonatheromatous stenoses may result from an inflammatory process (e.g., Takayasu arteritis), aortic dissections spreading into the origins of the cervicobrachial arteries, traumatic vascular injuries, and compression syndromes involving more distal portions of the subclavian artery. Long-segment stenoses of the common carotid artery have also been observed following radiation to the neck.

Clinical Presentation and Diagnosis

It is sometimes difficult to appreciate the relationship between clinical manifestations and a proximal stenosis. Of course, there are patients who manifest neurologic symptoms in the form of transient ischemic attacks or stroke. Because most patients have subclavian stenosis, it is more common to find symptoms relating to the posterior circulation such as rotary or staggering vertigo, dysarthria, diplopia, and visual field defects rather than hemispheric symptoms with hemiplegia or aphasia.

> **Caution**
>
> Many patients with subclavian stenosis complain of nonspecific dizziness, and even neurologists may find it difficult to establish a cause.

Imaging studies, preferably MRI, can make it easier to appreciate the clinical significance of a stenosis by demonstrating infarctions in the territory of the stenosed vessel. Diffusion-weighted MRI showing new lesions consistent with the patient's symptoms may even be diagnostic and aid in therapeutic decision-making (**Fig. 15.1**).

Most recent publications on proximal stenoses are aimed more at cardiologists than neurologists and contain little information on neurologic deficits. Stenoses that cause steal phenomena may present clinically with exercise-dependent syncope, vertigo, and impaired consciousness (Khurana et al. 2009). Some patients complain of pulsatile tinnitus due to the collateral recruitment of external carotid artery branches (Lehmann et al. 2005). Subclavian and innominate stenoses may also present with nonneurologic symptoms such as exercise-dependent arm pain. There have been recent reports of proximal subclavian stenosis and acute coronary syndrome in patients with a mammary artery bypass graft as well as steal phenomena induced by the stenosis (Lelek et al. 2008).

IV

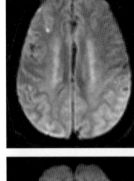
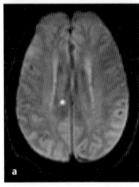
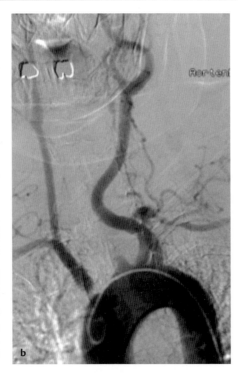
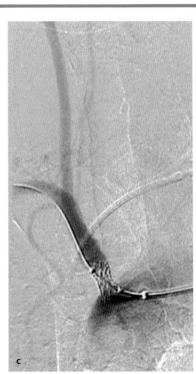

Fig. 15.1a–c Diagnostic imaging and intervention in a 67-year-old man with recurrent right hemispheric transient ischemic attacks.

a Two fresh microembolic infarctions are detected in the right carotid territory.

b Survey angiogram of the aortic arch demonstrates a stenosis of the brachiocephalic trunk.

c The stenosis is recanalized with a balloon-expandable stent delivered through a long transfemoral sheath.

IV

> ### Note
>
> Side-to-side comparison of blood pressures and pulses is an important screening aid for stenoses involving the subclavian artery. Blood pressure differences > 15 mmHg are suggestive of stenosis (Shadman et al. 2004). A strong radial artery pulse tends to exclude the presence of a high-grade ipsilateral subclavian stenosis.

Noninvasive screening with Doppler ultrasound is not as well standardized for proximal stenoses as it is for carotid bifurcation stenosis. Stenoses close to the aortic arch are difficult to evaluate with ultrasound. Accurate localization of the stenosis is difficult, and poststenotic flow changes such as decreased flow velocity or flow reversal are often the only demonstrable findings. Moderately severe stenoses that are not hemodynamically significant are difficult to detect with ultrasound (Widder and Görtler 2004). Accordingly, equivocal cases should additionally be evaluated by another vascular imaging modality. The standard method for this purpose is contrast-enhanced MRA. Although the degree of stenosis is occasionally distorted by flow artifacts arising near the aortic arch, contrast-enhanced MRA is still preferred to the less artifact-prone CTA owing to the lack of radiation exposure and greater

ease of image postprocessing (Cosottini et al. 2003). It appears that high-field imaging at 3 T and parallel image acquisition can largely offset the disadvantages of contrast-enhanced MRA, allowing stenoses to be evaluated as accurately as with CTA or conventional DSA (Nael et al. 2007).

Catheter angiography is performed in doubtful cases and to aid the planning of surgical and interventional procedures.

> ### Note
>
> Clinical manifestations and diagnostic studies:
> - Usually generalized atherosclerosis with localized arterial occlusive disease
> - Transient ischemic attacks or stroke, often in the posterior circulation
> - Exercise-dependent syncopal attacks due to stenosis causing a steal phenomenon
> - Acute coronary syndrome in patients with stenosis proximal to a mammary artery bypass
> - Caution: nonspecific dizziness
> - Side-to-side comparison of blood pressures and pulses, and Doppler ultrasound for screening
> - Diagnosis best confirmed by contrast-enhanced MRA including MRI (for detection of infarction)

Interventional Treatment Options

Although data with a high level of evidence are not currently available for the balloon angioplasty and stenting of proximal supra-aortic stenoses, interventional treatment is generally preferred for these lesions because it is effective and much less invasive than operative treatment. Nevertheless, a carotid–subclavian bypass and other vascular surgical reconstructions are still available as alternatives in patients who are difficult to treat by interventional therapy, and these techniques have yielded better long-term patency rates than stenting (AbuRahma et al. 2007). The proximal arterial trunks are elastic vessels that can offer significant resistance to balloon angioplasty when lined by fibrous or calcified plaque. The results of percutaneous transluminal angioplasty alone are often disappointing as a result of elastic recoil forces or intimal dissection. Primary stent placement yields better initial results and 1-year patency rates of ~90%, and has therefore become the preferred option at most centers (Sixt et al. 2009).

Balloon-expandable stents approved for use in peripheral vessels are most commonly used. They provide an effective scaffold for rigid plaques and can be accurately deployed at the desired location. Self-expanding stents, which conform better to changing vascular diameter, have also been used in selected cases (Pulido-Duque et al. 2005).

Most stenoses can be treated via femoral access. Retrograde recanalization via brachial access may be used for subclavian obstructions that are difficult to negotiate by the transfemoral route.

Note

Combined procedures involving surgical exposure of the carotid bifurcation and retrograde stent insertion into the common carotid artery are rarely necessary nowadays and are recommended only in exceptional cases, because there are differences in antithrombotic management for surgical and interventional procedures.

Accurate positioning and apposition of the stent are important considerations in the placement of balloon-expandable stents. Most short stents have a tendency to shift proximally or distally when the balloon is inflated. It is essential to know the exact position of the proximal and distal ends of the stent, the origins of important side branches (vertebral artery, internal mammary artery), and the upper circumference of the aortic arch when stenting a stenosis near the ostium. To avoid stent malplacement, it is helpful in the transfemoral approach to support and stabilize the lower end of the stent with the guide catheter or long sheath. Predilatation is recommended when dealing with angled vessel origins, a small residual lumen, or rigid calcified stenoses. Next, the sheath or guide catheter can be advanced into the stenosis to direct the placement of the coaxial stent (see **Fig. 15.1c**). When the stent delivery catheter has been positioned, the balloon should be inflated very slowly by an assistant while the operator holds the stent in the desired position.

The stent should completely cover the plaque and should be fully apposed to eliminate visible gaps between the stent scaffold and vessel wall. With ostial stenosis, care is taken to obtain good coverage by the proximal end of the stent, which should project no more than a few millimeters into the main vessel (**Fig. 15.2**).

Caution

Oversized stent diameters and overdilatation should be avoided because of the risk of vessel rupture. If pain occurs, the dilatation should be interrupted.

In addition to stenoses, proximal occlusions can also be recanalized, especially in the subclavian artery. Recanalization via femoral access is often difficult when dealing with a small stump and rigid occlusive material. Transbrachial recanalization is often easier and less risky in this situation. On the other hand, large-caliber stent delivery systems should be introduced by the femoral approach after crossing the lesion with a guidewire to avoid injuring the brachial artery by a large-bore sheath. With calcified occlusions that are difficult to cross, aggressive recanalization maneuvers with stiff wires should be avoided because of the risk of vessel rupture and bleeding, or obstruction of the vertebral artery origin by a dissected flap. Bypass surgery may be the less risky alternative in situations of this kind.

There is still controversy as to whether filters or balloon occlusion should be used to protect the distal vasculature in interventions for proximal stenoses. Since these procedures have a lower embolic risk than the treatment of carotid stenoses, most interventions are performed without protection. Filters and balloon occlusion techniques are technically feasible (Michael et al. 2009) but make the procedure more complex while providing uncertain benefit. On the other hand, embolic protection is advisable in high-risk situations such as nonocclusive thrombi or plaques with a very irregular surface (Körner et al. 1999). It was once believed that flow reversal in the vertebral artery would normalize over time following the correction of subclavian stenosis (Ringelstein and

IV

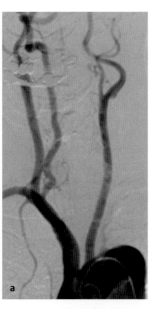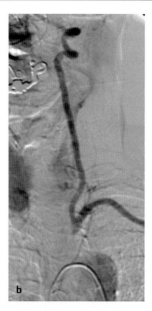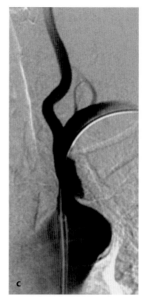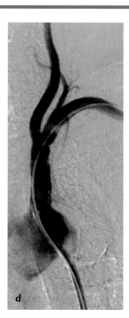

Fig. 15.2a–d   Angiography and intervention in a 72-year-old man with syncopal episodes during left arm exercise.

a Survey angiogram of the aortic arch shows a subtotal stenosis of the left subclavian artery.

b Steal phenomenon is evidenced by retrograde filling of the left vertebral artery and distal subclavian artery.

c The stenosis has been predilated with a balloon for percutaneous transluminal angioplasty. Subsequent angiogram shows a lateral

intimal flap and pseudoaneurysmal bulge on the lateral aspect of the vessel.

d The vessel is recanalized with a balloon-expandable stent, which extends slightly across the subclavian artery ostium. Antegrade flow has been restored in the left vertebral artery.

Zeumer 1984), but this assumption is no longer considered reliable.

Results of Interventional Therapy

Proximal stenoses can be treated by angioplasty or stenting with high technical success rates > 90%. Although some series report optimistic success rates of 70–80% or more for subclavian occlusions (Henry et al. 2007; Sixt et al. 2009), the rates are probably lower in cases with rigid obstructions and cases that require meticulous technique.

Most recent studies use immediate and long-term patency rates as their main criteria for a successful outcome, and it is difficult to extract neurologic event rates from published case reports. Complication rates are usually reported from an angiologic perspective, so they consist mainly of thromboembolisms, dissections, and hematomas at the vascular access site.

Based on published case data and personal experience, complications with neurologic deficits appear to be rare and probably occur at rates < 3%. In one series of 170 patients who underwent primary stent placement (Patel et al. 2008), only one stroke occurred (0.6%).

The rate of vascular complications was 5.3%, although 3 deaths from myocardial infarction occurred during the first 30 days.

Balloon angioplasty may cause dissections and ruptures leading to severe hemorrhage. It appears, however, that hemorrhagic complications do not always have serious clinical effects, suggesting that pseudoaneurysms and small mediastinal hematomas can also be managed conservatively (Broadbent et al. 2003). The primary patency rate, which is ~90% during the first year after stent placement, falls to 70–80% during follow-up periods of up to 5 years (Bates et al. 2004).

Besides a certain biologic tendency for stenosis to recur in the proximal arteries, stent fractures have also been identified as an occasional cause of restenosis (Periard et al. 2008). Regular clinical follow-ups with blood pressure measurement and Doppler scanning are recommended for the early detection of restenosis. Re-interventions are performed in ~15% of patients. They rely mainly on the technically simple and low-risk procedure of repeat balloon angioplasty and yield secondary patency rates of > 90%. Restenosis is asymptomatic in most patients, and strokes appear to be very rare during follow-up. Life expectancy in patients with generalized atherosclerosis is limited mainly by cardiac events and averaged only 8.4 years in a large case series (Patel et al. 2008).

Note

Interventional therapy:
- Standard method: balloon-expandable stents
- Low acute complications rates even without embolic protection
- Relatively high in-stent restenosis rates of up to 30% in the long term
- Follow-up examinations are required and may show need for repeat balloon dilatation
- Few strokes during follow-up, but life expectancy limited due to coronary heart disease

Indications for Interventional Treatment

Given the lack of study data with a high level of evidence, it is difficult to make a generally valid risk-benefit analysis for the interventional treatment of proximal supra-aortic stenoses. Based on the results summarized above, which are consistent with the author's own experience, stent-assisted angioplasty can be recommended for the following indications:

Note

Indications for interventional treatment:
- Stenoses causing neurologic symptoms
- Stenoses causing arm pain
- Stenoses causing syncopal episodes due to steal phenomena
- Stenoses causing a coronary syndrome in bypass patients
- Asymptomatic stenoses before proposed mammary artery bypass

The indications for other asymptomatic stenoses are less clear and should be decided on a case-by-case basis. Recanalization may be able to improve hemodynamics in obstructions involving multiple arteries supplying the brain. Given the high success rates and low complication rates, even asymptomatic stenoses should probably be treated if doubt exists, for the stenosis may progress to an occlusion, which will reduce the chance of a successful outcome and may necessitate a higher-risk operation. On the other hand, the relatively low event rates in untreated cases also suggest that it is better to avoid high-risk interventions in asymptomatic patients and especially in interventional high-risk cases with severe generalized atherosclerosis, as long as the benefit of these interventions remains unproven.

Summary

Proximal stenoses of the supra-aortic arterial trunks are not often symptomatic. Interventional treatment options with stent-assisted angioplasty can be performed with high success rates and little risk. Nevertheless, the indications should still be carefully weighed when we consider the somewhat unsatisfactory long-term patency rates and the potential for complications in any given case. Treatment of high-grade symptomatic stenoses is preferred to a blanket recommendation for the treatment of incidental findings.

References

Aboyans V, Criqui MH, McDermott MM, et al. The vital prognosis of subclavian stenosis. J Am Coll Cardiol 2007;49(14): 1540–1545

AbuRahma AF, Bates MC, Stone PA, et al. Angioplasty and stenting versus carotid-subclavian bypass for the treatment of isolated subclavian artery disease. J Endovasc Ther 2007;14(5):698–704

Bates MC, Broce M, Lavigne PS, Stone P. Subclavian artery stenting: factors influencing long-term outcome. Catheter Cardiovasc Interv 2004;61(1):5–11

Broadbent LP, Moran CJ, Cross DT III, Derdeyn CP. Management of ruptures complicating angioplasty and stenting of supra-aortic arteries: report of two cases and a review of the literature. AJNR Am J Neuroradiol 2003;24(10):2057–2061

Cosottini M, Calabrese R, Puglioli M, et al. Contrast-enhanced three-dimensional MR angiography of neck vessels: does dephasing effect alter diagnostic accuracy? Eur Radiol 2003;13(3):571–581

Henry M, Henry I, Polydorou A, Polydorou A, Hugel M. Percutaneous transluminal angioplasty of the subclavian arteries. Int Angiol 2007;26(4):324–340

Khurana V, Gambhir IS, Srivastava A, Kishore D. Dizziness and collapse? It's a steal! Lancet 2009;374(9699):1472

Körner M, Baumgartner I, Do DD, Mahler F, Schroth G. PTA of the subclavian and innominate arteries: long-term results. Vasa 1999;28(2):117–122

Lehmann MF, Mounayer C, Benndorf G, Piotin M, Moret J. Pulsatile tinnitus: a symptom of chronic subclavian artery occlusion. AJNR Am J Neuroradiol 2005;26(8):1960–1963

Lelek M, Bochenek T, Drzewiecki J, Trusz-Gluza M. Unstable angina as a result of coronary-subclavian steal syndrome. Circ Cardiovasc Interv 2008;1(1):82–84

Mazighi M, Labreuche J, Gongora-Rivera F, Duyckaerts C, Hauw JJ, Amarenco P. Autopsy prevalence of proximal extracranial atherosclerosis in patients with fatal stroke. Stroke 2009;40(3):713–718

Michael TT, Banerjee S, Brilakis E. Subclavian artery intervention with vertebral embolic protection. Catheter Cardiovasc Interv 2009;74(1):22–25

IV

Treatment of Supra-aortic Extra- and Intracranial Stenoses

Moran KT, Zide RS, Persson AV, Jewell ER. Natural history of subclavian steal syndrome. Am Surg 1988;54(11):643–644

Nael K, Villablanca JP, Pope WB, McNamara TO, Laub G, Finn JP. Supraaortic arteries: contrast-enhanced MR angiography at 3.0 T—highly accelerated parallel acquisition for improved spatial resolution over an extended field of view. Radiology 2007;242(2):600–609

Patel SN, White CJ, Collins TJ, et al. Catheter-based treatment of the subclavian and innominate arteries. Catheter Cardiovasc Interv 2008;71(7):963–968

Periard D, Haesler E, Hayoz D, Von Segesser LK, Qanadli SD. Rupture and migration of an endovascular stent in the brachiocephalic trunk causing a vertebral steal syndrome. Cardiovasc Intervent Radiol 2008;31(Suppl 2):S53–S56

Pulido-Duque JM, Carreira JM, Qian Z, Maynar M. Treatment of innominate arterial stenosis with self-expanding stent: long-term follow-up. Minim Invasive Ther Allied Technol 2005;14(1):19–22

Ringelstein EB, Zeumer H. Delayed reversal of vertebral artery blood flow following percutaneous transluminal angioplasty for subclavian steal syndrome. Neuroradiology 1984;26(3):189–198

Shadman R, Criqui MH, Bundens WP, et al. Subclavian artery stenosis: prevalence, risk factors, and association with cardiovascular diseases. J Am Coll Cardiol 2004;44(3):618–623

Sixt S, Rastan A, Schwarzwälder U, et al. Results after balloon angioplasty or stenting of atherosclerotic subclavian artery obstruction. Catheter Cardiovasc Interv 2009;73(3):395–403

Widder B, Görtler M. Doppler- und Duplexsonographie der hirnversorgenden Arterien. Berlin: Springer; 2004:205–214

IV

Summary and Recommendations Part IV

O. Jansen and H. Brueckmann

The endovascular treatment of carotid artery stenosis should be included in the repertoire of every interventional neuroradiologist. Despite the sometimes spirited and politically charged debate on the indications for carotid stenting as opposed to surgical endarterectomy, there is no good alternative to the stenting of a carotid stenosis during an acute stroke, and consequently this procedure should be mastered by anyone working in this specialty.

The elective interventional treatment of a carotid stenosis, whether symptomatic or asymptomatic, is always classified as a prophylactic procedure. For this reason, the complication rates that are associated with this treatment must meet rigorous standards. Even if the treatment is considered a "simple" neurointerventional procedure (compared with intracranial therapies), the special challenge is to keep complication rates at the necessary low level. In experienced centers the stenting of carotid stenosis always follows a highly standardized protocol, as this is the only way to achieve acceptably low treatment risks. Moreover, large therapeutic trials have clearly shown that in the comparison between surgical and endovascular treatment, the complication rate depends less on the type of therapy than on the therapist, and that the differences between different therapists are considerably greater than the difference between the two modes of treatment. Thus the main concern for the referring physician and for the patient is not the selection of treatment mode but the selection of a qualified therapist.

Available study data also show that the selection of materials and the identification of specific high-risk groups influence the complication rate. This emphasizes the importance of developing new stent technology specifically designed for the anatomy of the carotid bifurcation and the pathology of carotid stenosis. These developments have been lacking in the past, and peripheral stents have generally been adapted for more central use. Accordingly, there is still room for technological advances that could further reduce the complication rates of stent angioplasty and improve long-term results.

In summary, the stent angioplasty of carotid stenosis can be offered as an alternative to carotid surgery at experienced centers that have a track record of low complication rates, thereby broadening the range of treatment options available for carotid stenosis. Also, there are many situations in which stenting provides a first-line treatment option, and so mastering the procedure is an important element in the management of stroke patients.

In contrast to the treatment of extracranial carotid stenosis, relatively few data are available on the treatment of intracranial stenoses due to the much lower incidence of this vascular disease. Thus, balloon angioplasty and stenting are still in the testing stage as treatments for intracranial stenoses, and their superiority over drug therapy has yet to be proven in randomized studies. But the term "intracranial stenosis" falsely implies a single disease entity with a uniform risk profile for endovascular therapy. It is important to distinguish between lesions in the anterior and posterior circulations and especially between intra- and extradural stenoses. For example, while lesions in the petrous segment of the internal carotid artery can be treated relatively easily and with a low complication rate, the indications for treating a middle cerebral artery stenosis must be weighed much more carefully due to the significantly higher periprocedural complication rate on the one hand and a higher restenosis rate on the other. In principle, endovascular treatment would be indicated in patients with relatively high-grade intracranial stenoses who are still symptomatic on medical therapy. In all other cases, the indication for endovascular treatment should be decided on an individual basis because factors such as degree of stenosis, collateral supply, the morphology and location of the stenosis, and vascular access options play an important role. Given these challenges, endovascular treatment should generally be reserved for experienced neurointerventional centers.

The situation is quite different with regard to subclavian artery stenosis and proximal vertebral artery stenosis. In most cases these lesions are relatively easy to treat by the endovascular route and the treatments have a low complication rate, although restenosis rates after the treatment of proximal vertebral artery stenosis are still relatively high. In both diseases it is important to select patients carefully for stent angioplasty and avoid the temptation to treat every detectable stenosis. A discriminating approach should be taken so that patients are not endangered by unnecessary treatments.

Given the problem of restenosis, which may occur after any endovascular treatment, it is essential to offer treated patients a structured follow-up program that includes regular examinations using methods appropriate for the individual patient.

IV

Index

Illustrations are comprehensively referred to from the text. Therefore, significant material in illustrations have usually only been given a page reference in the absence of their concomitant mention in the text referring to that figure.